PENNINGTON CENTER NUTRITION SERIES

GEORGE A. BRAY, MD, *and* DONNA H. RYAN, MD, *Editors*

VOLUME 3

Vitamins and Cancer Prevention

PENNINGTON CENTER NUTRITION SERIES

Sponsored by the Pennington Biomedical Research Center

VOLUME 3

Vitamins and Cancer Prevention

Edited by

GEORGE A. BRAY, MD

and

DONNA H. RYAN, MD

LOUISIANA STATE UNIVERSITY PRESS
BATON ROUGE AND LONDON

Manufactured in the United States of America
First printing
02 01 00 99 98 97 96 95 94 93 5 4 3 2 1

Designer: Laura Roubique Gleason
Typeface: Palatino
Typesetter: G&S Typesetters, Inc.
Printer and binder: Thomson-Shore, Inc.

Published with the assistance of the Pennington Biomedical Research Foundation.

LIBRARY OF CONGRESS CATALOGING-IN-PUBLICATION DATA

Vitamins and cancer prevention / edited by George A. Bray and Donna H. Ryan.
p. cm. — (Pennington Center nutrition series ; v. 3)
"Published with the assistance of the Pennington Biomedical Research Foundation"—T.p. verso.
Includes index.
ISBN 0-8071-1789-7 (alk. paper)
1. Vitamins—Therapeutic use. 2. Cancer—Chemoprevention. I. Bray, George A. II. Ryan, Donna H. III. Pennington Biomedical Research Foundation. IV. Series.
RC271.V58V585 1992
616.99'4052—dc20 92-19677
CIP

The paper in this book meets the guidelines for permanence and durability of the Committee on Production Guidelines for Book Longevity of the Council on Library Resources. ∞

Contents

Preface

This text represents papers submitted as part of a conference held at the Pennington Biomedical Research Center from October 30 through November 1, 1991, entitled "Vitamins and Cancer Prevention." The major focus of these papers is the cancer-prevention potential of vitamin A and beta-carotene, vitamin C, and vitamin E. International epidemiologic investigations have consistently reported that the frequent ingestion of fresh fruits and vegetables reduces the risk of cancer. Although the exact mechanism of this association is not fully understood and both nutrients and non-nutrients may play a role, there is sufficient evidence to justify intervention research. Since 1981, the National Cancer Institute has funded nearly thirty chemoprevention programs and nutrition research in dietary patterns and food groups, single-nutrient chemoprevention, and non-nutrient chemoprevention. Because the level of evidence as reviewed in these papers differs between animal and clinical studies and across the various clinical studies, we have attempted to summarize the data as best we can see it. In Table 1 various types of cancer are listed, along with the three vitamins and an assessment of the strength of the evidence as we read it from the various papers. The dietary intake of these vitamins is below the recommended level for many Americans, and given the convincing experimental story on oxidative stress, there may well be individuals for whom supplemental vitamin therapy is appropriate as a cancer preventive. The large chemoprevention trials evaluating these agents are likely to provide within this decade the data we need to judge vitamin therapy as a cancer chemoprevention. This is certainly an exciting time for preventive oncologists, who are taking a second look at the role of these chemical compounds in cancer prevention.

The conference on vitamins and cancer prevention was made pos-

Table 1. Evidence for Chemopreventive Effect

Cancer Type	Vitamin A	Vitamin C	Vitamin E
Epidemiologic data			
Esophagus	+ +	+ + +	+ + +
Stomach	+ +	+ + +	+ + +
Colon	+ +	+	+ + +
Pancreas		+ + +	
Lung	+	+ + +	
Breast		+	
Animal data			
Oral cavity	+ + +	+ + +	+ + +
Lung	+ + +		
Colon		+ + +	+ + +
Breast	+ + +	+ + +	+ + +
Bladder	+ + +	+ + +	+ + +
Human data			
Colon		+ ?	+ ?
Oral cavity	+ + + [a]		
Skin	+ + + [a]		
Bladder	+ + + [b]		
Lung	+ + + [b]		
Cervix	+ + + [c]		

[a] 13-*cis*-retinoic acid.
[b] Etretinate.
[c] Transretinoic acid.

sible by the work of many people. We wish to thank in particular Mr. C. B. "Doc" Pennington, without whose support this conference would not have taken place. We are also grateful for financial support from the Hoffman LaRoche Company and for assistance from scientists in that company in planning the conference. Finally, we want to thank Ben Phillips and the many other diligent members of the Pennington Biomedical Research Center staff who were so helpful in making this conference a success.

Vitamins and Cancer Prevention

PETER GREENWALD and CAROLYN CLIFFORD

Diet and Cancer Prevention: A National Cancer Institute Priority

ABSTRACT

The National Cancer Institute invested in diet-related epidemiologic and carcinogenesis research in the 1970s and in 1980 commissioned the National Research Council to critically review this scientific information. This resulted in the National Research Council report *Diet, Nutrition, and Cancer* (1982). These efforts along with major advances in characterizing the process of carcinogenesis created new opportunities in prevention leading to a new commitment to two major nutrition-related programs: the diet and cancer program and the chemoprevention program. On the strength of consistent findings from multiple studies, randomized controlled dietary intervention trials have been started: a multi-institution dietary intervention trial is under way to test whether a low-fat, high-fiber, vegetable- and fruit-enriched diet will prevent the recurrence of large-bowel adenomatous polyps in high-risk females and males, and a National Institutes of Health Women's Health Initiative will test whether a similar eating pattern, hormone replacement, or calcium/vitamin D supplementation can reduce the risk of breast and colon cancer, cardiovascular disease, or osteoporosis.

The chemoprevention program parallels this effort and aims to identify and characterize specific anticarcinogenic substances through its preclinical agent development program; an organized series of steps leads to human clinical trials. From a modest beginning in 1982, now more than thirty clinical chemoprevention trials are studying the anticarcinogenic effects of several vitamins, synthetic analogues of vitamins, minerals, other natural substances, and pharmaceuticals. Increasingly important to this program is the variety of biological marker end points under evaluation to reduce the time involved to measure risk modulation by these agents. The progress in diet and cancer prevention and chemoprevention research has been greatly helped by the National Cancer Institute's support of extramural research in basic nutrition and carcinogenesis, clinical nutrition research units, and the recent establishment of an intramural Laboratory of Nutritional and Metabolic Regulation.

Introduction

Diet and cancer research had its beginnings more than fifty years ago when animal studies demonstrated a lower incidence of tumors in animals chronically restricted in caloric intake and an increased incidence of tumors in animals as the level of dietary fat increased (1, 2). However, there was little attempt to relate early research to humans until the 1960s, when the World Health Organization, after examination of life-style and environmental factors associated with cancer risk, concluded that the majority of human cancer is potentially preventable (3). With the exception of smoking, dietary habits are the single most significant life-style factor in cancer risk. Doll and Peto (4) estimated that approximately 35% of all cancer mortality in the United States is related to diet.

The National Cancer Institute (NCI) invested in carcinogenesis and epidemiologic research in the 1970s, which led to later diet and cancer research. Because diet and nutrition were recognized as major factors in the development of cancer, the National Cancer Advisory Board (NCAB) concluded that a need existed for a defined diet, nutrition, and cancer research program with goals made known to the scientific community. Also, NCI divisions would offer input into the goals, design, and specification of the overall program. The NCAB advised the director of the NCI to give top priority to diet, nutrition, and cancer research (5).

In 1982 the National Research Council (NRC), commissioned by the NCI, reviewed the epidemiologic and experimental data on diet and cancer and concluded that the evidence suggested that many of the most common cancers in humans are influenced by dietary patterns (6). Cancers of the esophagus, stomach, liver, colon/rectum, lung, breast, and prostrate all have been associated with dietary factors. More recently, both the Office of the Surgeon General and the NRC, recognizing that policy makers, scientists, health professionals,

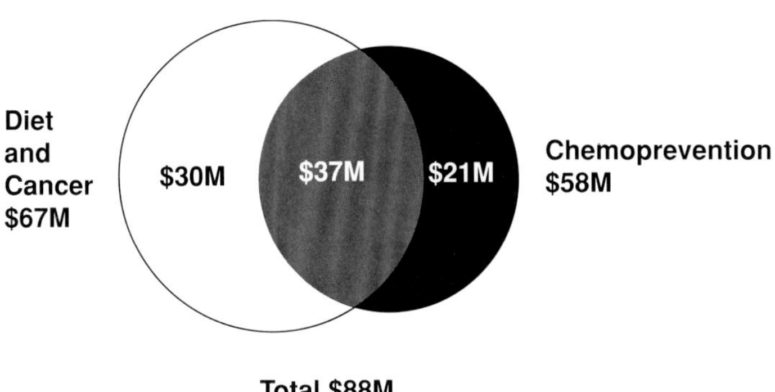

Figure 1. NCI Research Programs, 1990.

and the public need guidance in evaluating the abundance of available information on diet and chronic disease, including cancer, conducted comprehensive analyses of the scientific literature (3, 7). Both the NRC report and the surgeon general's report emphasized the need for further diet and cancer research. Basic nutritional research and clinical intervention trials were considered essential parts of the overall research effort to obtain definitive information on the role of diet in cancer prevention.

Over the past ten years, diet and chemoprevention research programs at NCI have grown in size and scope. The recommendations made in 1982 by the NCAB and the publication of the NRC's and surgeon general's expert reviews on factors that influence diet and cancer and diet and health (3, 6, 7) have served to foster the growth of the NCI diet and cancer budget from its modest beginnings in 1974 of under $3 million to $67 million in 1990. The 1990 budget for NCI chemoprevention programs was $58 million; however, as is shown in Figure 1, there is considerable overlap in the total $88 million budgeted for these two programs.

The effort being made in nutrition-related research at NCI includes activities in the areas of the basic biomedical and behavioral sciences, food sciences, nutrition monitoring and surveillance of populations, nutrition education, and research on socioeconomic factors that affect nutritional status and cancer risk. The two major program thrusts of diet and nutrition and chemoprevention research involve actions or interventions with implications for reducing human cancer risk. Pursued through extramural and intramural mechanisms, this research focus represents a major change from the first half of this century, when human nutrition studies were concerned primarily with the role of essential nutrients in human deficiency diseases (7). Although the precise role of diet in cancer etiology remains unclear, the objective of current research remains one of continued systematic evaluation of the scientific evidence relating diet to the cause and prevention of disease.

The goals of the diet and nutrition program discussed in this paper are to conduct research in nutritional and molecular regulation, prevention-related epidemiology, and clinical nutrition and dietary intervention trials to identify and evaluate cancer prevention dietary patterns. Finally, through education and information dissemination, health-promoting dietary changes are encouraged through behavioral modification research. The chemoprevention program has parallel goals, but its focus is to identify and assess specific chemical substances, many naturally occurring in foods, with the potential for cancer-inhibiting activity in humans. Research in chemoprevention at NCI systematically pursues the selection of chemical substances first for preclinical determinations of the agent's cancer-inhibiting efficacy and safety and finally through randomized placebo-controlled intervention trials concerned with the agent's broad effectiveness in humans.

Extramural Nutrition Research

Investigator-initiated research is the backbone of basic research sponsored by the National Institutes of Health (NIH). The NCI supports extensive research on the relationship between diet and cancer in a variety of areas, including cancer prevention, epidemiology, etiology, and basic cellular mechanisms. For example, through epidemiologic studies, assessments are being made about the effects of diet and nutritional status on cancer incidence and survival. Also, improved methods for assessing nutritional status, metabolic patterns, and genetic predisposition are being evaluated for use in epidemiologic studies. Chemopreventive and dietary trials are being conducted on the quantitative relationship between foods, nutrient intake, and cancer incidence. The relationship between dietary factors and cancer is largely the result of interactions occurring at the cellular and subcellular levels in specific tissues. However, nutrient levels in the blood may not necessarily reflect tissue or cell nutrient levels. Thus, NCI is sponsoring studies to identify the relationship between blood or serum and tissue micronutrient levels as well as the association between blood and tissue levels of vitamins A and E and carotenoids in persons at varying levels of risk of developing cancer. In addition, researchers are studying mechanisms by which both nutritive and nonnutritive dietary components affect carcinogen metabolism and in vitro tumor cell metabolism and growth.

Several extramural projects focus on breast cancer. An ongoing randomized feasibility study will examine the degree of compliance and the behavior modification patterns associated with a low-fat diet in stage II breast cancer patients in the Women's Intervention Nutrition Study. Another extramural project examining the relationship between diet and breast tissue morphology on mammograms is under way.

Clinical Nutrition Research Units

Another means by which NCI expands its knowledge base is through the Clinical Nutrition Research Unit (CNRU). The CNRUs bring together, on a cooperative basis, basic science and clinical investigators in a manner that strives to enrich the effectiveness of research in nutritional science and related metabolic disorders. These units are established at institutions that have in place a strong base of ongoing, independently supported, peer-reviewed research programs in nutritional science. In addition to conducting basic research in nutrition science, CNRUs strengthen and implement nutrition training and education programs for health professionals and enhance patient care and promote good health by emphasizing nutrition education and by disseminating nutritional information to the public. Three CNRUs in particular focus on the relationship between various dietary components and cancer.

By sharing resources from seven core laboratories and facilities, the CNRU at the University of Alabama supports more than 40 projects, 17 of which focus on nutrition and cancer. Recent research accomplishments include demonstrated improvement in preneoplastic lesions of the cervix and epithelium by folate and vitamin B_{12} supplementation and the synthesis and evaluation of new potential chemopreventive retinoids. Basic research projects under way at the CNRU at the University of California at Los Angeles primarily focus on the role of nutrients in cancer prevention and control. A second, related focus is the alteration in nutrition and metabolism in patients at risk of developing cancer. Areas of emphasis include vitamins and trace elements, lipids, hormones, and cellular and molecular biology. The CNRU based at Memorial Hospital for Cancer and Allied Diseases in New York represents collaborative efforts in nutrition research at five participating institutions. Methodological and conceptual advances in both basic and clinical nutrition are achieved through this CNRU's five shared core laboratories in biophysics, immunology, lipids, metabolic bone diseases, and metabolism and oncology; a sixth core laboratory in carcinogenesis and nutrition is planned. The Memorial Hospital CNRU also sponsors enrichment, training, and education programs for health professionals and supports a nutrition information center.

Intramural Nutrition Research

Laboratory of Nutritional and Metabolic Regulation

Investigators at NCI's newly established Laboratory of Nutritional and Metabolic Regulation at the Frederick Cancer Research and Development Center plan, develop, and conduct intramural basic research on cellular and molecular regulation relevant to nutrition and cancer. The major areas of research at the laboratory are cellular resistance to carcinogens and the modulation of this resistance by nutrients and hormones; the effects of nutrients on cell signaling mechanisms modulated by metal-dependent redox mechanisms, retinoids, and metabolic intermediates such as pyrroline 5-carboxylate; the effects of dietary levels of vitamin A and its analogues on the pharmacokinetics and physiological metabolism of radiolabeled retinol; the physiologic processing of dietary carcinogens, including the effects of dietary fat and fiber on the formation of DNA adducts in animals fed low doses of carcinogens; the metabolic regulation of post translational modification of oncoproteins, in particular, regulation of the cholesterol biosynthetic pathway and its effects on farnesylation of $p21^{ras}$; and the identification and characterization of fiber components and fermentation products as agonists or antagonists of colonic mucosa cell proliferation.

Clinical Metabolic Studies

The role of dietary factors in cancer prevention has been evaluated in animal experiments, in human epidemiologic studies, and most recently in clinical trials. For many of these agents, however, information on safety, toxicity, dosage, form, bioavailability, pharmacokinetics, and mechanisms of action is incomplete. To define these parameters in humans further, cooperative research efforts between the Beltsville Human Nutrition Research Center of the United States Department of Agriculture (USDA) and NCI's Division of Cancer Prevention and Control and its Cancer Prevention Studies Branch have been developed. Initial efforts in this collaboration focused on three nutrients that have a role in cancer prevention: selenium, fat, and beta-carotene. More recent studies have evaluated the metabolic effects of alcohol, omega-3 fatty acids, and vitamin C.

Selenium is being considered for use in intervention trials. However, because information on the kinetics of selenium is limited, estimating optimum dosage and time and route of administration has been difficult. Therefore, a study examining the pharmacokinetics of a single oral dose of two forms of stable, radiolabeled selenium (sodium selenite [inorganic form] and selenomethionine [organic form]) was conducted. Results suggest two distinct multicompartmental models to describe the kinetics of these two forms of selenium; the data also indicate that fasting status modulates the appearance of selenite in the plasma and that there is a greater first pass effect when the dose is given with food. Another aspect of this study involves analyzing variations in total selenium levels in the plasma, urine, and feces, both within and between individuals living in regions of the United States with high-selenium soil content.

Studies examining the metabolic effects of changes in dietary fat and fiber have been conducted separately in premenopausal women, postmenopausal women, and men. The relationships between dietary modifications and serum lipids, hormonal status, bile acid metabolism, and fecal mutagenicity are being assessed. In the first study, premenopausal women consumed a controlled diet containing 40% or 20% fat calories at two different ratios of polyunsaturated to saturated (P:S) fats for eight menstrual cycles. Results analyzed thus far indicate that the low-fat diet was associated with a significant increase in serum triglycerides, a lengthening of the menstrual cycle, lower plasma levels of DHEA-S and cortisol and higher levels of plasma insulin, changes in bile acid levels specific to the P:S ratio, cycle phase– and fat level–dependent changes in lipoproteins and red blood cell fluidity, and reduction in percent body fat. The second study compared a variety of metabolic parameters in healthy men on a controlled high-fat, low-fiber reference diet with those for the same group of individuals consuming a controlled low-fat, high-fiber experimental diet. Results of lipid determinations indicate that total cholesterol, low-density lipoprotein cholesterol, and high-density lipoprotein cholesterol were 17% to 20% lower for the experimental diet as compared with the reference diet, regardless of initial cholesterol level. Results also supported the hypothesis that changes in dietary lipids can substantially alter the in vivo production of E-series prostaglandins. The third study of fat compared serum lipids and hormones in free-living postmenopausal women on an uncontrolled diet with those on a controlled, low-fat (20% of calories) diet. Preliminary results indicate no differences between the two groups.

Another NCI-sponsored study will evaluate the effect of a fat-modified diet on sex hormones during adolescence. This is an ancillary study to the Diet Intervention Study in Children, which is being sponsored by the National Heart, Lung, and Blood Institute (NHLBI). The NCI study also will characterize factors of adolescents that influence sex hormone levels and bioavailability, such as age, Tanner stage, anthropometric measures, physical activity, and diet, and evaluate the effect of dietary intervention on sex hormone levels in parents of the children.

Epidemiologic studies and some small clinical trials have suggested an inverse association between cancer risk and carotenoids. However, several questions concerning the metabolism of carotenoids remain unanswered. For example, it is not known whether the consistently low serum beta-carotene levels found in men and in individuals who smoke and consume alcohol are due to low intakes of carotenoids, to differences in metabolism of carotenoids, or to both. There are also individuals whose blood levels of carotenoids do not increase appreciably in response to large oral doses of carotenoids given either in food or in pills, and the reasons for this lack of "normal" response are unknown. Two human studies have examined plasma carotenoid levels following ingestion of various forms of selected carotenoids. The first study examined plasma responses after a single oral dose; the second study assessed responses of prescribed doses administered daily over a six-week period. Results indicate that beta-carotene in carrots or broccoli is poorly absorbed compared with beta-carotene in capsules. Carotenodermia (yellowing of the skin) was observed in all five individuals given 30 mg of beta-carotene but in none of the five given 12 mg of purified beta-carotene daily. Additional studies on the absorption and metabolism of carotenoids using carbon-13 stable isotopes are being designed.

The potential role of alcohol consumption in the etiology of breast cancer has been the focus of several recent epidemiologic studies. This relationship needs further characterization, and NCI has initiated a clinical metabolic study to examine the effects of alcohol consumption on steroid hormone status, lipid status, bile acid metabolism, and constituents of breast fluid in premenopausal women. In this study one group of women will be in a controlled diet study in which they will consume 35% to 37% energy from fat, 12 g of fiber per day, and either no alcohol or the equivalent of two glasses of wine per day; in a cross-sectional study, 150 women on a self-selected diet will consume various amounts of alcohol. The results are anticipated to provide information on the influence of dietary components and alcohol on the bioavailability of hormones and, subsequently, on breast cancer. Defining the relationship between alcohol and breast cancer is important because alcohol intake is a risk factor that can be modified.

Several animal and human studies suggest that omega-3 polyunsaturated fatty acids may prevent or inhibit carcinogenesis. To understand the underlying mechanisms of this proposed protective role, NCI has initiated a controlled feeding study in humans that will evaluate the effect of consuming omega-3 fatty acids from fish oils on several metabolic parameters including prostaglandin synthesis, oxidant stress, and immune function.

Consistently strong evidence from epidemiologic studies indicates that vegetables and fruits have a significant protective effect against cancer. However, it is not clear which constituents of these foods are most critical to cancer prevention. In addition to carotenoids, vitamin C is considered one of the prime candidates among the potentially protective nutrients in vegetables and fruits, and NCI has initiated a controlled feeding study that will compare the bioavailability of vitamin C from vegetables, fruits, and supplements.

Controlled dietary studies provide a unique opportunity to identify possible markers of dietary-induced mechanisms of cancer or of compliance to dietary modifications. For example, circulating steroid hormones, which appear to be affected by fat and fiber intake, have been proposed as possible markers for breast cancer risk. Assays have been developed for the isolation and quantification of metabolic products of estradiol, such as 16-hydroxyestrone. Measuring these metabolites in subjects participating in controlled dietary studies is expected to provide some insights into diet-induced changes in metabolic pathways that may direct or inhibit carcinogenesis. Biological markers being assessed in dietary trials with previous colon cancer patients include the multiplicity of new colon adenomas, [^{3}H] thymidine-labeling index determinations of epithelial cell proliferation, and prostaglandin synthetase and ornithine decarboxylase activities. Several animal and human studies conducted thus far indicate that fecal mutagens and bile acid profiles change significantly in response to dietary modifications and that examination of bile acid fractions as well as total bile acids may provide a greater understanding of the relationship between diet and cancer. These data have encouraged NCI to consider conducting a study that will evaluate fecal mutagens following ingestion of putative carcinogens from cooked meats. Identifying markers for dietary compliance will be especially useful in large intervention trials with cancer or a premalignant condition as an end point. Results of completed and ongoing studies suggest that certain carotenoids may be good markers of vegetable intake in general or of intake of specific vegetables.

Dietary Intervention Trials

Dietary intervention studies evaluate the relationship between dietary modification and cancer incidence and/or mortality. The NCI has sponsored several extramural intervention studies and supports intramural intervention trials as well.

Because of the potential protective role of fiber in the development of certain cancers, NCI has sponsored several controlled feeding studies and metabolic studies in humans to investigate the physiochemical effects of dietary fiber, such as that present in vegetables, grains, cereals, and fruits. These studies will attempt to define the metabolic and physiologic functions of dietary fiber, identify potential biochemical markers for colon cancer risk, and elucidate the possible protective role of dietary fiber in carcinogenesis. Two small clinical trials have suggested a protective role of fiber in the recurrence of rectal polyps. In one study, a decreased number of adenomatous rectal polyps was seen in patients with familial polyposis who consumed more than 11 g of wheat bran fiber per day (8). The rate of polyp recurrence also was assessed in this group of individuals following administration of vitamin C and vitamin E supplements alone and in conjunction with a diet enriched with wheat bran fiber. Although no significant protective effect was observed with the vitamin supplements, the combination of vitamin supplements with wheat bran fiber showed a significant protective effect when adjusted for compliance (8). Alberts *et al.* (9) reported that consumption of a wheat bran fiber supplement of 13.5 g per day for two months inhibited DNA synthesis and epithelial cell proliferation within the rectal mucosa crypts of patients with resection for colorectal cancers.

The Polyp Prevention Trial

The NCI is conducting a multi-institution randomized control trial to assess the association between dietary fat and fiber and colon cancer. The Polyp Prevention Trial is designed to test whether a low-fat, high-fiber, and vegetable- and fruit-enriched eating plan will prevent the recurrence of large-bowel adenomatous polyps in otherwise healthy women and men who have had a polypectomy. This clinical trial is based on the strong association between colon polyps and the development of colon cancer.

This dietary intervention trial will enroll a total of 2000 male and female patients over the age of 25 at eight clinical centers across the United States. Half will be randomized to a control group with no intervention except for information on basic nutrition, and the other half will be assigned to the diet intervention group. The daily intervention target goals are 20% of calories from fat, 18 grams of fiber per 1000 calories, and increased vegetable and fruit intake. The participants will be individually counseled on how to meet their target goals, with a strong emphasis on behavior modification. The recurrence of polyps as the end point will be assessed in both groups at years 1 and 4 to determine the effect of this dietary intervention.

Women's Health and Women's Health Trial Initiative

On the strength of a large body of epidemiology and carcinogenesis research, the NIH is planning a major women's health initiative to address the prevention of health problems of women. This study will take a comprehensive approach to three major sources of morbidity and mortality: cancer, cardiovascular disease, and osteoporosis in women of diverse ethnicity and socioeconomic status. Although distinctly different problems, these diseases are now linked through potential preventive regimens. The NIH proposes to address these issues by a study of the effects of disease risk on changes in diet, the use of hormones, and calcium supplementation. Components of this study include a large intervention trial with an associated cohort epidemiologic study and a community study. Coordinated by the NIH Office of Research on Women's Health and the NIH Associate Director for Disease Prevention, in collaboration with the NCI, the NHLBI, the National Institute on Aging, the National Institute of Arthritis and Musculoskeletal and Skin Diseases, and the National Institute of Child Health and Human Development, the Women's Health Initiative will be the largest community-based clinical prevention and intervention trial ever conducted in the United States.

The lack of knowledge about the feasibility of such a comprehensive trial for underserved populations has led the NCI to request proposals for a low-fat dietary intervention in minority populations. The results of this Women's Health Trial minority study should help refine the Women's Health Initiative and be useful in other efforts aimed at dietary modification in minority groups. The overall objective of the study is to determine whether a low-fat (less than 20% of calories from fat) diet and an increased intake of vegetables, fruits, and grain products reduce the incidence of breast and colon cancer and the mortality from cardiovascular disease in this study population.

Women's Intervention Nutrition Study

The Women's Intervention Nutrition Study is a multi-institutional randomized clinical trial to test the effects of a low-fat diet in stage II breast cancer patients. The proposed study will examine adherence to a dietary modification program for 300 postmenopausal stage II breast cancer patients in conjunction with chemotherapy or hormonal therapy. The primary objective of this study is to determine the degree to which patients will adhere to the dietary modification. The secondary objectives include identifying a set of behavioral and psychosocial variables that can be used as predictors of dietary change. This study is believed to be a critical intermediate step in the effort to determine whether a full-scale outcome study evaluating dietary modification as an adjunct to standard breast cancer therapy is justified.

Chemoprevention and Phytochemical Research

Chemoprevention Research

In addition to dietary modification trials, NCI has established a program in chemoprevention that involves natural or synthetic cancer-inhibiting substances to reduce cancer incidence. The NCI Chemoprevention Program, established in 1982, uses a systematic strategy to identify and characterize potential new agents that have either proven efficacy in preventing carcinogenesis in animal models or a high probability of preventing human cancer, based on epidemiological studies; conduct preclinical efficacy and toxicity testing of candidate agents; and conduct clinical intervention trials with safe and effective agents that may reduce human cancer incidence.

Chemopreventive Agent Development

Laboratory efforts and human studies, most supporting research leads from epidemiologic studies, have identified more than 1000 natural compounds and synthetic agents that appear to have cancer-inhibitory effects (10, 11). Agents of interest are diverse with respect to source, chemical structure, and physiological effects and include micronutrients (vitamins A, C, E, selenium, molybdenum, calcium), natural products (carotenoids, isothiocyanates, flavonoids), and synthetics (Piroxicam, tamoxifen, difluoromethylornithine [DFMO], and retinoid derivatives). Of special interest is the development of combinations of chemopreventives that may be more effective and less toxic than agents used singly. Several priority agents include Oltipraz, a synthetic antischistosomal drug that enhances electrophilic detoxification while increasing glutathione levels in tissues; the mucolytic drug N-acetylcysteine, which promotes glutathione formation and protects against free radical damage; the natural food constituent glycyrrhetinic acid, shown to have nonsteroidal anti-inflammatory properties; and the prostaglandin synthesis inhibitor, ibuprofen, a nonsteroidal anti-inflammatory drug.

Preclinical Testing

In the preclinical research arm of NCI's Chemoprevention Program, compound efficacy is assessed through in vitro cell screening systems and in vivo assays using animal model systems that evaluate agent efficacy at specific target sites. Of primary interest are models representing target organs relevant to human cancer, including lung, breast, colon, bladder, skin, and connective tissues. If results are promising, toxicological and safety evaluations are conducted in animal studies to assess acute, subchronic, chronic, and developmental effects.

Chemoprevention Clinical Trials

Because the predictive value of animal models in the evaluation of chemopreventive agents in humans is limited, the Chemoprevention Program has a clinical arm that tests agents for efficacy and toxicity in clinical intervention trials, mostly in medical settings. A phase I clinical trial provides data on pharmacokinetics, preliminary information on safe and effective dose ranges, and toxicity patterns. Phase II trials determine whether an agent affects some stage or aspect of the carcinogenic process. Based on results from phase I and phase II trials and concerns about perceived risks and benefits, a decision is made as to the advisability of conducting a large-scale clinical intervention trial (phase III).

Phase II trials increasingly incorporate into the study design modulation of biological intermediate end points, that is, the biologic events that take place between carcinogenic exposure and development of malignancy (12). The reliability and sensitivity of these intermediate end points can be determined only from these clinical assessments. Tissue and cellular intermediate end points under consideration include sputum metaplasia/dysplasia, cervical dysplasia, gastric metaplasia, and colonic cell proliferation, as evaluated by histology and rate of cellular incorporation of [^{3}H]thymidine. Inhibition of ornithine decarboxylase and/or prostaglandin synthetase and changes in fecal mutagens and concentrations of fecal bile acids also are being assessed as potential biochemical markers. Several genetic indexes are being studied, including oncogene activation and suppression, nuclear aberrations (micronuclei, sister chromatic exchange), and quantitative DNA analysis and DNA ploidy (13). In several trials, a variety of markers are being evaluated.

Nearly forty clinical chemoprevention trials sponsored by NCI are in progress, mostly in high-risk populations in medical settings. Table 1 summarizes data for trials being conducted in the United States and includes information on study population, site, agent, and dosage. Several completed and ongoing trials are discussed below.

A phase II trial was recently completed, testing the hypothesis that exposure to cigarette smoke results in folic acid deficiency, rendering the bronchial epithelium more susceptible to neoplastic transformation. Preliminary data from this trial, using folic acid and vitamin B_{12} supplements in men who are heavy smokers and at high risk for lung cancer, indicate significantly greater reduction in cellular atypia of the bronchial epithelium in vitamin-supplemented smokers than in the placebo group. Although these results suggest that sputum atypia may serve as an intermediate end point for lung cancer, they must be confirmed by further research (14).

Other phase II clinical trials, particularly those using retinoids as the chemopreventive agent, also have been encouraging. Isotretinoin was markedly effective in preventing new skin cancers in patients with xeroderma pigmentosum, an inherited condition in which the defective repair of ultraviolet-damaged DNA results in a thousand-fold increase in skin cancer incidence compared with the general population (15). Another study demonstrated temporary remission of oral leukoplakia and reversal of oral dysplasia by 13-*cis*-retinoic acid, indicating the potential of this retinoid to prevent oral cancer in this high-risk population (16). A recent chemoprevention trial found that 13-*cis*-isotretinoin prevented the occurrence of second primary head and neck tumors in high-risk patients (17). Patients who were disease free after primary treatment for squamous-cell cancers of the larynx, pharynx, or oral cavity received daily for 12 months either a placebo or 50 to 100 mg of isotretinoin per square meter of body surface. Al-

Table 1. Selected Current Chemoprevention Intervention Trials

Target Site(s)	Study Population Characteristics	Study Agent(s), Dosage
All	Physicians	Beta-carotene, 50 mg every other day
Breast	High risk	4-HPR (Fenretinide), 200 mg/day
Breast	High risk	Tamoxifen, 20 mg/day
Cervix	Women, mild/moderate dysplasia	Beta-transretionic acid, .372%
Cervix	Women, cervical dysplasia	Folic acid, 5 mg/day
Cervix	Women, cervical dysplasia	Beta-carotene, 30 mg/day
Colon	Previous colon adenoma	Beta-carotene, 30 mg/day Ascorbic acid, 1 g/day Alpha-tocopherol, 400 mg/day
Colon	Previous colon adenoma	Calcium carbonate, 3 g/day
Colon	Previous adenoma of colon	Wheat bran, 13, 5, or 2 g/day Calcium carbonate, 0.25 or 1.50 g/day
Colon	Previous adenoma of colon	Piroxicam, 20, 10, 7.5, or 5 mg/day
Colon	High risk	DFMO
Colon	High risk	Calcium carbonate, 3 or 5 g/day
Colon	Familial adenomatous polyposis	Sulindac, 150 mg twice a day
Colon	Previous colon cancer	Beta-carotene, 30 mg/day
Colon	Previous colon polyp	Calcium, 1,200 mg
Lung	Men exposed to asbestos	Retinol, 25,000 IU every other day Beta-carotene, 50 mg/day
Lung	High-risk women	Beta-carotene, 50 mg QOD Retinol, 25,000 IU/day
Lung	Chronic smokers	13-*cis*-retinoic acid, 1.0 mg/kg daily
Lung	Cigarette smokers	Beta-carotene, 30 mg/day Retinol, 25,000 IU/day
Lung	High-risk women	Beta-carotene, 50 mg QOD Vitamin E, 600 mg QOD
Oral cavity	Oral leukoplakia	13-*cis*-retionic acid, 1.5 mg/kg daily for 3 months, then .5 mg/kg daily for 9 months Beta-carotene, 30 mg/day for 9 months

Table 1. (continued)

Target Site(s)	Study Population Characteristics	Study Agent(s), Dosage
Oral cavity	Oral leukoplakia	Bowman Birk Inhibitor
Skin	Albinos in Tanzania	Beta-carotene, 100 mg/day
Skin	Previous basal cell carcinoma of skin	Beta-carotene, 50 mg/day
Skin	Previous basal cell carcinoma of skin	Retinol, 25,000 IU/day 13-*cis*-retinoic acid, .15 mg/kg daily
Skin	Actinic keratosis patients	Retinol, 25,000 IU/day

though this treatment significantly prevented second primary tumors, isotretinoin did not prevent recurrences of the initial cancer (17).

The synthetic retinoid compound 4-HPR (Fenretinide), appearing to be an effective modifier of mammary carcinogenesis, is significantly less toxic than other retinoids. A phase III randomized clinical trial of breast cancer chemoprevention with 4-HPR was implemented at the Milan Tumor Institute in 1987 to evaluate the effect of 4-HPR on the incidence of contralateral breast cancer in disease-free, surgically treated patients.

Phytochemical Research

Phytochemicals, or plant food chemicals, are under study in a new project initiated by NCI. This research aims to increase understanding of the relationship between edible plants and human cancer prevention. In the developmental phase, it focuses on vegetables, grains, fruits, herbs, and spices reported in the scientific literature to have epidemiologic links to cancer prevention. Plant foods of interest are conventional foods that are readily available, easily grown, and normally consumed, for example, cruciferous vegetables, umbelliferous vegetables, citrus fruits, garlic, and onions. This project will focus on identifying and quantifying the phytochemicals and the sources that have potential for cancer prevention studies in high-risk populations.

To explore systematically the influence of phytochemicals in human diets on cancer prevention, NCI-sponsored studies are being conducted in four research areas: analytical studies to quantify phytochemicals in foods and biological fluids; clinical-metabolic studies to determine the influence of phytochemicals on metabolic processes related to carcinogenesis (*e.g.*, metabolism of steroids, prostaglandins, and toxins); experimental animal studies to evaluate synergistic or antagonistic effects of combinations of edible plant foods; and safety evaluation studies.

Dietary Guidance

Although many questions remain about diet and cancer, NCI believes enough data are available to support dietary guidance while the research continues; thus, NCI provides current information to the public on the role of dietary factors in cancer (18). The 1982 NRC committee concluded that although the scientific evidence was not definitive, it was sufficiently strong to support interim guidelines for the United States public (5). Specifically, the NRC recommended the following dietary practices: reduce both saturated and unsaturated fat from 40% of calories to 30%; include fruits, vegetables, and whole-grain cereal products in the daily diet; minimize consumption of salt-cured, salt-pickled, and smoked foods; consume alcoholic beverages in moderation. At about this time other health organizations were issuing dietary guidelines to the American public for disease prevention and health promotion (19–21). Most of these guidelines are consistent in advocating a lower-fat diet, increased intake of fiber-rich grains and fruits and vegetables, and moderate alcohol intake, while maintaining a desirable body weight.

The scientific rationale for the NCI dietary guidelines, developed in 1985 and published in 1988, is based on the 1982 NRC report on diet, nutrition, and cancer and is augmented by reports of expert workshops, literature reviews, and meta-analyses (22). NCI dietary guidelines are consistent with those of most other organizations that advocate reduction in total fat; however, NCI also provides a quantitative guideline for dietary fiber. As with the more general diet and health guidelines of other agencies and organizations, the NCI guidelines also emphasize eating a varied diet rich in vegetables and fruits. The NCI reviews and reissues diet and cancer guidelines periodically, based on information derived from the continuous critical appraisal of the scientific literature, and coordinates this effort with the Department of Health and Human Services and, through them, with the USDA.

In regard to the NCI's recommendation to eat a variety of vegetables and fruits daily, an explanatory statement following this guideline reads: "To obtain an adequate intake of substances protective against cancer, consume a variety of vegetables and fruits." Although it was recognized that the effects of dietary fiber cannot be fully separated from those of other protective food components such as beta-carotene, vitamin C, and phytochemicals, the importance of identifying vegetables and fruits rich in these chemopreventive factors was stressed.

Five a Day Program

In 1988, with major funding from NCI, the Five a Day for Better Health campaign was launched by the California Department of Health Services and the California Public Health Foundation. The goal of this program, a cooperative effort between public health groups and private industry, was to promote the importance of eating at least five servings of fruits and vegetables daily as a way to improve health and possibly reduce disease risk. The program was targeted to adults and focused on three main channels for message delivery: retail groceries, mass media, and community organizations.

To continue to promote the benefits of eating fruits and vegetables as part of a low-fat, high-fiber eating pattern, NCI is expanding the program nationally, with the overall goal of increasing the per capita consumption of fruits and vegetables to five servings a day by the year 2000. The Produce for Better Health Foundation, Inc., was incorporated in May, 1991, after receiving industry commitments. The new foundation will coordinate the national Five a Day program in cooperation with NCI. The NCI's role will be to maintain the scientific integrity and nutritional accuracy of the program. The national Five a Day program will begin very much like the California program by having educational brochures, point-of-purchase signs, food demonstrations, and print advertising used by retailers in stores and in newspapers to help educate consumers.

The NCI develops, implements, and evaluates cancer information and education programs for cancer patients and their families, the general public, and health professionals. The Five a Day program is one example of an effort designed to assist Americans in changing their diets to decrease their risk for certain types of cancer. Additional efforts to reduce cancer risk through dietary changes focus on the development of nutrition education materials for people of low literacy and for culturally and ethnically diverse groups. A primary care physician's manual on nutrition entitled *How to Help Your Patients Improve Their Eating Habits* is in production for pilot testing with approximately one thousand physicians.

Conclusion

The effort that began as carcinogenesis and epidemiologic studies at NCI has now developed into a major program of diet and cancer research. The evidence from analytic epidemiology studies suggests that a large portion of the cancer burden is influenced by diet and chemical metabolites of diet. Emphasis on basic nutritional research will help in the interpretation of this evidence and in understanding of mechanisms. Controlled randomized trials in humans, when feasible, are being implemented to demonstrate the efficacy and strength of a wide variety of factors for their anticarcinogenic properties. Concurrently, other research studies on the biochemical and biological mechanisms of carcinogenesis at the molecular level may resolve some of the etiologic issues concerning diet-related cancers.

REFERENCES

1. Tannenbaum A. The initiation and growth of tumors: introduction. I: effects of underfeeding. *Am J Cancer.* 1940;38:335–350.
2. Tannenbaum A. The genesis and growth of tumors. III: effects of a high fat diet. *Cancer Res.* 1942;2:468–475.
3. *Prevention of cancer. WHO Tech Rep Ser.* 1964:276.
4. Doll R, Peto R. The causes of cancer: quantitative estimates of avoidable risks of cancer in the United States today. *J Nat Cancer Inst.* 1981;66:1191–1308.
5. National Cancer Advisory Board. *Report of the National Cancer Advisory Board and Ad Hoc Sub-committee on Nutrition and Cancer.* February 3, 1982.
6. National Academy of Sciences, National Research Council, Committee on Diet, Nutrition, and Cancer, Assembly of Life Sciences. *Diet, Nutrition and Cancer.* Washington, DC: National Academy Press; 1982.
7. National Academy of Sciences, National Research Council, Food and Nutrition Board, Council on Life Sciences. *Diet and Health:*

Implications for Reducing Chronic Disease Risk. Washington, DC: National Academy Press; 1989.

8. DeCosse J, Miller HH, Lesser ML. Effect of wheat fiber and vitamins C and E on rectal polyps in patients with familial adenomatous polyps. *J Nat Cancer Inst.* 1989;81:1290–1297.
9. Alberts DS, Einsphar J, Rees-McGee S, *et al.* Effects of dietary wheat bran fiber on rectal epithelial cell proliferation in patients with resection for colorectal cancers. *J Nat Cancer Inst.* 1990;82: 1280–1285.
10. Greenwald P, Nixon DW, Malone WF, Kelloff GJ, Stern HR, Witkin KM. Concepts in cancer chemoprevention research. *Cancer.* 1990;65(7):1483–1489.
11. Malone WF. Studies evaluating antioxidants and beta-carotene as chemopreventives. *Am J Clin Nutr.* 1991;53:3055–3135.
12. Schatzkin A, Freedman LS, Schiffman MH, Dawsey SM. Validation of intermediate endpoints in cancer research. *J Nat Cancer Inst.* 1990;82(22): 1746–1752.
13. Kelloff GJ, Malone WF, Boone CW, Sigman CC, Fay JR. Progress in applied chemoprevention research. *Semin Oncol.* 1990;17: 438–455.
14. Heimburger DC, Alexander DB, Birch R. Improvement in bronchial squamous metaplasia in smokers treated with folate and B_{12}. *JAMA.* 1988;259:1525–1530.
15. Kraemer KH, DiGiovanna JJ, Moshell AN, Tarone RE, Peck GL. Prevention of skin cancer in xeroderma pigmentosum with the use of oral isotretinoin. *N Engl J Med.* 1988;318:1633–1637.
16. Hong WK, Endicott J, Itri LM, *et al.* Thirteen-cis-retinoic acid in the treatment of oral leukoplakia. *N Engl J Med.* 1986;315: 1501–1505.
17. Hong WK, Lippman SM, Itri LM, Karp DD, Lee JS, Byers RM. Prevention of second primary tumors with isotretinoin in squamous-cell carcinoma of the head and neck. *N Engl J Med.* 1990;323: 795–801.
18. Greenwald P, Light L, McDonald S, Stern HR. Strategies for cancer prevention through diet modification. *Med Oncol Tumor Pharmacother.* 1990;7($\frac{2}{3}$): 199–208.
19. US Select Committee on Nutrition and Human Needs. *Dietary Goals for the United States.* 2nd ed. Washington, DC: Government Printing Office; 1977.
20. US Department of Agriculture, US Department of Health and

Human Services. *Nutrition and Your Health: Dietary Guidelines for Americans.* 2nd ed. Washington, DC: Government Printing Office; 1985. Home and Garden bulletin 232.

21. American Cancer Society. Nutrition and cancer: cause and prevention: an American Cancer Society special report. *CA.* 1984;34: 121–126.
22. Butrum RR, Clifford CK, Lanza E. Dietary guidelines: rationale. *Am J Clin Nutr.* 1988;48:888.

PART I

Mechanisms of Vitamin Action in Cancer Prevention

WILLIAM A. PRYOR

The Antioxidant Vitamins as Pharmoprotective Agents

ABSTRACT

There are potential benefits in viewing the antioxidant nutrients (such as vitamin E and beta-carotene) as both vitamins and pharmoprotective agents against chronic diseases like cancer and ischemic heart disease. There is much to be gained by continuing and extending human trials to establish whether these nutrients play a dual role. Their classic role, the prevention of deficiency diseases, has little importance in developed countries. The newer role of these nutrients, the optimization of health and prevention of disease, is relatively inexpensive and one of the most promising avenues for nutrition research in the coming decade. The simultaneous monitoring of oxidative stress status among participants in the ongoing trials could shorten the end point for future trials, as well as provide mechanistic insight into how the antioxidant vitamins can protect against disease.

The Antioxidant Vitamins—A Bifurcated Role in Health

Over the past decade, nutritional experts have recognized that micronutrients, and especially antioxidant vitamins, serve two purposes. The first is their classic role, the prevention of deficiency diseases. For example, scurvy, which is caused by an insufficient intake of vitamin C, was one of the earliest diseases attributed to a simple vitamin deficiency (1). And deficiency in vitamin E may result in fat malabsorption, muscular dystrophy, and neurological abnormalities (2, 3).

The recommended dietary allowance (RDA) for the various vitamins is designed "to be adequate to meet the known nutrient needs of practically all healthy persons" and includes a reasonable "safety factor" (2). A problem is that "there are only limited data on which estimates of nutrient requirements can be based" (2). For this reason, the RDA typically has been set at an intake that is just safely above the intake that will prevent known vitamin deficiency diseases; for example, the RDA for vitamin C is set at a level that will safely prevent scurvy. For vitamin E, human deficiency diseases are rare, so the Food and Nutrition Board has set the RDA for vitamin E as an intake that "protects the lipids from peroxidation, permits normal physiological function, and allows for individual variations in [the intake of dietary] lipids." In practice, this means that the intake is set as equal to the "amounts of vitamin E and polyunsaturated fatty acids (PUFA) consumed by normal individuals ingesting balanced diets in the United States" (2). This process, which under the accepted definition of the RDA may be the only one available, has a certain tautology about it: We assume that no one is deficient in vitamin E, and everyone is "normal"; and we recommend that everyone just continue to eat as they do and they will continue to be "normal." But what is normal? Under this reasoning, normal is what we now observe. But if these antioxidant vitamins have a role in preventing cancer, emphysema (especially in smokers), ischemic heart disease (IHD), cataracts, and perhaps other degenerative processes, then clearly there is no certainty that an RDA that is calculated to continue the status quo will serve this added function. That is, since persons eating today's typical diet do develop cataracts, for example, an intake of vitamin E equal to that in today's diet will not prevent or retard cataract development beyond what we observe in today's population. But it seems likely that an elevated intake of vitamin E or vitamin C might prevent or retard the development of cataracts (4).

And thus we come to a paradox: If we assume that everyone who is normal ingests enough vitamins, then we are assuming that no one who is normal needs more; but normal people develop degenerative diseases that we would like to prevent, and there is some evidence that elevated intakes of vitamins play a role in this prevention.

The thoughts outlined above are commonly known and are even something of a consensus; yet some nutritionists and physicians continue to treat vitamin supplementation, and particularly supplementation above the RDA, as controversial. This seems odd. For example, niacin is now used both at the RDA level as a vitamin and at much higher levels to lower blood cholesterol; although this is accepted and common practice among health professionals, some of those same health professionals would regard taking a vitamin supplement as extreme.

Nutrition in the 1990s

In 1900 the majority of deaths in America and similar developed nations resulted from infectious diseases. Today a small number of chronic diseases such as cancer and heart and blood vessel diseases are responsible for the majority of all deaths (5). This gives us an enormous opportunity: If these diseases can be prevented or even postponed, the health of persons in developed countries can be maintained well into the seventh and eighth decades of life.

This possibility is recognized by many nutritionists. For example, Hegsted in his 1985 Atwater Award address (6) stated: Chronic diseases are now the "primary health concern. . . . Most of us will die from one or more of these diseases—coronary heart disease, cancer, stroke, hypertension or diabetes. . . . Improvements in the health of Americans depend upon bringing these diseases under control. The major opportunities in nutrition lie in this area." Weisburger (7) made a similar point: "It is clear that the prevailing chronic diseases worldwide stem from lifestyles, specifically the use of . . . tobacco and the local prevailing nutritional traditions and habits."

These insights have led the National Institutes of Health (NIH) to fund a number of prospective, double-blind human trials involving nutritional additives. Malone (8) has pointed out that of 21 human efficacy trials currently sponsored by the National Cancer Institute (NCI), 10 involve antioxidants, including beta-carotene.

Resistance Toward Antioxidant Vitamins

Some health professionals reject the concept that vitamins can serve a second function, that of optimizing health, and that levels considerably above the RDA are necessary for this second function. This idea clearly is not extreme. One can hardly call a concept extreme that leads the NIH to sponsor a large number of expensive human trials. Furthermore, some physicians are more positive in their view of vitamins than others; for example, pediatricians routinely recommend vitamin supplements of micronutrients for children in their care. The health professionals that reject this concept believe that the evidence does not conclusively support a benefit from vitamin supplementation.

Two arguments are often made to support vitamin supplementation. First, many segments of the population, even in developed countries, do not get even the RDA in their food (9–11). Second, the antioxidant vitamins may play a role in preventive medicine, and because they are completely nontoxic, it is a prudent and reasonable plan to begin taking them now, before conclusive evidence is at hand (12–14).

Some health professionals nevertheless reject arguments for vitamin supplements such as those given above. Persons who argue against supplementation with vitamins appear to have two principal grounds for objection. First, health professionals (especially physicians) have been trained to "do no harm." The natural conservatism of their training that goes with this admonition leads them to believe that a balanced diet provides all the necessary nutrients. Thus when a patient asks a physician whether it is wise to take vitamin supplements, the physician often says no, believing this is scientific. In fact, this advice would be scientific if the physician first carefully probed the diet of the patient and/or did laboratory work to determine whether the patient was sufficient in various micronutrients. Such things are, however, seldom done. Second, it is human nature (and it also is consistent with Occam's Razor) to simplify problems. Since a particular vitamin deficiency disease can be prevented by a particular level of a vitamin, it is assumed that all conditions that might be influenced by this vitamin would require the same intake of that vitamin. However, that is simply not the case.

Figure 1 shows two different associations between the protective effect of vitamin E and its daily intake. Line A shows the situation that will occur if the RDA provides an intake such that the effect of vitamin E is fully realized, and more will not lead to any improvement in the protective effect of vitamin E against this particular pathological condition. In condition B, the protective effect of vitamin E against a particular type of disease or insult continues to increase as more vitamin E is taken, even up to very high levels (12, 15, 16).

The different responsiveness to vitamin E by different pathological conditions is known to occur. Bendich and colleagues (17) have found that the protection that vitamin E affords against hemolysis of the rat red blood cell (RBC) reaches a plateau at a low intake of vitamin E. However, the rat immune system continues to show benefits of increased intake of vitamin E over the unusually wide range of serum

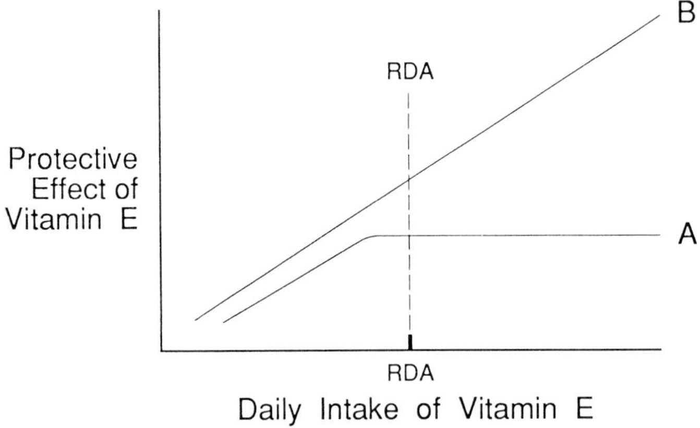

Figure 1. Two potential relationships between the daily intake of vitamin E and the protective effect of vitamin E against a given pathological condition (16, 17).
From Pryor (16) and Bendich *et al.* (17).

concentrations of 0.04 to 18 μg/mL (17). Thus, RBC hemolysis, which is the test often used to determine human sufficiency in vitamin E, may behave like trace A in Figure 1, whereas immune system competency behaves like trace B. The improvement of the immune system is often observed in animals given high levels of vitamin E (18, 19); since vitamin E is sometimes implicated as an anticarcinogen, clearly this observation could be of enormous importance (20–22).

This observation by Bendich *et al.* is not unique. For example, Lemoyne *et al.* (23) have shown that the vitamin E daily intake of humans correlates with the inverse of the amount of pentane excreted in their exhaled breath. Breath pentane is thought to be a measure of the degree to which lipids undergo autoxidative damage (24–26).

Leibovitz and coworkers (27) have reported somewhat similar effects using rat liver, kidney, heart, and spleen slices. They investigated a complex cocktail of antioxidants including RRR-alpha-tocopherol, selenium, coenzyme Q_{10}, and beta-carotene. In one experiment they maintained most of the antioxidants at rather constant levels and varied vitamin E and found an excellent correlation between the dietary intake of vitamin E by the rats and the tissue autoxidation rates for all organs studied, as measured by thiobarbituric acid reactive substances (TBARS). It might be argued that the rates of autoxidation ex vivo by sensitive, accessible tissue (such as the RBC) could be an easy probe of the antioxidant status for humans. (See the discussion of oxidative stress status below.)

The Significance of Disease Prevention by Dietary Means

In the United States, heart and blood vessel diseases account for almost half of all deaths, and cancer for about another quarter (5). The opportunity to control such diseases through micronutrients is, perhaps, the most exciting prospect for preventive medicine in the coming decade. As W. F. Malone, head of the chemopreventive branch of NCI, has said, "Given that no or very low toxicity can be tolerated in most intervention opportunities, a safe agent . . . has a dramatic . . . potential for public health benefits" (8). Malone went on to stress the potential usefulness of the antioxidant nutrients in this role: "Selective investigation should proceed to establish a safe dose and determine whether antioxidants are efficacious in cancer prevention."

Oxidative Stress Status of Persons Enrolled in Clinical Trials

As remarked above, about thirty prospective trials are currently under way, sponsored by the NIH (28). Some of these are designed to probe the effects of vitamin E supplementation (at levels of 100 IU to 800 IU per day) or of beta-carotene on cancer or heart disease. Trials of these types produce data that are generally presented only in terms of the effect of nutritional supplement on the total population of the trial. However, there may be groups of responders and nonresponders, and it would be helpful to separate the effects of supplements on these two groups. For example, in a study of the effect of vitamin E supplementation on IHD, it is possible that certain subsets of the population might be helped and others not. Thus, the potential benefit of antioxidant supplementation on the responders may be diluted by the nonresponsiveness of many of the persons in the trial.

It is likely that the oxidizability of the low-density lipoprotein (LDL) of persons contributes to their susceptibility to IHD (29, 30). If so, the existence of responders and nonresponders to a lessening of IHD by antioxidant therapy may be possible. That this might occur may be indicated, for example, by the enormous variance in antioxidant content of LDL in humans. In 21 humans studied by Esterbauer *et al.* (31), alpha-tocopherol varied from 1.3 nmol/mg to 3.5 nmol/mg and beta-carotene from 0.05 nmol/mg to 0.36 nmol/mg. If these differences are due to different metabolic processing of antioxidants by different persons, and not merely to differing dietary intake, then persons with low "native" antioxidant protection might show greater improvement in a trial than persons with naturally high levels of protection. Thus, it is wise to test the antioxidant protection levels of subjects before, during, and after trials.

In addition, certain persons may be more responsive to oxidative stress, and these persons might respond more strongly to antioxidant therapy. We have previously discussed the usefulness of establishing a routine method for measuring the oxidative stress status (OSS) of humans using a simple noninvasive test (26, 32). If a routine method were available, we could ask, Does taking antioxidant supplements lower OSS, at least for certain groups of responders? And if the answer to this question is affirmative, then we could ask, Are humans with lower OSS at a lower risk for chronic diseases such as cancer and IHD?

These questions suggest that it would be wise to add relatively inexpensive OSS measurements to prospective clinical trials. Most of the trials now in progress take years for the end point—often heart disease or cancer—to develop. If OSS could be measured throughout the clinical trial, and if a correlation were found between OSS and the outcome of the trial, then a method would have been developed that would have predictive value. In addition, if persons taking vitamin E supplements were found to develop cancer at lower rates, and if they also were found to have lower OSS, then the hypothesis that oxidative stress contributes to cancer etiology in some manner (21, 22, 33–39) would be supported.

Methods of Measuring OSS

There are several methods of measuring OSS that are potentially inexpensive and routine and that could be practical candidates for use in clinical trials. One is the evaluation of exhaled breath. Pentane in exhaled breath is reported to be significantly lower in a preliminary study of patients with myocardial infarction than in hospital controls without infarction (40). Similarly, hydrogen peroxide in exhaled breath is increased for patients with adult respiratory distress syndrome (41). (For a discussion of the role of oxidative stress in adult respiratory distress syndrome, see reference 42.)

Several types of ex vivo studies of the oxidizability of blood components could be proposed. One relatively inexpensive study could involve the measurement of volatile products such as pentane from the in vitro oxidation of red blood cells from patients suspected of having various diseases (43). Another possible ex vivo study would be the oxidizability of LDL particles of patients enrolled in clinical trials testing the relationship between diet and IHD. The oxidizability of the LDL particle and the role of vitamin E in preventing LDL oxidation have been studied in detail by Esterbauer *et al.* (31, 44, 45), and there are similar reports for vitamin C (46). Some pilot studies with relatively few patients have in fact already been reported. For example, the yields of TBARS in the plasma and LDL were examined in 17 smokers, and dietary vitamin C was found to have a protective role (46).

It would seem particularly attractive to couple some measure of OSS that involves the oxidizability of the LDL particle with trials that study the role of antioxidant supplements on the occurrence of heart disease. Another possibility is suggested by Janero (47), who recommends that a controlled clinical trail of the effect of vitamin E supplementation on heart disease might be useful for patients undergoing elective coronary revascularization. This trial also could be coupled with a measure of OSS. For example, patients undergoing coronary revascularization could have their OSS measured before and after the surgery; the hypothesis to be tested then would be that only those patients with elevated OSS benefit from vitamin E supplementation prior to revascularization.

Although criticism of the thiobarbituric acid (TBA) test to measure lipid peroxidation is based on concerns about the specificity, interferences, and reliability of TBARS yields as a measure of lipid peroxidation, the TBA test remains one of the easiest methods applicable to complex biological samples. The group led by Yagi in Japan continues to show that elevated TBARS values often are associated with diseases in humans (48–56). In particular, Yagi and his colleagues have shown that the TBA test on blood plasma and on blood lipoprotein fractions can be used to study heart-disease patients in a relatively routine clinical setting (48, 53–56).

The TBA test has been used to compare patients having cancer or heart disease with controls. For example, TBA-reactive substances are reported to be elevated in the urine of women with evidence of mammographic dysplasia relative to controls without such radiological evidence (57).

Conclusion

There is considerable evidence that the antioxidant nutrients play a dual role in human health. The classic role of vitamins and similar micronutrients is the prevention of deficiency diseases. The newer role of these nutrients, the optimization of health and prevention of disease, is one of the most promising avenues for nutrition research in the coming decade.

The simultaneous monitoring of OSS among participants in ongoing clinical trials of the antioxidant vitamins would be wise. Technology would allow the addition of OSS measurements to the trials. The discovery of correlations between OSS and the trial outcomes would provide mechanistic insight into how the antioxidant vitamins help prevent diseases. Furthermore, if OSS was correlated with trial outcomes, OSS could be used as a shorter end point in future trials.

ACKNOWLEDGMENT

Research in our laboratory is supported in part by grants from the National Institutes of Health.

REFERENCES

1. Block G, Menkes M. Ascorbic acid in cancer prevention. In: Moon TE, Micozzi MS, eds. *Nutrition and Cancer Prevention.* New York: Marcel Dekker, Inc; 1989:341–388.
2. National Research Council. *Recommended Dietary Allowances.* Washington, DC: National Academy Press; 1989:1–285.
3. Diplock AT, Machlin LJ, Packer L, Pryor WA, eds. *Vitamin E: Biochemistry and Health Implications.* New York, NY: New York Academy of Sciences; 1989:1–555.
4. Taylor A, Jahngen-Hodge J, Huang LL, Jacques P. Aging in the

eye lens: roles for proteolysis and nutrition in formation of cataract. *Age*. 1991;14:65–71.

5. Leaf A. The aging process: lessons from observations in man. *Nutr Rev*. 1988;46:40–44.
6. Hegsted DM. Nutrition: the changing scene. *Nutr Rev*. 1985;43: 357–367.
7. Weisburger JH. Nutritional approach to cancer prevention with emphasis on vitamins, antioxidants, and carotenoids. *Am J Clin Nutr*. 1991;53(suppl):226S–237S.
8. Malone WF. Studies evaluating antioxidants and β-carotene as chemopreventives. *Am J Clin Nutr*. 1991;53(suppl):305S–313S.
9. Murphy SP, Subar AF, Block G. vitamin E intakes and sources in the United States. *Am J Clin Nutr*. 1990;52:361–367.
10. Block G. Vitamin C and cancer prevention: the epidemiologic evidence. *Am J Clin Nutr*. 1991;53(suppl):270S–282S.
11. Block G. Dietary guidelines and the results of food consumption surveys. *Am J Clin Nutr*. 1991;53(suppl):356S–357S.
12. Pryor WA. Views on the wisdom of using antioxidant vitamin supplements. *Free Radic Biol Med*. 1987;3:189–191.
13. Diplock AT. Dietary supplementation with antioxidants: is there a case for exceeding the recommended dietary allowance? *Free Radic Biol Med*. 1987;3:199–201.
14. Diplock AT. Antioxidant nutrients and disease prevention: an overview. *Am J Clin Nutr*. 1991;53(suppl):189S–193S.
15. Pryor WA. Vitamin E: the status of current research and suggestions for future studies. *Ann N Y Acad Sci*. 1989;570:400–405.
16. Pryor WA. The antioxidant nutrients and disease prevention—what do we know and what do we need to find out? *Am J Clin Nutr*. 1991;53(suppl):391S–393S.
17. Bendich A, Gabriel E, Machlin LJ. Dietary vitamin E requirement for optimum immune responses in the rat. *J Nutr*. 1986;116: 675–681.
18. Bendich A, Phillips M, Tengerdy RP, eds. *Antioxidant Nutrients and Immune Functions*. New York: Plenum Press; 1990:1–171.
19. Pryor WA. Can vitamin E protect us against the pathological effects of ozone in smog? *Am J Clin Nutr*. 1991;53:702–722.
20. Meyskens FL Jr, Prasad KN, eds. *Vitamins and Cancer*. Clifton, NJ: Humana Press; 1986:1–481.
21. Tryfiades GP, Prasad KN, eds. *Nutrition, Growth, and Cancer*. New York: Alan R. Liss, Inc; 1988:1–428.

22. Moon TE, Micozzi, MS, eds. *Nutrition and Cancer Prevention*. New York: Marcel Dekker, Inc; 1989:1–588.
23. Lemoyne M, Van Gossum A, Kurian R, Ostro M, Axler J, Jeejeebhoy KN. Breath pentane analysis as an index of lipid peroxidation: a functional test of vitamin E status. *Am J Clin Nutr.* 1987; 46:267–272.
24. Tappel AL, Dillard CJ. In vivo lipid peroxidation: measurement via exhaled pentane and protection by vitamin E. *Fed Proc.* 1981; 40:174–178.
25. Dillard CJ, Sagai M, Tappel AL. Respiratory pentane: a measure of in vivo lipid peroxidation applied to rats fed diets varying in polyunsaturated fats, vitamin E, and selenium and exposed to nitrogen dioxide. *Toxicol Lett.* 1980;6:251–256.
26. Pryor WA, Godber SS. Noninvasive measures of oxidative stress status in humans. *Free Radic Biol Med.* 1991;10:177–184.
27. Leibovitz B, Hu M-L, Tappel Al. Dietary supplements of vitamin E, β-carotene, coenzyme Q_{10} and selenium protect tissues against lipid peroxidation in rat tissue slices. *J Nutr.* 1990;120:97–104.
28. Brown M, Desai M, Traber LD, Herndon DN, Traber DL. Dimethylsulfoxide with heparin in the treatment of smoke inhalation injury. *J Burn Care Rehabil.* 1988;9:22–25.
29. Palinski W, Rosenfeld ME, Yia-Herttuala S, *et al.* Low-density lipoprotein undergoes oxidative modification in vivo. *Proc Natl Acad Sci U S A.* 1989;86:1372–1376.
30. Steinbrecher UP, Parthasarathy S, Leake DS, Witztum JL, Steinberg D. Modification of low-density lipoprotein by endothelial cells involves lipid peroxidation and degradation of low-density lipoprotein phospholipids. *Proc Natl Acad Sci U S A.* 1984;81: 3883–3887.
31. Esterbauer H, Striegl G, Puhl H, *et al.* The role of vitamin E and carotenoids in preventing oxidation of low-density lipoproteins. *Ann NY Acad Sci.* 1989;570:254–267.
32. Pryor WA, Godber SS. Oxidative stress status: an introduction. *Free Radic Biol Med.* 1991;10:173.
33. Copeland ES, Borg DC, Cerutti P, Kaufman DG, Birnboim HC, Pryor WA. Free radicals in promotion—a chemical pathology study section workshop. *Cancer Res.* 1983;43:5631–5637.
34. Pryor WA, Uehara K, Church DF. The chemistry and biochemistry of the radicals in cigarette smoke: ESR evidence for the binding of the tar radical to DNA and polynucleotides. In: Bors W, Saran

M, Tait D, eds. *Oxygen Radicals in Chemistry and Biology.* Berlin: Walter de Gruyter and Co; 1984:193–201.
35. Pryor WA. Cancer and free radicals. In: Shankel D, Hartman P, Kada T, Hollaender A, eds. *Antimutagenesis and Anticarcinogenesis Mechanisms.* New York: Plenum Press; 1986:45–59.
36. Pryor WA. Cigarette smoke and the involvement of free radical reactions in chemical carcinogenesis. *Br J Cancer.* 1987;55:19–23.
37. Pryor WA. The involvement of free radicals in chemical carcinogenesis. In: Cerutti PA, Nygaard OF, Simic MG, eds. *Anticarcinogenesis and Radiation Protection.* New York: Plenum Press; 1987: 1–11.
38. Halliwell B, Borish ET, Pryor WA, *et al.* Oxygen radicals and human disease. *Ann Intern Med.* 1987;107:526–545.
39. Pryor WA. Commentary. In: Pryor WA, ed. *Free Radicals and Peroxides in the Etiology of Cancer.* Washington, DC: Government Printing Office; 1987:v–xiii.
40. Weitz ZW, Birnbaum AJ, Sobotka PA, Zarling EJ, Skosey JL. High breath pentane concentrations during acute myocardical infarction. *Lancet.* 1991;337:933–935.
41. Sznajder JI, Fraiman A, Hall JB, *et al.* Increased hydrogen peroxide in the expired breath of patients with acute hypoxemic respiratory failure. *Chest.* 1989;96:606–612.
42. Cochrane CG, Spragg R, Revak SD. Pathogenesis of the adult respiratory distress syndrome. *J Clin Invest.* 1983;71:754–761.
43. Frankel EN, Tappel AL. Headspace gas chromatography of volatile lipid peroxidation products from human red blood cell membranes. *Lipids.* 1991;26:479–484.
44. Esterbauer H, Dieber-Rotheneder M, Striegl G, Waeg G. Role of vitamin E in preventing the oxidation of low-density lipoprotein. *Am J Clin Nutr.* 1991;53(suppl):314S–321S.
45. Esterbauer H, Jürgens G, Quehenberger O, Koller E. Autoxidation of human low density lipoprotein: loss of polyunsaturated fatty acids and vitamin E and generation of aldehydes. *J Lipid Res.* 1987;28:495–509.
46. Jialal I, Vega GL, Grundy SM. Physiologic levels of ascorbate inhibit the oxidative modification of low-density lipoprotein. *Atherosclerosis.* 1990;82:185–191.
47. Janero DR. Therapeutic potential of vitamin E against myocardial ischemic-reperfusion injury. *Free Radic Biol Med.* 1991;10:315–324.

48. Yagi K. Increased serum lipid peroxides initiate atherogenesis. *Bioessays*. 1984;1:58–60.
49. Yagi K. A simple fluorometric assay for lipoperoxide in blood plasma. *Biochem Med*. 1976;15:212–216.
50. Sato Y, Hotta N, Sakamoto N, Matsuoka S, Ohishi N, Yagi K. Lipid peroxide levels in plasma of diabetic patients. *Biochem Med*. 1979;21:104–107.
51. Ohkawa H, Ohishi N, Yagi K. Assay for lipid peroxides in animal tissue by thiobarbituric acid reaction. *Anal Biochem*. 1979;95: 351–358.
52. Komura S, Yoshino K, Kondo K, Yagi K. Lipid peroxide levels in the skin of the senescence-accelerated mouse. *J Clin Biochem Nutr*. 1988;5:255–260.
53. Yagi K. A biochemical approach to atherogenesis. *Trends Biochem Sciences*. 1986;11:18–19.
54. Hagihara M, Nishigaki I, Maseki M, Yagi K. Age-dependent changes in lipid peroxide levels in the lipoprotein fractions of human serum. *J Gerontol*. 1984;39:269–272.
55. Yagi K. Lipid peroxides and human disease. *Chem Phys Lipids*. 1987;45:337–351.
56. Yamauchi T, Inagaki T, Ohishi N, Yagi K. Rapid preparation of subfractions of low density lipoprotein from hypercholesterolemic rabbit serum. *J Clin Biochem Nutr*. 1990;8:9–19.
57. Boyd NF, McGuire V. Evidence of lipid peroxidation in premenopausal women with mammographic dysplasia. *Cancer Lett*. 1990; 50:31–37.

ADRIANNE BENDICH

Vitamins and Tumor Immunity

ABSTRACT

The major functions of the immune system are to protect us from pathogens and to protect us from cancer. The immune system utilizes several strategies to destroy cancer cells. The three major classes of white blood cells that can kill tumor cells directly are cytotoxic T lymphocytes, macrophages, and natural killer cells. In addition, activated macrophages secrete tumor necrosis factor, which kills tumor cells. Several cytokines can enhance the activities of immune cells capable of killing tumor cells.

Data from laboratory studies show that certain carotenoids and vitamin E boost the activities of the cancer-fighting white blood cells, resulting in decreased tumor burden. Vitamin A, vitamin C, vitamin B_6, and folic acid have been shown to enhance many aspects of immunity. Cancer incidence and mortality have been inversely associated with vitamin and carotenoid intakes in many studies. Enhancement of tumor immunity by certain vitamins and carotenoids may be an important factor in cancer prevention.

Tumor Immunity

The immune system protects us from infection by environmental pathogens such as bacteria, viruses, and protozoan parasites. These agents are recognized as invaders of the body and as "nonself" and are destroyed by immune cells and their secretions. The immune system responds similarly to cells of the body that have undergone changes that may lead to cancer. The body's immune system no longer recognizes certain precancerous cells as "self." In essence, the altered cells are considered invaders and are destroyed. Conditions that depress immune functions consequently increase the risk of certain cancers. Conversely, factors that can enhance immunity may lower the risk of cancer (1).

Evidence that immunosuppression increases risk of cancer comes from many laboratory studies as well as from clinical investigations. For example, patients undergoing kidney transplants are given immunosuppressive drugs to prevent the rejection of the transplant. The incidence of skin cancer, especially squamous-cell carcinoma, is significantly higher in these patients. Skin cancer cells are normally strong stimulators of immune responses, which destroy the transformed cells. However, in the immunosuppressed patient, the loss of tumor immunity is considered an increased risk factor for the development of skin cancer (2).

Immune Mechanisms of Killing Tumor Cells

Three types of white blood cells of the immune system are capable of killing tumor cells directly. Cytotoxic T lymphocytes, macrophages, and natural killer cells can recognize and destroy tumor cells by several mechanisms. Natural killer cells bore a hole in the tumor cell, in effect bursting the cell membrane. Macrophages and cytotoxic T lymphocytes also destroy the outer membrane of the cancerous cell upon direct contact.

Macrophages secrete tumor necrosis factor, which can kill tumor cells without direct cell contact. Other factors synthesized and secreted by immune cells can also damage cellular components, resulting in decreased replication of the cancerous cell and/or cellular sterility.

Many cells of the body are capable of synthesizing factors that stimulate the activity of immune cells. Examples of such factors include the interleukins, the interferons, growth factors, and other small, hormonelike molecules that are critical in the development of immune responses to precancerous conditions (3).

Anticarcinogenic and Immunoenhancing Functions of Certain Vitamins and Carotenoids

The activities of the cells of the immune system are affected by a number of factors, including immunosuppressive, oxygen-containing free radicals and molecules that interfere with DNA synthesis. However, there are essential micronutrients that can inactivate free radicals and there are others that are essential in the synthesis of DNA.

Vitamin C, vitamin E, and beta-carotene are antioxidants and quench reactive oxygen species, including free radicals. Vitamin A, with some antioxidant potential, is critical for normal cellular differentiation. Folic acid and vitamin B_6 (pyridoxine) are essential for the synthesis of nucleic acids (4).

Because these micronutrients have been implicated in cancer chemoprevention (5) and are the focus of many of the following papers, the present discussion is limited to these even though single deficiencies of any of the vitamins adversely affects some aspect of immunity and most likely results in increased risk of malignancy.

Free Radicals and Immune Cell Function

The fluidity of leukocyte cell membranes is in part dependent upon the degree of unsaturation of its fatty acids. As the level of polyunsaturated fatty acids is increased, the potential for free radical–mediated membrane lipid peroxidation is also increased. Lipid peroxidation causes a decrease in membrane fluidity, which adversely affects immune responses. Mice fed oxidized lipids show marked atrophy of the thymus as well as T-cell dysfunction. Loss of membrane fluidity has been directly related to the decreased ability of lymphocytes to respond to challenges to the immune system (6).

The degree of unsaturation of the lipids incorporated into leukocyte membranes alters the exposure of membrane receptors and their activities. The synthesis of metabolites of arachidonic acid, such as immunosuppressive prostaglandins, is increased as the degree of unsaturation of membrane lipids increases and/or the concentration of antioxidants decreases (7).

Factors Affecting Tumor Immunity

Among the many factors that adversely affect tumor immunity are environmental exposure and genetic predisposition. External factors include exposure to ultraviolet (UV) light, cigarette smoking, and infection with viruses such as human immunodeficiency virus (HIV), and human papilloma virus (HPV). Genetic factors significantly influence the aging process, which is associated with a loss of cell-mediated immune responses and a concomitant increase in cancer incidence.

UV Exposure

Exposure to UV light has been shown to decrease immune responses, especially cell-mediated responses, and significantly increase the risk of skin cancer (8). Experimental studies have clearly linked the immunosuppressive effects of UV exposure with increased development of skin and other tumors (9).

Many carotenoids have the capacity to block the formation of UV-induced singlet oxygen. Singlet oxygen can initiate the generation of immunosuppressive, reactive oxygen species. Recent studies have shown that dietary intake of beta-carotene or canthaxanthin, a carotenoid lacking vitamin A activity, can significantly reduce the immunosuppressive effects of UV exposure. Supplemental intakes of canthaxanthin and vitamin A blocked the loss of tumor immunity in UV-exposed mice and reduced the growth of experimentally implanted tumors (10). Beta-carotene supplementation prior to exposure to UV light prevented UV-induced depression of cell-mediated immune responses in adult males (11) (Fig. 1).

Long-term consumption of foods rich in beta-carotene has repeatedly been shown to lower the risk of many cancers, especially lung cancer (12). One possible mechanism for carotenoid cancer prevention may be immunoenhancement (13). The finding that beta-carotene supplementation did not prevent the recurrence of skin cancer in a recent intervention trial (14) suggests that the length of supplementation may have been insufficient and/or the skin cancers have reached a point at which enhancement in tumor immunity may have been too late to overcome years of UV insult.

Exposure to UV light directly increases the free radical burden imposed upon the body. Antioxidants, such as beta-carotene, vitamin E, vitamin C, and to some extent vitamin A, may enhance tumor immunity by lowering the exposure to immunosuppressive reactive oxygen species.

Human Immunodeficiency Virus and Human Papilloma Virus

Viruses are intracellular parasites that usually result in immunosuppression of the host. Bacterial or other infections often follow viral infection because of the decreased protection from leukocytes. Hu-

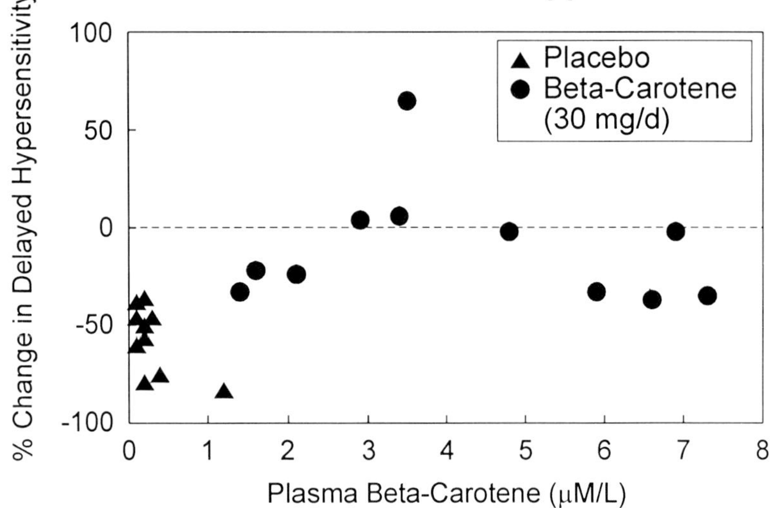

Figure 1. Twenty-four male subjects were randomly divided into two groups. Those in one group were given a placebo; those in the other group were given 30 mg of beta-carotene per day. All subjects then consumed diets excluding carotenoids for the study period. Delayed hypersensitivity skin test responses (DTH) were determined at three time points: at the onset of the study, after 4 weeks, at which time exposure to UV light began, and after exposure to UV. DTH were unchanged following the first 4 weeks. UV exposure involved anterior and posterior body surfaces exposed to a solar simulator for 10–12 days at a dosage of 15.9–19.3 J/cm^2. UV exposure caused a significant decrease in DTH in the placebo group, but DTH responses were maintained in the supplemented group.
From Fuller *et al.* (11).

man immunodeficiency virus is particularly devastating because the virus infects and inactivates the cells of the immune system. The link between depressed immunity and greater risk of cancer is clearly seen in the HIV infected, who are at increased risk of developing cancers such as Kaposi's sarcoma. Not as clear currently is the link between lowered vitamin B_{12}, B_6, folic acid, and beta-carotene levels seen in HIV-infected patients and the immunosuppression and increased cancer risk in this population. Greater emphasis is beginning to be given to the nutritional status of HIV-infected subjects prior to the development of overt symptoms. Elimination of marginal micronutrient deficiencies could help lower the risk of secondary infections, which are a leading cause of HIV-related mortalities (15, 16).

Another viral infection associated with a greater risk of cancer is HPV. Women with cervical cancer or the precancerous condition cervical dysplasia are far more likely to have HPV than not. In several epidemiological studies, women with cervical dysplasia had significantly reduced serum levels of folic acid, beta-carotene, and/or vitamin C (17, 18, 19, 20). Intervention studies, discussed below, suggest that folic acid supplementation may lower the risk of cervical dysplasia in HPV-infected women.

Cigarette Smoking

The risk of lung cancer is approximately fifteen times greater in smokers compared with nonsmokers (21). Along with many other known harmful chemicals found in cigarette smoke, there are thousands of free radicals per puff. Reports from the second National Health and Nutrition Examination Survey (1976–1980) show that in the American population ascorbic acid levels in serum are consistently lower in smokers than in nonsmokers. Smokers need to consume well over twice the recommended daily allowance of vitamin C to have similar concentrations of vitamin C in serum as nonsmokers (22).

Levels of folic acid and beta-carotene in serum as well as vitamin E concentrations in the lung are significantly lower in smokers compared with nonsmokers (23, 24, 18). Smokers have greater damage to chromosomes in their lymphocytes than nonsmokers, which may be in part due to their significantly decreased folic acid status (25, 26). Increased lymphocyte chromosome fragility is used as an index of systemic chromosome damage, which can represent the first step in the multistep carcinogenesis process. Damage to lymphocyte DNA may also indicate an enhanced risk of cancers that affect the immune system, such as leukemia and lymphoma. Decreased folate status seen in smokers may facilitate chromosome damage. The reduction of antioxidant status also seen in smokers may favor cellular damage because of the increased free radical burden imposed by smoking (22).

Chronic exposure to cigarette smoke significantly lowers lymphocyte functions such as proliferation and antibody production. Decreased natural killer cell activity and significantly increased risk of infection and precancerous lesions are well documented in chronic smokers. Cigarette smoke also contributes to the development of local inflammation in the lung, with resultant increased production of reactive oxygen radicals from activated leukocytes. Several laboratories have found that experimentally induced tumors grow faster in animals exposed to cigarette smoke; concomitant immunosuppression has also been documented in a number of the animal models (27). The combined effects of increased free radical burden and increased damage to DNA as well as decreased status of vitamins C, E, and folic acid and beta-carotene in smokers may interfere sufficiently with normal tumor immunity to result in increased carcinogenesis in smokers.

Aging

Of the many factors that affect immunocompetence and risk of carcinogenesis, the aging process has been investigated to the greatest extent. Cancer is a disease of aging; it is the second leading cause of death in United States populations including individuals over the age of 65 (28). As an example, the risk of cancer of the large intestine increases 1000 times between the ages of 30 and 80, with the majority of the increased risk occurring after 65 (29).

Table 1. Effects of Vitamin Supplementation on Immune Responses in the Elderly

Oral Supplement, Dose/Day	Duration	Immune Effects	Reference
Vitamin E, 800 IU	30 days	Enhanced DTH[a], enhanced IL_2[b], enhanced proliferation	7
Beta-carotene, 45–60 mg	60 days	Increased markers for helper-T cells, NK[c] cells, and IL_2 receptors	32
Vitamin A, 800 IU; vitamin E, 50 mg; vitamin C, 100 mg	28 days	Increased markers for helper-T cells and total T cells; enhanced proliferation	33
Multivitamin/mineral supplement	16 months	Enhanced DTH, enhanced proliferation	15

Note: All studies were double-blind and placebo controlled, and, other than Penn *et al.*, used healthy elderly individuals.

[a] DTH = delayed type hypersensitivity.

[b] IL_2 = interleukin 2.

[c] NK = natural killer.

One of the possible factors affecting the increased occurrence of cancer in the elderly could be the well-established decrease in immune functions seen as individuals age (30). The cell-mediated immune responses, involving T lymphocyte functions (cytotoxicity, interleukin 2 production, proliferation), are the most sensitive to the age-related decline in immune responses. As a consequence, delayed type hypersensitivity (DTH) responses to skin-test antigens are significantly diminished in the elderly, resulting in anergy—a complete lack of skin-test responses—in the most immunosuppressed.

Recent studies have shown that DTH can be used as a predictor of morbidity and mortality in the elderly; that is, elderly with reduced DTH responses (anergy) had twice the risk of death as elderly that responded to the antigens (31). Of great importance are recent data from four placebo-controlled, double-blind studies that indicate that certain micronutrient supplements can significantly enhance DTH responses and/or T-cell subpopulations and proliferative responses as well as interleukin 2 activities in the elderly (Table 1; Fig. 2). Vitamin E supplementation (800 IU/d) for one month increased DTH re-

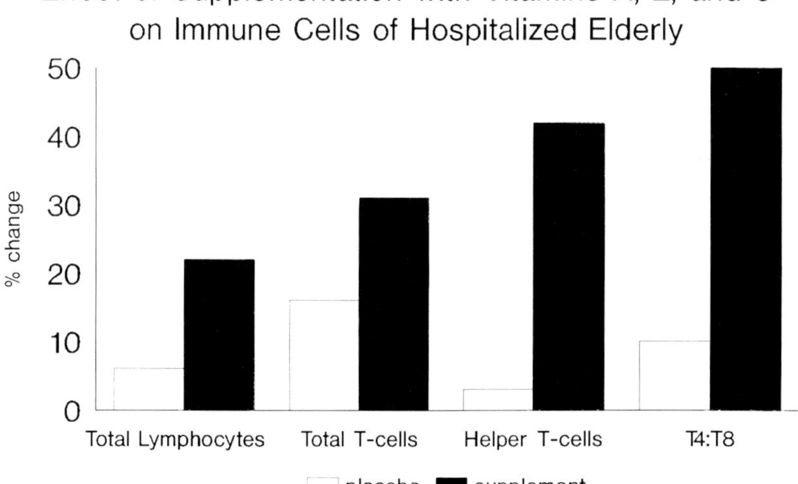

Figure 2. Thirty long-term hospitalized elderly patients were randomly divided into two groups: those receiving placebo and those being supplemented. Lymphocyte parameters were determined after 28 days of the study. From Penn *et al.* (33) by permission of Oxford University Press.

sponses of healthy elderly individuals (7). Beta-carotene supplementation of 45 or 60 mg per day for two months increased leukocyte markers for natural killer cells and interleukin 2 receptors in healthy elderly individuals (32). A high-potency multivitamin and mineral supplement taken for 16 months enhanced DTH in healthy elderly persons (15). A supplement of 8000 IU of vitamin A, 50 mg of vitamin E, and 100 mg of vitamin C taken for twenty-eight days increased total T lymphocyte numbers as well as helper T-cell markers in a group of long-term, hospitalized elderly patients (33).

These data strongly suggest that supplementation with certain vitamins and/or beta-carotene provides a safe, cost-effective, and practical approach for delaying or reversing the rate of decline of certain immune functions in the elderly. To lower the rates of cancer occurrence, adoption of preventive dietary and supplementation programs may have to begin in early adulthood.

Carotenoids, Vitamin A, and Tumor Immunity

Carotenoids are naturally occurring red and yellow pigments found in all photosynthetic plants and organisms. Of the more than six hundred characterized compounds, less than 10% can serve as precursors of vitamin A. Beta-carotene, the most commonly available carotenoid in human diets, has the greatest potential vitamin A activity (34). The importance of vitamin A to immune function is well accepted. In fact, vitamin A has been called the anti-infective vitamin for many decades (35). Vitamin A has also been shown to be critical for the development of immune responses to tumors (36).

Nutritionists have traditionally viewed carotenoids solely as sources of vitamin A activity in the diet. However, several studies have shown that carotenoids can enhance immune functions independent of any provitamin A activity (13). The mechanisms of immunoenhancement may include the antioxidant and singlet oxygen quenching capacities of a number of carotenoids. In contrast, vitamin A is a relatively poor antioxidant and cannot quench singlet oxygen (34).

Antioxidants may enhance many immune functions by lowering the concentrations of immunosuppressive free radicals and their products (6). Increased exposure to hydroxyl radicals and lipid peroxides as well as other reactive oxygen species has been associated with increased risk of certain cancers (37). Carotenoid immunoenhancement may be part of the explanation for the cumulative evidence from epidemiological studies that high carotenoid status is strongly associated with lowered risk of many cancers (12).

In laboratory studies, comparisons between beta-carotene and the nonvitamin A carotenoid canthaxanthin have shown that both carotenoids enhanced T and B lymphocyte proliferative responses to mitogens (38), increased cytotoxic T-cell (39) and macrophage tumor killing activity, and stimulated the secretion of tumor necrosis factor alpha, and at the same time lowered the tumor burden (40). As discussed earlier, dietary supplementation with canthaxanthin and vitamin A significantly overcame the immunosuppressive effects of UV light exposure and decreased the tumor burden in mice (10).

Supplementation of healthy elderly individuals for two months with 45 or 60 mg per day of beta-carotene increased the concentration of peripheral blood cells bearing markers for natural killer cells as well as three markers of mononuclear cell activation (transferrin, HLA-Dr, and interleukin 2 receptors) (32).

In another study, vegetarians were found to have serum vitamin levels similar to those of a matched nonvegetarian population. However, serum beta-carotene levels were two times higher in the vegetarian group. Natural killer cells from the vegetarian group lysed twice the number of tumor cells as natural killer cells from the nonvegetarian group, suggesting that beta-carotene may enhance natural killer cell functions (41).

Folic Acid

Human papilloma virus infects the cells of the cervix, resulting in a significantly increased risk of precancerous cervical dysplasia and cervical cancer. Recent studies suggest that lower than normal cervical cell folic acid concentrations enhance the infectivity of the cells with HPV (42).

Oral contraceptive users have been shown to have lower circulating folic acid levels than nonusers consuming similar diets. Folic acid was given for three months to oral contraceptive users with cervical dysplasia and initially lower folate status. This group showed a significant decrease in dysplasias, whereas a placebo group with cervical dysplasia either remained stable or had a worsening of the dysplasias (17). As mentioned above, smokers also have lower folic acid levels, which increases the risk for DNA damage. Smoking, therefore, may further exacerbate the folic acid–lowering effects of oral contraceptive use and add to the risk of infection with HPV, precancerous lesions, and cancer.

Smokers with precancerous bronchial metaplasia, when given 10 mg of folate and 500 μg of vitamin B_{12} per day for four months, had a significant reduction in atypical bronchial cells compared with subjects in the placebo group (43). These data point to the importance of maintaining optimal folic acid concentrations in the epithelial tissues of smokers.

Low folate status adversely affects many immune parameters. There is enhanced susceptibility to bacterial and viral infections, depressed antibody responses, reduced circulating levels of leukocytes, decreased cytotoxic T-cell responses, and hypersegmentation of the nucleus of the neutrophils (44–46). More research is needed, however, to link folic acid status to tumor immunity in animal models as well as in humans.

Vitamin B_6

Vitamin B_6, like folic acid, is important in the synthesis of components of DNA. Vitamin B_6 deficiency also adversely affects cell-mediated immune responses, cytotoxic T-cell functions, and antibody synthesis in animal models (45). Chandra and Sudhakaran (47) showed that vitamin B_6-deficient mice had significantly decreased natural killer cell lysis of tumor cells compared with pair-fed controls; antibody-dependent cell-mediated cytotoxicity, however, was unaffected by the deficiency in the same mice.

In a small placebo-controlled, double-blind study, elderly subjects given 50 mg daily of vitamin B_6 for eight weeks had significantly increased lymphocyte proliferation and enhanced levels of total and helper T cells (48). As discussed above, several well-controlled studies have shown that elderly persons supplemented with other vitamins showed consistent enhancement of certain immune functions associated with the destruction of tumor cells.

Conclusions

The immune system has many components capable of identifying and destroying cancerous cells. The optimal functioning of the immune system can be diminished by external factors, such as exposure to UV light, infection with pathogenic viruses, and cigarette smoking, as well as by low intakes of micronutrients including vitamins A, C, and E, folic acid, vitamin B_6, and beta-carotene. The aging process includes the reduction of cell-mediated immune responses that are required for tumor immunity.

Data from laboratory experiments and controlled clinical studies show immunoenhancement and/or decreased loss of immune responses in vitamin-supplemented groups. Some of the data indicate that the supplemented groups have enhanced tumor immunity, resulting in decreased tumor size, number, and/or reversal of the precancerous state. Immunoenhancement, with optimal intake of vitamins and carotenoids, may be a critical factor in lowering cancer risk.

REFERENCES

1. Roitt IM, Brostoff J, Male DK, eds. *Immunology.* New York: Gower Medical Publishing; 1985.
2. Streilein WJ. Immunogenetic factors in skin cancer. *N Engl J Med.* 1991;325:884–887.
3. Oppenheim JJ, Shevach EM, eds. *Immunophysiology: The Role of Cells and Cytokines in Immunity and Inflammation.* New York: Oxford University Press, Inc; 1990.
4. Machlin LJ, ed. *Handbook of Vitamins.* New York: Marcel Dekker, Inc; 1991.
5. Knekt P, Aromaa A, Maatela J, *et al.* Serum micronutrients and risk of cancers of low incidence in Finland. *Am J Epidemiol.* 1991; 134:356–361.
6. Bendich A. Antioxidant vitamins and their functions in immune responses. In: Bendich A, Phillips M, Tengerdy RP, eds. *Antioxidant Nutrients and Immune Functions.* New York: Plenum Press; 1990:33–35.
7. Meydani SN, Barklund MP, Liu S, *et al.* Vitamin E supplementation enhances cell-mediated immunity in healthy elderly subjects. *Am J Clin Nutr.* 1990;52:557–563.
8. Donawho CK, Kripke ML. Evidence that the local effect of ultraviolet radiation on the growth of murine melanomas is immunologically mediated. *Cancer Res.* 1991;51:4176–4181.
9. Punnonen K, Autio P, Kiistala U. In-vivo effects of solar-simulated ultraviolet irradiation on antioxidant enzymes and lipid peroxidation in human epidermis. *Br J Dermatol.* 1991;125:18–20.
10. Gensler HL. Reduction of immunosuppression in UV-irradiated mice by dietary retinyl palmitate plus canthaxanthin. *Carcinogenesis.* 1989;10:203–207.

11. Fuller CJ, Faulkner H, Roe DA. Effect of beta-carotene on the photosuppression of cellular immune function in normal males. *FASEB J.* 1991;5:A1323.
12. Ziegler RG. A review of epidemiologic evidence that carotenoids reduce the risk of cancer. *J Nutr.* 1989;119:116–122.
13. Bendich A. Carotenoids and immunity. *Clin Appl Nutr.* 1991; 1:45–51.
14. Greenberg RE, Baron JA, Stukel TA, *et al.* A clinical trial of beta carotene to prevent basal-cell and squamous-cell cancers of the skin. *N Engl J Med.* 1990;323:789–801.
15. Bogden JD, Oleske JM, Lavenhar MA, *et al.* Effects of one year of supplementation with zinc and other micronutrients on cellular immunity in the elderly. *J Am Coll Nutr.* 1990;9:214–225.
16. Boudes P, Zittoun J, Sobel A. Folate, vitamin B_{12}, and HIV infection. *Lancet.* 1991;325:1401–1402.
17. Butterworth CE, Hatch KD, Gore H, Muller H, Krumdiek CL. Improvement in cervical dysplasia associated with folic acid therapy in users of oral contraceptives. *Am J Clin Nutr.* 1982;35:73–82.
18. Stryker WS, Kaplan LA, Stein EA, Stampfer M, Sober A, Willett WC. The relation of diet, cigarette smoking, and alcohol consumption to plasma β-carotene and alpha-tocopherol levels. *Am J Epidemiol.* 1988;127:283–296.
19. Romney SL, Duttagupta C, Basu J, *et al.* Plasma vitamin C and uterine cervical dysplasia. *Am J Obstet Gynecol.* 1985;151:976–980.
20. Verreault R, Chu J, Mandelson M, Shy K. A case-control study of diet and invasive cervical cancer. *Int J Cancer.* 1989;43:1050–1054.
21. Byers TE, Graham S, Haughey BP, Marshall JR, Swanson MK. Diet and lung cancer risk: findings from the western New York diet study. *Am J Epidemiol.* 1987;125:351–363.
22. Bendich A, Machlin LJ, Scandurra O, Burton GW, Wayner DDM. The antioxidant role of vitamin C. *Adv Free Rad Biol Med.* 1986: 2:419–444.
23. Heimburger DC, Krumdieck CL, Butterworth CE. Role of folate in prevention of cancers of the lung and cervix. *J Am Coll Nutr.* 1987;6:425.
24. Pacht ER, Kasek H, Mohammed JR, Cromwell DG, Davis WB. Deficiency of vitamin E in the alveolar fluid of cigarette smokers: influence on alveolar macrophage cytotoxicity. *J Clin Invest.* 1986; 77:789–796.

25. Chen ATL, Reidy JA, Annest JL, Welty TK. Relationship between chromosome fragility, smoking, and folate. *Environ Sci Res.* 1987; 36:369–374.
26. Chen ATL, Reidy JA, Annest JL, Welty TK, Zhou H. Increased chromosomes fragility as a consequence of blood folate levels, smoking status, and coffee consumption. *Environ Mol Mutagen.* 1989;13:319–324.
27. Johnson JD, Houchens DP, Kluwe WM, Craig DK, Fisher GL. Effects of mainstream and environmental tobacco smoke on the immune system in animals and humans: a review. *Crit Rev Toxicol.* 1990;20:369–395.
28. National Center for Health Statistics. Births, marriages, divorces, and deaths for June 1991. *Monthly Vital Statistics Report.* 1991; 40:1–23.
29. Visek WJ. Diet and cancer. In: Prinsley DM, Sandstead HH, eds. *Nutrition and Aging.* New York: Alan R. Liss, Inc; 1990:301–320.
30. Goodwin JS, Burns EL. Aging, nutrition, and immune function. *Clin Appl Nutr.* 1991;1:85–94.
31. Wayne SJ, Rhyne RL, Garry PJ, Goodwin JS. Cell-mediated immunity as a predictor of morbidity and mortality in subjects over 60. *J Gerontol.* 1990;45:M45–M48.
32. Watson RR, Prabhala RH, Plezia PM, Alberts DS. Effect of β-carotene on lymphocyte subpopulations in elderly humans: evidence for a dose-response relationship. *Am J Clin Nutr.* 1991; 53:90–94.
33. Penn ND, Purkins L, Kelleher J, Heatley RV, Mascie-Taylor BH, Belfield PW. The effect of dietary vitamin-supplementation with vitamin-A, C and E on cell-mediated immune function in elderly long-stay patients: a randomized controlled trial. *Age Ageing.* 1991;20:169–174.
34. Bendich A, Olson JA. Biological actions of carotenoids. *FASEB J.* 1989;3:1927–1932.
35. Nauss KM. Influence of vitamin A status on the immune system. In: Bauernfeind CJ, ed. *Vitamin A Deficiency and Its Control.* Orlando, Fla: Academic Press, Inc; 1986:207–284.
36. Moon RC. Comparative aspects of carotenoids and retinoids as chemopreventive agents for cancer. *J Nutr.* 1989;119:127–134.
37. Krinsky NI. Carotenoids and cancer in animal models 1, 2. *J Nutr.* 1989;119:123–126.

38. Bendich A, Shapiro SS. Effect of beta-carotene and canthaxanthin on the immune responses of the rat. *J Nutr.* 1986;116:2254–2262.
39. Tomita Y, Himeno K, Nomoto K, *et al.* Augmentation of tumor immunity against syngeneic tumors in mice by beta carotene. *J Natl Cancer Inst.* 1987;78:679–680.
40. Schwartz JL, Shklar G, Flynn E, *et al.* The administration of beta carotene to prevent and regress oral carcinoma in the hamster cheek pouch and the associated enhancement of the immune response. In: Bendich A, Phillips M, Tengerdy RP, eds. *Antioxidant Nutrients and Immune Functions: Advances in Experimental Biology and Medicine.* New York: Plenum Press; 1990:77–93.
41. Malter M, Schriever G, Eilber U. Natural killer cells, vitamins, and other blood components of vegetarian and omnivorous men. *Nutr Cancer.* 1989;12:271–278.
42. Butterworth CE. Folate deficiency and cancer. In: Bendich A, Butterworth CE, eds. *Micronutrients in Health and in Disease Prevention.* New York: Marcel Dekker, Inc; 1991:165–183.
43. Heimburger DC, Alexander CB, Birch R, Butterworth CE, Bailey WC, Krumdiek CL. Improvement in bronchial squamous metaplasia in smokers treated with folate and vitamin B_{12}: report of a preliminary randomized double-blind intervention trial. *JAMA.* 1988;259:1525–1530.
44. Beisel WR, Edelman R, Nauss K, Suskind RM. Single-nutrient effects of immunologic functions. *JAMA.* 1981;245:53–58.
45. Bendich A, Cohen M. B Vitamins: effects on specific and nonspecific immune responses. In: Chandra RK, ed. *Nutrition and Immunology.* New York: Alan R. Liss, Inc; 1988:101–123.
46. Dhur A, Galan P, Christides J-P, Potier De Courcy G, Perziosi P, Hercberg S. Effect of folic acid deficiency upon lymphocyte subsets from lymphoid organs in mice. *Comp Biochem Physiol.* 1991; 98A:235–240.
47. Chandra RK, Sudhakaran L. Regulation of immune responses by vitamin B_6. In: Dakshinamurti K, ed. *Vitamin B_6.* New York: *Ann N Y Acad Sci;* 1990:404–423.
48. Miller LT, Kerkvliet NI. Effect of vitamin B_6 on immunocompetence in the elderly. In: Bendich A, Chandra RK, eds. *Micronutrients and Immune Functions.* New York: *Ann N Y Acad Sci;* 1990: 49–54.

MOHAMMAD Z. HOSSAIN, LI-XIN ZHANG, DAVID F. C. GIBSON, and JOHN S. BERTRAM

A Mechanistic Basis for the Actions of Retinoids and Carotenoids as Chemopreventive Agents

ABSTRACT

In clinical and experimental situations, retinoids and carotenoids have proved promising as chemopreventive agents, causing delays in cancer development or regression of premalignant lesions at several anatomic sites. In the 10T½ cell system of in vitro carcinogenesis, retinoids and carotenoids reversibly inhibit the development of carcinogen-induced transformation in the postinitiation phase of carcinogenesis. Both of these chemopreventive compounds induce gap junctional communication in 10T½ cells in a time- and dose-dependent manner. This induction of communication is strongly correlated with the inhibition of transformation. The observed increases in gap junctional communication were a result of elevations in the junctional protein connexin 43 at the mRNA and protein levels. In treated cells, extensive phosphorylation of connexin 43 was observed, together with an increased number and size of immunofluorescent junctional plaques in regions of cell-cell contact. These studies provide a mechanistic basis for the actions of retinoids and carotenoids. In this model, carcinogen-initiated cells are blocked in the promotional phase of carcinogenesis and therefore are unable to progress to full malignant transformation, by virtue of growth-controlling signals from surrounding normal cells mediated through gap junctions. The existence of such signals is implied by other studies in which the growth of neoplastic cells is arrested when communication is established with neighboring normal cells.

Introduction

Epidemiological studies have indicated that the chemoprevention of tumor development by agents that occur naturally in the diet is a realistic aim. The agents of most promise are the retinoids (natural and synthetic compounds with vitamin A activity) (1) and the carotenoids (plant pigments found in vegetables and fruits) (2). In clinical trials, retinoids delay neoplasia or cause a reversion of preneoplastic pathology at several anatomic sites (3, 4). Individuals with a high dietary intake of beta-carotene, a carotenoid with a high degree of vitamin A activity, have a reduced risk of cancer at various sites (5, 6). In a recent intervention trial, encouraging results have been reported in the regression of oral leukoplakia (7). It was important to reproduce these effects in the more controlled environment of the laboratory. This has been achieved, with both retinoids and carotenoids demonstrating antineoplastic effects in in vivo experimental animal systems and in vitro cell culture models (8–13). The carotenoid beta-carotene, demonstrating a high degree of provitamin A activity, was assumed to exert inhibitory effects upon transformation through a conversion to vitamin A (14). However, canthaxanthin, a carotenoid without any provitamin A activity in mammals, also exhibits such antineoplastic effects in the laboratory (11–13), suggesting a direct antitumor action for both retinoids and carotenoids.

Central to chemoprevention is a knowledge of carcinogenesis. An insight into the mechanism of action of chemopreventive agents and the development of novel compounds can be achieved only with a detailed knowledge of the conversion of a normal cell to one with a malignant phenotype. Advances in molecular biology have provided the scientist with new insights into the genetic changes that occur during carcinogenesis. Of most importance is the concept that carcinogenesis is a multistep process, requiring both the activation of oncogenes (15) and the inactivation or deletion (16, 17) of tumor-suppressor genes. The entire sequence of events is beginning to be unraveled in human colon carcinoma (18) and a variety of other tissues (19). There are three main stages to the carcinogenic process.

1. *Initiation.* Genetic damage is induced by a carcinogen or occurs spontaneously. Although many tissues have the ability to repair the chemical damage, it appears that this damage is converted into a stable biological lesion during DNA replication. This explains the high frequency of tumors in proliferating tissues and suggests that chemoprevention (for

example, blocking carcinogen metabolism and activation, stimulating DNA repair, inhibiting DNA replication) must occur before or shortly after the initiating events. This obviously requires a thorough knowledge of the type and timing of the initiating insult.

2. *Promotion.* The initiated cells are converted into phenotypically malignant cells. This is a prolonged process, lasting decades in humans. An interruption of this process at any point up to the appearance of frank malignancy would be expected to delay the onset of disease and lead to a decrease in tumor incidence. This phase of the carcinogenic process offers the best prospects for clinical intervention, and it is during the promotional stage that retinoids and carotenoids exert their antineoplastic effects.
3. *Progression.* Transformed cells grow to form a progressively malignant tumor. Within in vitro cell culture systems, the progression of malignant cells results in a transformed focus.

The C3H/10T$\frac{1}{2}$ Fibroblast Cell Line as an In Vitro Model of Carcinogenesis

The choice of an in vitro system with which to study the actions of chemopreventive agents is dependent upon several important requirements. In simple terms, it is crucial that the stages of carcinogenesis (initiation, promotion, progression) known to occur in vivo faithfully occur within the in vitro model. More specifically for the aims of our research efforts, it is also important that structure/function relationships determined in vivo for known chemopreventive agents be maintained, in addition to a responsiveness to a diverse class of agents. Our group has extensively used the C3H/10T$\frac{1}{2}$ cell line, which satisfies the above criteria (20), for the study of retinoids and carotenoids and the inhibition of transformation.

The 10T$\frac{1}{2}$ mouse embryo fibroblast cell line was originally developed for basic carcinogenesis investigations (21, 22). The cells are nontumorigenic in syngeneic immunosuppressed hosts, have a very low spontaneous transformation rate, and exhibit a high degree of postconfluence inhibition of cell division. These criteria make the cell line an ideal model in the study of transformation and chemoprevention.

The use of the 10T½ cell line in transformation assays by our group is essentially as originally described (22). Cells are seeded at low density and treated with carcinogenic hydrocarbons for 24 hours. It can be estimated that this insult results in a small percentage (up to 2%) of initiated cells. Approximately ten days after treatment, cultures become confluent and growth is arrested. For a three- to four-week posttreatment period, cultures appear morphologically normal. After this time, microscopic foci of transformed cells can be observed. One week later (approximately thirty-five days after seeding), these foci have attained macroscopic size. When these cells are injected into syngeneic mice, sarcomas appear at the site of injection. In contrast, a tenfold excess of the parental line results in no such in vivo tumor formation.

The Inhibition of In Vitro Neoplastic Transformation by Retinoids and Carotenoids

A diverse range of retinoids and carotenoids has been tested in in vitro chemoprevention assays (10, 11, 23, 24). One important observation was that those retinoids known to have activity in epithelial models of differentiation (25) were also found to have antineoplastic effects in the 10T½ cell transformation system (10). In contrast, compounds with certain side-chain or ring modifications that were without provitamin A activity in epithelial differentiation assays were also unable to inhibit the formation of foci of transformed 10T½ cells. Data of this kind are crucial in establishing the relevance of the 10T½ system in the study and development of chemopreventive agents that are ultimately aimed at the inhibition of epithelial carcinogenesis.

Of the compounds discussed in this paper, three are retinoids and two are carotenoids (Fig. 1). The retinoids are retinol (the principal retinoid in blood), retinoic acid (the metabolite responsible for growth and differentiation), and tetrahydrotetramethylnaphthalenylpropenyl benzoic acid (TTNPB, a stable benzoic acid analogue of retinoic acid). The carotenoids include beta-carotene (displaying the highest degree of provitamin A activity in mammals) and canthaxanthin (with no provitamin A activity). The compounds under investigation were added to 10T½ cultures seven days after the removal of the carcinogen 3-methylcholanthrene and maintained for the remaining four weeks of the experiment. The retinoids completely inhibited

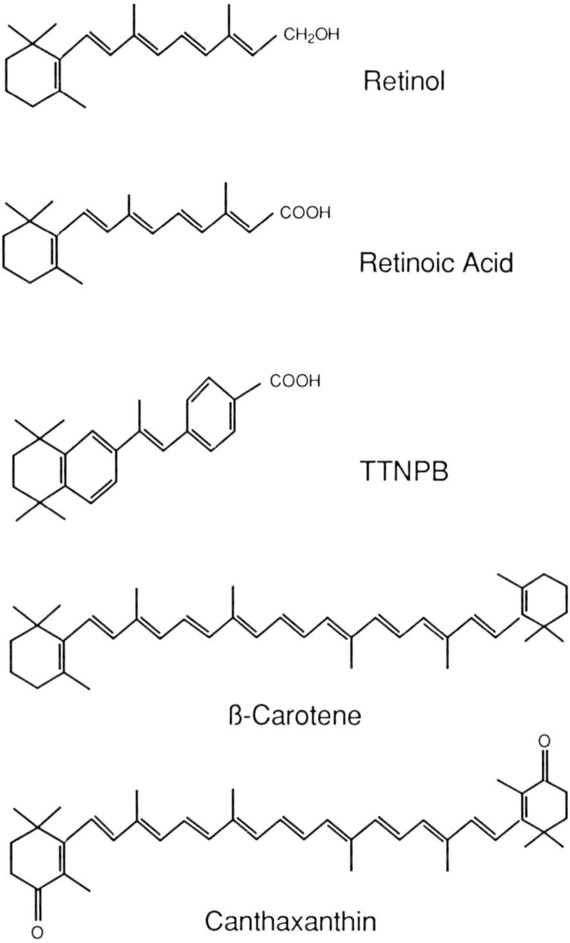

Figure 1. Structures of retinoids and carotenoids tested.

the formation of transformed foci (26) (Fig. 2A), with TTNPB being the most potent (10^{-9}M). Both retinol and retinoic acid also caused a complete inhibition of foci formation at 10^{-7}M and 10^{-6}M respectively. In addition to displaying antineoplastic effects, the retinoids also affected growth control. All three retinoids caused a decrease in cell density at confluence (27), considered a measure of growth control. These effects of retinoids are not a reflection of mere cytotoxicity, as both are reversible upon removal of the compound (9, 27). The carotenoids, beta-carotene and canthaxanthin, were also able to completely suppress foci formation (Fig. 2B). As noted with retinoids, this

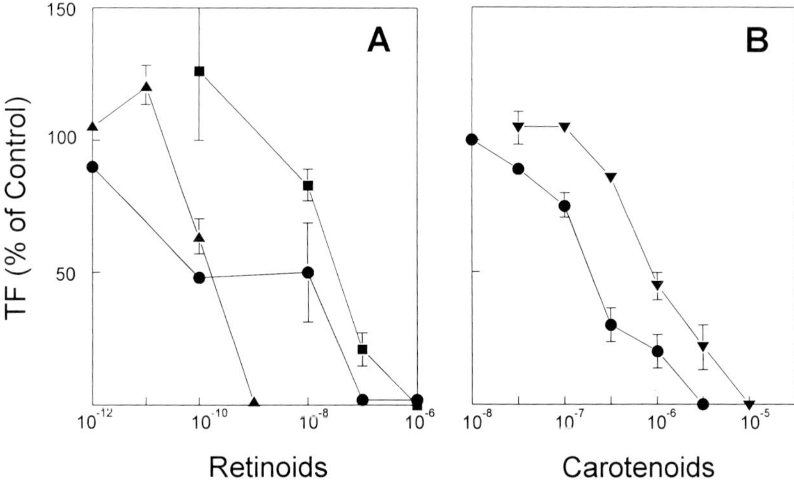

Figure 2. Inhibition of 3-methylcholanthrene–induced transformation by retinoids (A: ●, retinol; ■, retinoic acid; ▲, TTNPB) and carotenoids (B: ▼, beta-carotene; ●, canthaxanthin). 10T½ cultures were initiated with 3-methylcholanthrene, then received retinoids or carotenoids for 7 days after the removal of the carcinogen. The drug treatments were given every 3 days (retinoids) or every 7 days (carotenoids) with weekly medium changes for the remaining 35 days of the experiment. Results are expressed as a percentage of the transformation frequency (TF) observed in cultures exposed to methylcholanthrene than with solvent control.

Figures 2A and 2B are reproduced from Hossain *et al.* (26) and Pung *et al.* (11), respectively, by permission of Oxford University Press.

effect was reversible. However, these effects were achieved in the range of 10^{-5}M (11), a dose somewhat higher than necessary with the retinoids. The activity of canthaxanthin and other structurally diverse carotenoids such as lycopene and lutein (23), also lacking provitamin A activity, suggests that activity is not a reflection of any provitamin A–like qualities (11).

In summary, these studies (9, 11, 27) demonstrated three main points.

1. Retinoids and carotenoids are able to inhibit the formation of foci of transformed 10T½ cells. This effect is upon initiated cells in the promotional phase of carcinogenesis and is reversible upon drug removal. Thus, selective toxicity of initiated cells is not involved.
2. These compounds are able to reduce the proliferation of den-

sity arrested cells, resulting in a reduced confluent saturation density. However, they are unable to affect the proliferation of nontransformed or transformed cells in the logarithmic phase, using those doses that completely inhibit transformation.

3. In reconstruction experiments, in which established transformed cells (isolated from foci) were overlaid upon confluent parental 10T½ cells, retinoids had no inhibitory effects upon the expression of the transformed phenotype as expressed in focus formation. Therefore, these compounds are not merely causing growth inhibition of transformed cells, thereby preventing focus formation. These observations indicate that initiated cells are sensitive to retinoids and carotenoids in the promotional phase of carcinogenesis only. These compounds appear to stabilize the initiated cell phenotype (9, 11, 27) by a cytostatic mechanism. Extrapolations made to the clinical situation suggest that both retinoids and carotenoids should be administered for extended periods to maintain effectiveness.

Mechanism of Action of Retinoids and Carotenoids as Chemopreventive Agents

Induction of Junctional Communication

The central observation that retinoids and carotenoids exhibit antineoplastic effects upon confluent cells suggests that cell-cell communication is important. Indeed, a role for gap junctional communication has been proposed in growth control and carcinogenesis (28).

Put simply, gap junctions are direct hydrophilic channels that connect adjacent cells (28). The inner diameter of 16 to 20 angstroms allows the passive diffusion of small ions and molecules up to 1000 daltons in size. Each channel, called a connexon, is composed of two hemiconnexons, one from each of the communicating cells. The hemiconnexon is a hexagonal structure, composed of six proteins called connexins. A family of connexins has been described, displaying tissue and cell type specificity (29). Functions for gap junctions in nutrient exchange and tissue homeostasis are well established (29, 30). However, we have proposed that another important role of gap junctions is the regulation of growth and development; central to this concept is the transfer of growth regulatory signals via the junctional pore (26, 28, 31). Ideas of this kind obviously suggest a role of junctional communication in carcinogenesis. Indeed, communication is frequently lost in tumors (32, 33) and often inhibited by oncogenes, tumor promoters, and growth factors (34–36). Of central importance to these concepts is our demonstration that neoplastic cells undergo reversible growth arrest when made to establish communication via gap junctions with growth-arrested normal cells (31). We therefore examined the effects of retinoids and carotenoids upon gap junctional communication in 10T½ cells. Junctional communication was measured as previously described (26). Briefly, single cells within a confluent monolayer were microinjected with a fluorescent junctionally permeable dye (lucifer yellow), and the number of surrounding cells that became fluorescent after ten minutes was counted.

Retinoid and Carotenoid Induction of Cellular Communication by Gap Junctions

When the retinoids were added at doses equipotent as inhibitors of transformation to 10T½ cells for the period of time of a typical transformation assay, gap junctional communication was increased over the 35-day experimental duration (Fig. 3A). Although all three retinoids were active, retinol and retinoic acid required a thousandfold higher concentration than TTNPB to achieve comparable enhancement. The induction of junctional communication by the potent retinoid TTNPB (10^{-9}M) required at least 18 hours of treatment (Fig. 3A inset) (26); at this time, communication was significantly different from controls ($P < 0.001$), and it continued to increase thereafter. As with the effects upon transformation and growth control, this increased intercellular communication was reversible (37). Similarly, the two carotenoids also elevated junctional communication in a time-dependent manner (38) (Fig. 3B). In contrast to retinoids, the carotenoids required four days to induce increased communication (Fig. 3B inset). The dose dependency of the retinoid effects upon junctional communication is shown in Figure 4A. Retinoic acid appears to cause a biphasic response, actually inhibiting communication at the lowest concentration tested (10^{-10}M). At the same concentration, retinoic acid also enhanced transformation (Fig. 2A). The correlation sug-

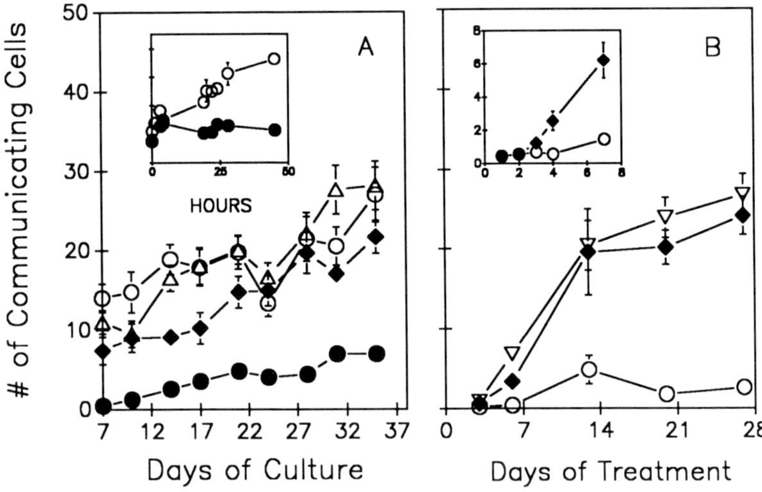

Figure 3. Effects of retinoids and carotenoids on junctional communication in 10T½ cells. *A. Retinoid effects.* Cells were seeded, and treated with retinoids on day 1 and every 3 days thereafter. Junctional communication was indexed by the number of cells to which lucifer yellow was transferred within 10 minutes of microinjection into a test cell (represents the number of communicating cells). Cultures were assayed at the intervals shown. Data points represent the mean ± SEM of at least 10 microinjection assays, performed in each of 2 dishes. ●, acetone control 0.2%; △, retinol 10^{-6}M; ♦, retinoic acid 10^{-6}M; ○, TTNPB 10^{-9}M. Inset: time course of enhancement of junctional communication by TTNPB 10^{-9}M. The cultures were assayed at the indicated times. The y-axis of the inset is as main figure (scale 0–20). The results represent the mean ± SEM of at least 20 microinjections in 2 dishes each. *B. Carotenoid effects.* Cells were treated with carotenoids dissolved in tetrahydrofuran (THF), or with 0.5% THF control, when the cultures were confluent (day 7) and weekly thereafter. Data points represent the mean ± SEM of 15 microinjections performed in 2 dishes each. ○, THF control; ▽, beta-carotene 10^{-5}M; ♦, canthaxanthin 10^{-5}M. Inset: expanded scale, axes as main graph.

Figures 3A and 3B are reproduced from Hossain *et al.* (26) and Zhang *et al.* (38), respectively, by permission of Oxford University Press.

gested by these data in a positive and negative sense between communication and transformation is demonstrated in Figure 5A. Statistical analysis showed a strong negative correlation between the two parameters (Pearson correlation coefficient of −0.86; $P < 0.001$); that is, enhanced communication resulted in an inhibition of transformation, whereas reduced communication led to increased cell transformation (26). The other reported effect of retinoids, namely, a decrease

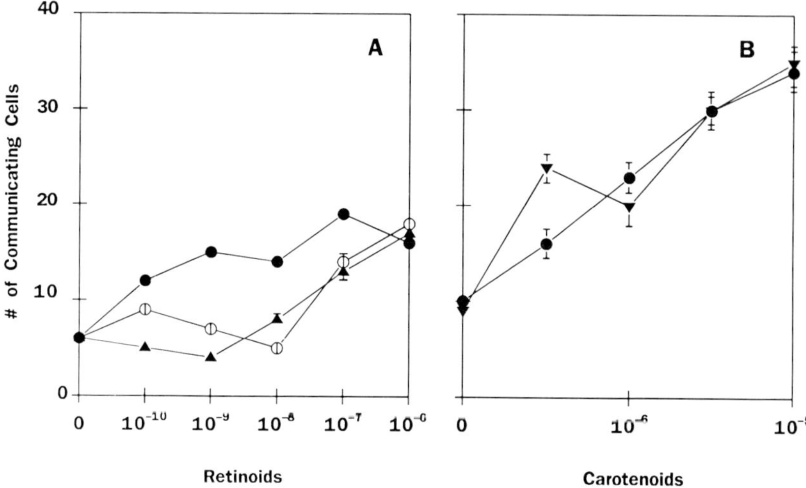

Figure 4. Dose-response for the induction of junctional communication by retinoids (*A*) and carotenoids (*B*). *A.* Cultures were treated as in Figure 3A, and were probed 2 days after reaching confluence. Data points represent the mean ± SEM of 2 experiments each involving about 20 microinjections in 2 separate dishes. ○, retinol; ▲, retinoic acid; ●, TTNPB. Dose-response relationships were significant for TTNPB ($P = 0.002$) and for retinol ($P = 0.03$). If the zero dose treatment for retinoic acid is excluded (as 10^{-10}M retinoic acid inhibits communication), the dose-response relationship is significant ($P = 0.0003$). *B.* Cells were treated as in Figure 3B and probed after 2 weeks of treatment. ▼, beta-carotene; ●, canthaxanthin.

Figures 4A and 4B are reproduced from Hossain *et al.* (26) and Zhang *et al.* (38), respectively, by permission of Oxford University Press.

in the cell density at confluence, was itself negatively correlated with the induction of junctional communication (37).

Similar experiments and subsequent data analysis were carried out with the two carotenoids (38). As predicted from the previous results in transformation assays, both compounds were less potent than the retinoids in communication assays (Fig. 4B). As with the retinoids, the elevation of intercellular communication was strongly correlated with the inhibition of transformation (Fig. 5B).

A Molecular Mechanism for the Actions of Retinoids and Carotenoids upon Gap Junctional Communication

A possible site of action of retinoids and carotenoids in their abilities to affect gap junctions is the connexin proteins that make up the junc-

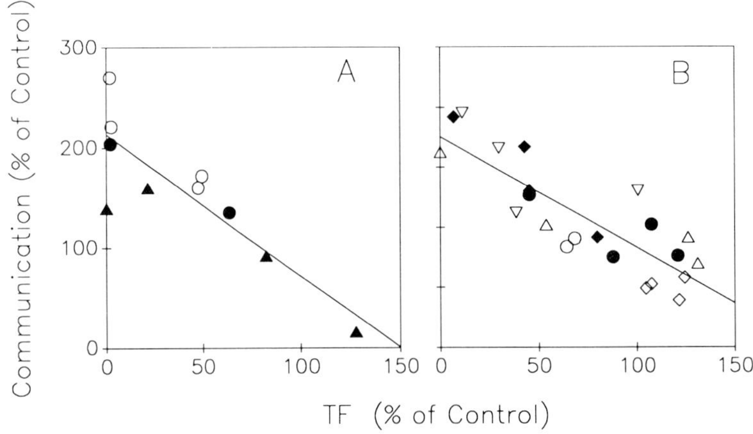

Figure 5. *A.* Correlation between transformation and junctional communication. The Pearson correlation coefficient was −0.86, indicating a strong negative association. This was also highly significant ($P = 0.001$). *B.* Correlation between inhibition of carcinogen-induced neoplastic transformation and induction of junctional communication by carotenoids. The Pearson correlation coefficient was −0.823 ($P = 0.005$).

Figures 5A and 5B are reproduced from Hossain *et al.* (26) and Zhang *et al.* (38), respectively, by permission of Oxford University Press.

tional complex (28, 29). The 10T½ cells express connexin 43 (Cx43) (39), a protein initially described in the intercalated disc of heart tissue (29). Northern blot analysis demonstrated that Cx43 mRNA levels were increased within 6 hours of TTNPB treatment and continued to rise over the 72-hour duration of the experiment (Fig. 6). Microinjection of similarly treated cultures with lucifer yellow demonstrated that the retinoid-induced increase in Cx43 mRNA levels clearly preceded the increases in communication (39). In addition, Cx43 message induction was direct and required no prior protein synthesis (unpublished observation). As expected, the TTNPB induction of Cx43 message was reversible, with the levels falling below those detectable within six hours of retinoid removal (39). The carotenoids beta-carotene and canthaxanthin also induced comparable elevations in Cx43 message levels in 10T½ cells (manuscript in preparation). This increase in Cx43 message was followed by an increase in Cx43 protein. We used a rabbit polyclonal antibody against a 15-mer polypeptide located in the predicted C-terminal cytoplastic domain of the protein to probe Western blots of total cellular proteins. Retinoid treatment induced a dramatic increase in immunoreactive protein in

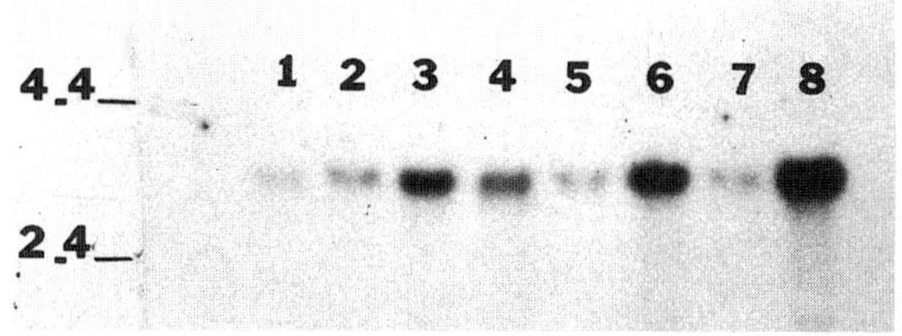

Figure 6. Time course of TTNPB-induced increase in connexin 43 mRNA. Confluent 10T½ cells were treated with TTNPB 10^{-8}M for the times indicated. 10 μg of total RNA were loaded per lane, electrophoresed, and transferred to nitrocellulose. The blot was hybridized with ^{32}P-labeled Cx43 DNA. Lane 1, acetone 6 hours; lane 2, TTNPB 6 hours; lane 3, TTNPB 12 hours; lane 4, TTNPB 24 hours; lane 5, acetone 48 hours; lane 6, TTNPB 48 hours; lane 7, acetone 72 hours; lane 8, TTNPB 72 hours. The positions of the RNA standards (kb) are shown.

the appropriate 43 to 45 kDa region of the gel (Fig. 7). This increase was observed within 6 hours of TTNPB (10^{-8}M) and increased progressively over the 96 hours of the experiment (Fig. 7A). A dose dependency in the increase in Cx43 protein was also observed (Fig. 7B). These effects of TTNPB at 10^{-8}M upon Cx43 protein levels were mirrored by retinol and retinoic acid at 10^{-6}M (unpublished data).

The carotenoids under investigation also dramatically increased Cx43 protein levels (Fig. 7C), although a longer period of time (seven days) was required compared with the three days for TTNPB action. This Cx43 elevation induced by the carotenoids was also time and dose dependent.

Both retinoids and carotenoids resulted in increases in immunoreactive protein bands of 43 and 45 kDa (Fig. 7). The higher Mr band represents a phosphorylated form of Cx43 (39). Connexon 43 phosphorylation at Ser/Thr residues has been shown to be associated with junctional competence (40), and it is possible that the Cx43 phosphorylation observed in 10T½ cells is required for the proper assembly of connexins into gap junctions in the cell membrane (39).

The retinoid-induced Cx43 protein could be observed in situ after double immunofluorescence staining as fluorescent plaques in regions of cell-cell contact (Fig. 8). This demonstrates that the increased Cx43 protein becomes localized in regions of the cell membrane

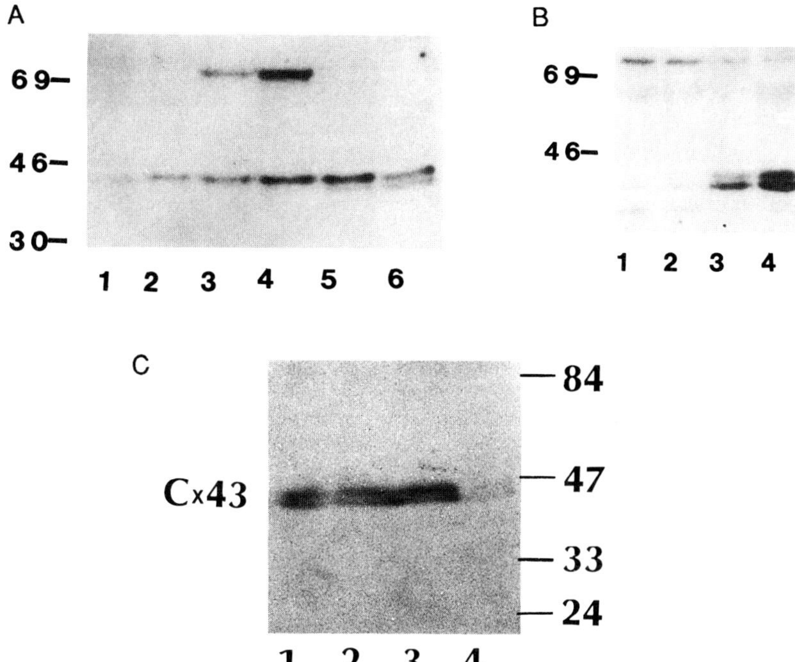

Figure 7. Up-regulation of Cx43 by TTNPB and carotenoids. *A.* Time course of TTNPB-induced increase in Cx43. Confluent cultures of 10T$\frac{1}{2}$ cells were treated with TTNPB 10^{-8}M for the indicated times. Cell lysates were reduced prior to electrophoresis, equal amounts of protein were loaded to each lane, and Western blotting was performed. Cx43 protein was detected using a rabbit polyclonal antibody. Lane 1, solvent control 0 hours; lane 2, TTNPB 6 hours; lane 3, TTNPB 24 hours; lane 4, TTNPB 48 hours; lane 5, TTNPB 96 hours; lane 6, solvent control 96 hours. The 70 kDa bands (lanes 3 and 4) are believed to represent Cx43 dimers. The molecular weight markers are expressed in kDa. *B.* Dose response for Cx43 induction by TTNPB. Confluent cultures were treated with TTNPB of acetone control for 96 hours. Levels of Cx43 were examined as before. Lane 1, acetone control; lane 2, TTNPB 10^{-10}M; lane 3, TTNPB 10^{-9}M; lane 4, TTNPB 10^{-8}M. *C.* Induction of Cx43 by carotenoids. Cultures were treated with 10^{-5}M beta-carotene or canthaxanthin for 7 days and the Cx43 levels examined as before. For comparison, cell lysates from TTNPB-treated cells were loaded in the same gel. Lane 1, TTNPB 10^{-8}M; lane 2, beta-carotene 10^{-5}M; lane 3, canthaxanthin 10^{-5}M; lane 4, THF control 0.5%.

Figures 7A and 7B are reproduced from Rogers *et al.* (39), with permission of Wiley-Liss, a division of John Wiley & Sons, Inc.

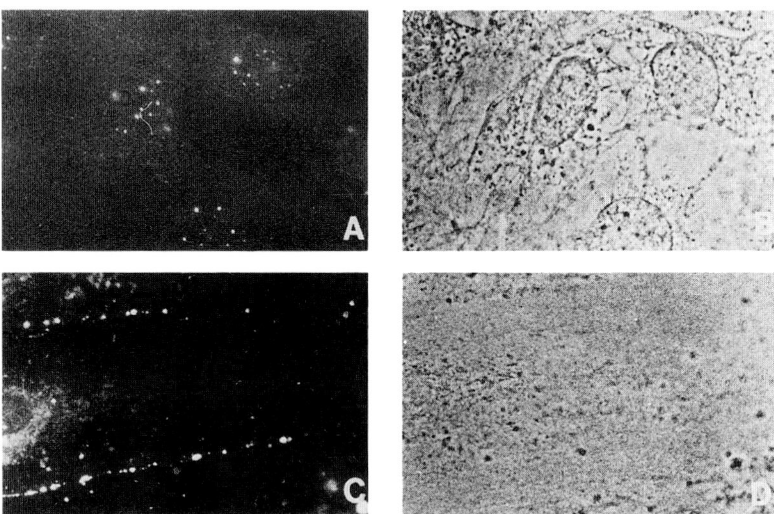

Figure 8. Cx43 is localized in regions of cell-cell contact. 10T½ cells were grown on Permanox culture slides and treated with TTNPB or acetone control for 96 hours. Cultures were fixed and labeled with Cx43 antiserum and then with FITC-labeled goat antirabbit IgG F(ab`)$_2$ fragment. Panels A and B, acetone control, fluorescent and respective phase image; panels C and D, TTNPB 10^{-8}M, fluorescent and respective phase image.

where gap junctions would be expected to form. Carotenoids induce similar increases in junctional plaques (41).

Conclusions

Retinoids and carotenoids are cancer-chemopreventive compounds that in in vitro models, experimental animal systems, and clinical situations delay the process of carcinogenesis (5). An understanding of their mode of action may ultimately lead to the improved clinical use of these compounds and the rational design of novel agents. Central to the ideas of retinoid and carotenoid action discussed here is the role of gap junctions as conduits for growth-regulatory signals (28). Our results indicate that retinoids and carotenoids are able to block the progression of initiated 10T½ cells to malignancy by inducing communication between growth-arrested normal cells. It was also demonstrated that the expression of the transformed phenotype by initiated cells was inhibited when the transformed cells were induced to communicate with normal cells (31). Retinoids and carotenoids only suppress neoplastic transformation in 10T½ cells when applied before the phenotypic expression of transformation (*i.e.*, during promotion). Indeed, when applied after transformation, retinoids act to inhibit communication and stimulate the growth of the transformed cells (9, 31). This may explain some of the deleterious actions of retinoids in experimental animals (5). Furthermore, in clinical studies of retinoic acid, many primary tumors in existence before treatment are not influenced by treatment (4).

We propose that the signals that traverse the gap junctional complexes are antiproliferative in nature, originating from normal growth-arrested cells and influencing neighboring initiated cells. We would predict that these signals are electrically charged so as to limit membrane diffusion, be hydrophilic, and display low protein binding. To pass through the junctional pore, they must be no greater than 1000 daltons in size. Cyclic adenosine monophosphate, inositol trisphosphate, and free Ca^{2+} all traverse gap junctions (42, 43) and represent potential candidates as regulatory signals.

ACKNOWLEDGMENTS

This work has been supported by grants CA 39947 from the National Institutes of Health and BC 686 from the American Cancer Society.

REFERENCES

1. Roberts AB, Sporn MB. Cellular biology and biochemistry of the retinoids. In: Sporn MB, Roberts AB, Goodman DW, eds. *The Retinoids.* New York: Academic Press; 1984;2:209–286.
2. Goodwin TW. The biochemistry of the carotenoids. 2nd ed. London: Chapman and Hall; 1980:79–95.
3. Alfthan O, Tarkkanen J, Grohn P, Heinonen E, Pyrhonen S, Saila K. Tigason (etretinate) in prevention of recurrence of superficial bladder cancer. *Eur Urol.* 1983;9:6–9.
4. Hong WK, Lippman SM, Itri LM, *et al.* Prevention of secondary tumors with isotretonin in squamous-cell carcinoma of the head and neck. *N Engl J Med.* 1990;323:795–801.
5. Bertram JS, Kolonel LN, Meyskens FL Jr. Rationale and strategies for chemoprevention of cancer in humans. *Cancer Res.* 1987; 47: 3012–3031.

6. Connett JE, Kuller LH, Kjelsberg MO, *et al.* Relationship between carotenoids and cancer: the multiple risk factor intervention trial (MRFIT) study. *Cancer.* 1989;64:126–134.
7. Stich HF, Rosin MP, Hornby AP, Mathew B, Sankaranarayanan R, Nair MK. Remission of oral leukoplakias and micronuclei in tobacco/betel quid chewers treated with β-carotene and with β-carotene plus vitamin A. *Int J Cancer.* 1988;42:195–199.
8. Moon RC. Comparative aspects of carotenoids and retinoids as chemopreventive agents for cancer. *J Nutr.* 1989;119:127–134.
9. Merriman RL, Bertram JS. Reversible inhibition by retinoids of 3-methylcholanthrene-induced neoplastic transformation in C3H/10T$\frac{1}{2}$ clone 8 cells. *Cancer Res.* 1979;39:1661–1666.
10. Bertram JS. Structure-activity relationships among various retinoids and their ability to inhibit neoplastic transformation and to increase cell adhesion in the C3H/10T$\frac{1}{2}$ CL8 cell line. *Cancer Res.* 1980;40:3141–3146.
11. Pung A, Rundhaug J, Yoshizawa CN, Bertram JS. β-carotene and canthaxanthin inhibit chemically- and physically-induced neoplastic transformation in 10T$\frac{1}{2}$ cells. *Carcinogenesis.* 1988;9:1533–1539.
12. Mathews-Roth MM. Antitumor activity of β-carotene, canthaxanthin and phytoene. *Oncology.* 1982;39:33–37.
13. Schwartz J, Shklar G. Regression of experimental oral carcinomas by local injection of β-carotene and canthaxanthin. *Nutr Cancer.* 1988;11:35–40.
14. Stich HF, Stich W, Rosin MP, Vallejera MO. Use of the micronucleus test to monitor the effect of vitamin A, β-carotene and canthaxanthin on the buccal mucosa of betel nut/tobacco chewers. *Int J Cancer.* 1984;34:745–750.
15. Storm RW, Bose HR Jr. Oncogenes, protooncogenes, and signal transduction: toward a unified theory. *Adv Virus Res.* 1989;37:1–34.
16. Sager R. Tumor suppressor genes: the puzzle and the promise. *Science.* 1989;246:1406–1412.
17. Green MR. When the products of oncogenes and antioncogenes meet. *Cell.* 1989;56:1–31.
18. Fearon ER, Cho KR, Nigro JM, *et al.* Identification of a chromosome 18q gene that is altered in colorectal cancer. *Science.* 1990;247:49–56.
19. Doll R, Peto R. *The Causes of Cancer.* Oxford: Oxford University Press; 1981.

20. Bertram JS. Neoplastic transformation in cell culture: in vivo correlations. *IARC Sci Publ.* 1985;67:77–91.
21. Reznikoff CA, Brankow DW, Heidelberger C. Establishment and characterization of a cloned line of C3H mouse embryo cells sensitive to postconfluence inhibition of division. *Cancer Res.* 1973;33:3231–3238.
22. Reznikoff CA, Bertram JS, Brankow DW, Heidelberger C. Quantitative and qualitative studies of chemical transformation of cloned mouse embryo cells sensitive to postconfluence inhibition of cell division. *Cancer Res.* 1973;33:3239–3249.
23. Bertram JS, Pung A, Churley M, Kappock TJ IV, Wilkens LR, Cooney RV. Diverse carotenoids protect from chemically-induced neoplastic transformation. *Carcinogenesis.* 1991;12:671–678.
24. Mass MJ, Nettesheim P, Beeman DK, Barrett CJ. Inhibition of transformation of primary rat tracheal epithelial cells by retinoic acid. *Cancer Res.* 1984;44:5688–5691.
25. Newton DL, Henderson WR, Sporn MB. Structure-activity relationships of retinoids in hamster tracheal organ culture. *Cancer Res.* 1980;40:3413–3425.
26. Hossain MZ, Wilkens LR, Mehta PP, Loewenstein WR, Bertram JS. Enhancement of gap junctional communication by retinoids correlates with their ability to inhibit neoplastic transformation. *Carcinogenesis.* 1989;10:1743–1748.
27. Mordan LJ, Bertram JS. Retinoid effects on cell-cell interactions and growth characteristics of normal and carcinogen-treated C3H/10T$\frac{1}{2}$ cells. *Cancer Res.* 1983;43:567–571.
28. Loewenstein WR. Junctional communication and the control of growth. *Biochim Biophys Acta.* 1979;560:1–65.
29. Yancey SB, John SA, Lal R, Austin BJ, Revel J-P. The 43 kD polypeptide of heart gap junctions: immunolocalization, topology and functional domains. *J Cell Biol.* 1989;108:2241–2254.
30. Caveney S. The role of gap junctions in development. *Ann Rev Physiol.* 1985;47:319–335.
31. Mehta PP, Bertram JS, Loewenstein WR. Growth inhibition of transformed cells correlates with their junctional communication with normal cells. *Cell.* 1986;44:187–196.
32. Klaunig JE, Ruch RJ. Role of intercellular communication in carcinogenesis. *Lab Invest.* 1990;62:135–145.
33. Yamasaki H. Gap junctional intercellular communication and carcinogenesis. *Carcinogenesis.* 1990;11:1051–1058.

34. Atkinson MM, Menko AS, Johnson RG, Sheppard JR, Sheridan JD. Rapid and reversible reduction of junctional permeability in cells infected with a temperature-sensitive mutant of avian sarcoma virus. *J Cell Biol.* 1981;91:573–578.
35. Enomoto T, Yamasaki H. Phorbol ester mediated inhibition of intercellular communication in BALB/c 3T3 cells: relationship to enhancement of cell transformation. *Cancer Res.* 1985;45:2681–2688.
36. Madhukar BV, Oh SY, Chang CC, Wade M, Trosko JE. Altered regulation of intercellular communication by epidermal growth factor, transforming growth factor-β and peptide hormones in normal human keratinocytes. *Carcinogenesis.* 1989;10:13–20.
37. Mehta PP, Bertram JS, Loewenstein WR. The actions of retinoids on cellular growth correlate with their actions on gap junctional communication. *J Cell Biol.* 1989;108:1053–1065.
38. Zhang L-X, Cooney RV, Bertram JS. Carotenoids enhance gap junctional communication and inhibit lipid peroxidation in C3H/10T$\frac{1}{2}$ cells: relationship to their cancer chemopreventive action. *Carcinogensis.* 1991;12:2109–2114.
39. Rogers M, Berestecky JM, Hossain MZ, *et al.* Retinoid-enhanced gap junctional communication is achieved by increasing levels of connexin 43 mRNA and protein. *Mol Carcinog.* 1990;3:334–343.
40. Musil LS, Cunningham BA, Edelman GM, Goodenough DA. Differential phosphorylation of the gap junction protein connexin 43 in junction communication-competent and -deficient cell lines. *J Cell Biol.* 1990;111:2077–2088.
41. Zhang L-X, Cooney RV, Bertram JS. Enhancement of gap junctional communication by carotenoids correlates with inhibition of neoplastic transformation. *Proc Am Assoc Cancer Res.* 1991;32:124.
42. Fletcher WH, Byus CV, Walsh DA. Receptor-mediated action without receptor occupancy: a function for cell-cell communication in ovarian follicles. *Adv Exp Med Biol.* 1987;219:299–323.
43. Saez JC, Connor JA, Spray DC, Bennett MVL. Hepatocyte gap junctions are permeable to the second messenger, inositol 1, 4, 5-trisphosphate and to calcium ions. *Proc Natl Acad Sci U S A.* 1989;86:2707–2712.

PART II

Epidemiologic Aspects of Vitamin Use in Cancer Prevention

PELAYO CORREA and ELIZABETH T. H. FONTHAM

Vitamins and Cancer Prevention: An Epidemiologic Overview

ABSTRACT

The inverse association between cancer occurrence and ingestion of fresh fruits and vegetables is one of the most consistent findings in the international epidemiologic literature. The high content of antioxidant vitamins in these foods has been documented. Indexes of their intake have been developed and also found inversely related to certain cancers. Blood measurement of antioxidant vitamins and their precursors has shown lower levels in persons who later developed cancer. Although the antineoplastic mechanism of action of the antioxidant vitamins needs further elucidation, it seems clear that chemoprevention trials in humans should be encouraged.

Introduction

The role of vitamins in cancer prevention is being investigated actively throughout the world, as reflected in recent international conferences (1). This paper provides a summary of research activity, focusing on those sites for which most recent epidemiologic evidence has been provided. Some emphasis is given to lung cancer and to studies conducted in Louisiana.

Historical Perspective

Chemical and viral theories dominated research on cancer etiology for many years. Research on the role of diet in carcinogenesis has been a more recent development. In the 1940s Albert Tannenbaum published a series of studies based on the records of life insurance companies showing that overweight policyholders had higher cancer death rates, leading to the hypothesis that over-nutrition could be a cause of cancer (2). More recently, international correlations between death rates and food consumption have shown that certain cancers, especially those of the breast and large intestine, are positively associated with fat intake and inversely correlated with the intake of cereals (3, 4). This is in contrast with stomach cancer, for which the correlations are in the opposite direction. Most of the early activity looked for positive associations between diet and cancer. As the studies progressed, it became evident that a number of inverse associations were prominent. A rather large number of case-control studies have now been conducted in many countries, showing an inverse association between cancer of several sites and the ingestion of fresh fruits and vegetables (5–8). Prospective studies of large cohorts have been conducted in Japan (9), Great Britain (10), and the United States (11). They have also shown inverse associations between cancer and indicators of antioxidant micronutrients.

Although the antioxidant vitamins are suspected to be partially responsible for the inverse correlation, it is not at all clear what their relative role is. Plants contain a large number of nonnutrient substances that may influence cancer risk. The "more than 10 000 mutagens" they contain have led Ames to consider their role as carcinogens (12). The multitude of inhibitors of carcinogenesis they contain have led Wattenberg and other investigators to study their potential role in cancer prevention (13). The epidemiologic evidence indicates that the preventive role prevails.

It has been estimated that approximately 35% of all cancers are directly related to diet, and the proportion seems considerably greater for certain cancer sites (14). There is much hope that dietary intervention will substantially reduce cancer incidence and mortality.

Recent Case-Control Studies

Table 1 shows examples of recent case-control studies reporting on the association between the intake of fruits and vegetables and the risk of cancer (5–7, 15–24). Protective effects are reported against cancer of the oral cavity, larynx, esophagus, stomach, pancreas, and bladder. This table represents studies in white and black residents of the continental United States, Italy, and Hawaii. Other reports have documented similar findings in populations of diverse racial and geographic origin (25). The consistency of the results leaves little doubt

Table 1. Recent Case-Control Studies of Cancer Risk with Intake of Fruits and Vegetables

Authors	Site(s)	Exposure	Relative Risk (high intake)
Winn *et al.* U.S. Multicenter (5)	Oral cavity, pharynx	Fruits and vegetables	0.50 (0.30–0.80)
McLaughlin *et al.* (15)	Oral cavity, pharynx	Fruits	0.40 ($P < 0.05$)
Gridley *et al.* (16) Multicenter U.S. (New Jersey, Atlanta, Los Angeles, northern Calif.)	Oral cavity, pharynx	Noncitrus fruits	0.40 ($P < 0.01$)
		Green, leafy, raw vegetables	0.20 ($P < 0.001$)
LaVecchia *et al.* (17) (Italy)	Larynx	Green vegetables	0.40 (nonsignificant trend)
Ziegler *et al.* (6)	Esophagus	Vegetables	0.62 ($P < 0.10$)
		Fruits	0.50 ($P < 0.05$)
Mettlin *et al.* (18)	Esophagus	Fruits and vegetables	0.52 ($P = 0.001$)
Decarli *et al.* (19)	Esophagus	Green vegetables	0.62 (0.26–1.48)
		Fresh fruits	0.29 (0.13–0.62)
Correa *et al.* (7)	Stomach	Fruits	0.47 (0.24–0.92) whites
			0.33 (0.16–0.66) blacks
		Vegetables	0.50 (0.25–1.00) blacks
Chyou *et al.* (20)		Vegetables	0.60 (0.30–0.90)
		Fruits	0.60 (0.40–1.00)
Falk *et al.* (21)	Pancreas	Fruits and juices	0.40 (males $P < 0.05$) 0.46 (females $P < 0.05$)
Olsen *et al.* (22)	Pancreas	Cruciferous vegetables	0.57 (0.31–1.04)
LaVecchia *et al.* (23)	Bladder	Green vegetables	0.49 ($P < 0.05$)
Mills *et al.* (24)	Bladder	Fruit juice	0.31 (0.09–1.00)

about the potential of frequent intake of fruits and vegetables in reducing the risk of cancer of the upper respiratory and digestive organs.

Table 2 focuses on lung cancer, for which smoking is known to be the overriding etiologic factor (26–30). It is clear, however, that sub-

Table 2. Recent Case-Control Studies of Lung Cancer

Authors	Exposure	Relative Risk (high intake)
Pisani *et al.* (26)		0.77 (0.40–1.42)
(Italy)	Leafy green vegetable index	0.34 (0.19–0.62)
Ziegler *et al.* (27)		
(New Jersey)	Vegetable and fruit index	0.77 ($P = 0.04$)
Koo (28)	Fresh, leafy green vegetables	0.48 ($P = 0.24$)
(Hong Kong)	Fresh fruit	0.42 (0.55–0.91)
Fontham *et al.* (29)		
(Louisiana)	Fruit and vegetable index	0.70 (0.55–0.91)
LeMarchand *et al.* (30)		0.37 (males ($P < 0.001$)
(Hawaii)	All vegetables	0.14 (females $P < 0.01$)

stantially lower rates are observed in subjects who consume adequate amounts of fruits and vegetables.

Prospective Cohort Studies

A limited number of prospective cohort studies on the effects of the ingestion of fresh fruits and vegetables is available. The large census-based Japanese cohort reported by Hirayama found a significant negative correlation between cancer of all sites and the daily intake of green-yellow vegetables (31). Colditz *et al.* also reported a negative association between the two (32). A 1991 report from the Adventist Health Study, a cohort study of over 34 000 Seventh-day Adventists, provides a unique opportunity to evaluate the role of diet in lung cancer risk in a population composed primarily of never-smokers, with only 4% current smokers (33). During six years of follow-up, 61 incident lung cancer cases were diagnoses. Associations between risk of lung cancer and frequency of consumption of foods, particularly those foods for which the consumption pattern differs between vegetarians and nonvegetarians, were examined in an effort to explain the lower risk of lung cancer in Adventists than in nonsmoking non-Adventists. Fruit consumption showed a strong, significant protective effect. Compared with persons consuming fruit fewer than three times per week, persons who ate fruit three to seven times per week had a relative risk of 0.30 (0.16–0.58), and those who ate fruit two or more times per day had a relative risk of 0.26 (0.10–0.70), p trend

< 0.0006. The protective effect was similar against Kreyberg I and Kreyberg II tumors and for never-smokers and ever-smokers. With a few exceptions, notably Koo's study in Hong Kong (28) and Hirayama's in Japan (9), most studies of fruits and vegetables have found protective effects against lung cancer only in smokers. The results from this Adventist cohort study support the findings of Koo and Hirayama that the protective effect of these food groups against lung cancer risk is shared by nonsmokers as well as smokers.

Vitamin A and Carotenoids

Many of the studies that have evaluated the effects of fruits and vegetables on the carcinogenic process have also explored the possibility that the protective effects were attributable to the action of a specific nutrient. Which one of several micronutrients is targeted for report often reflects the particular research interest of the investigator. The early studies concentrated on preformed vitamin A (retinol) and lung cancer, prompted by the 1975 report of Bjelke (34). Because retinol is necessary for the normal differentiation of tissues and because cancer is characterized by loss of cell differentiation, the protective effect of fruits and vegetables (the principal dietary sources of beta-carotene and other carotenoids capable of conversion to vitamin A) was initially attributed to this vitamin A activity. The weight of the evidence in humans, however, does not support this contention. The dietary sources of retinol are primarily animal, especially organ meats and dairy products. Analytic studies of diet have not found the same consistent protective effect from retinol-containing foods as from fruits and vegetables. The antioxidant property of beta-carotene and other carotenoids, as well as a number of other micronutrients found in fruits and vegetables, provides a mechanism whereby these foods may confer protection unrelated to vitamin A activity. Prospective studies have reported a negative association between carotenoid intake and cancer of all sites (35) and lung cancer (36).

Prospective studies of blood levels of beta-carotene, which is a good indicator of dietary intake, have supported the findings of dietary studies (Table 3) (37–45). Low levels of serum or plasma beta-carotene have consistently been associated with increased risk of total cancers and lung cancer as well as cancers of other sites, including the stomach and the colon. A 1991 report of a 12-year follow-up of the

Table 3. Prospective Studies of Beta-Carotene Blood Levels

Authors	Year	Site(s)	Trend
Kark *et al.* (38) (Georgia)	1981	All	—[a]
Nomura *et al.* (39) (Hawaii)	1985	Colon	—
		Lung	—
		Stomach	—
Salonen *et al.* (40) (Finland)	1985	All	0[b]
		Lung	—
Menkes *et al.* (41) (Maryland)	1986	Lung	—
		Colon	0
Wald *et al.* (10) (U.K.)	1988	All	—
		Skin	0
		Lung	—
		Colorectum	—
		Stomach	—
Connett *et al.* (MRFIT) (42)	1989	Lung	—
		Colon	—
Knekt *et al.* (43) (Finland)	1991	All	0
		Lung	—
Stähelin *et al.* (44) (Switzerland)	1991	Lung	—
		Stomach	—

[a]— = Inverse trend.
[b]0 = No trend detected.

Basel study examined cancer mortality and its relation to several plasma antioxidants, including carotene (44). Both cancer of the lung and cancer of the stomach were associated with low mean plasma levels of carotene. Excluding mortality within the first two years of follow-up, low plasma carotene was associated with an 80% increased risk of lung cancer death. Low plasma levels of vitamin A were also associated with increased risk of lung cancer death, but only in older men (> 60 years of age).

Vitamin C

Block recently reviewed the findings of epidemiologic studies of dietary intake of vitamin C, as shown in Table 4 (45). A total of 33 studies on non-hormone-dependent cancers reported a statistically significant protective effect out of 46 such studies in which an index of dietary

Table 4. Number of Studies on Vitamin C Index

Site(s)	Protective	Total	Relative Risk (low intake)
All	33	46	—
Mouth	3	3	2.0
Larynx	1	1	2.4
Esophagus	4	4	2.2
Lung	5	10	1.6
Pancreas	1	1	2.2
Stomach	7	7	2.0
Cervix and precursors	4	5	2.0
Colorectum	4	8	1.1

Source: Block (45). © Am. J. Clin. Nutr. American Society for Clinical Nutrition.

vitamin C was derived. An approximate doubling of risk associated with low consumption is apparent for cancers of the oral cavity, esophagus, stomach, and cervix. There is also evidence of a protective effect against cancers of the larynx, rectum, pancreas, lung, and breast.

The Basel study is one of the few prospective studies, and certainly the largest, to measure plasma levels of vitamin C, which is unstable, is affected by recent intake and fasting, and is best measured in fresh blood samples.

Vitamin E

Vitamin E, a lipid antioxidant and free radical scavenger, is found in a wide variety of foods. Because it is ubiquitous in the food supply, measurement of dietary intake of vitamin E has not been used successfully to characterize persons at high or low risk of cancer. Serum levels have been examined in more than ten prospective studies, as illustrated in Table 5 (45–47). Protective effects are suggested against cancers of the stomach, pancreas, bladder, and central nervous system, and melanomas. The human data supporting an association between vitamin E and cancer are not as strong as the data for carotenoids and vitamin C. The lack of association between lung cancer and vitamin E may obscure any effect of vitamin E on less common cancers when the association between total cancer and vitamin E

Table 5. Low Serum Levels of Alpha-Tocopherol: Prospective Studies in Men

Site(s)	Relative Risk
All	1.4
Stomach	2.1
Colorectum	1.0
Pancreas	4.8
Lung	1.0
Melanoma	5.0
Bladder	5.6
Prostate	1.0
Skin	1.6
Central Nervous System	2.6
Lymphoma-leukemia	1.0

is examined, as is often the case when the total number of cancers is small. The role of vitamin E in human carcinogenesis at this time remains to be established.

Dietary Studies in South Louisiana

A number of studies have been conducted in south Louisiana, known for its unique diet and life-style. In the Atlases of Cancer Mortality, 1950–1969, a clustering of high mortality rates in south Louisiana was noted for cancer of the lung in black and white males, cancer of the stomach in blacks of both sexes, and cancer of the pancreas in white males. This geographic area was then targeted by the National Cancer Institute for studies to investigate the factors associated with excess risk.

Three case-control studies were conducted by Louisiana State University Medical Center in 26 high-risk Louisiana parishes from 1979 to 1983. Interviews were completed with 1253 lung cancer patients and 1274 matched controls, 391 stomach cancer cases and 390 matched controls, and 363 pancreatic cancer cases and 363 matched controls. The interview schedule included a 59-item food frequency section designed to estimate the usual adult diet, as well as a residential and occupational history, a medical history, detailed information on alcohol and tobacco use, and various demographic factors.

The Louisiana diet was examined as a risk factor for lung cancer (29). No significant protective or adverse effects were associated with consumption of dairy products, pork, nitrite-preserved meats, seafood, all meats, breads, grains and cereals, or use of spices. Low intake of fruits and vegetables, major sources of carotene and vitamin C, was associated with increased risk of lung cancer, especially squamous- and small-cell carcinomas. Fruit consumption adjusted for vegetable intake remained a strong protective factor against lung cancer, cutting the risk approximately in half. However, the protective effect of vegetable intake was weakened by adjustment for fruit consumption. Indexes of dietary intake of carotene, retinol, and vitamin C were calculated. Inverse gradients by vitamin C and carotene intake, that is, increasing risk with decreasing intake, were found for both whites and blacks, whereas an inverse relationship between dietary intake of retinol and risk of adenocarcinoma of the lung was strongest for blacks.

Diet was found to be the main determinant of gastric risk in south Louisiana (7). Both dietary patterns and dietary risk factors differed for blacks and whites. Two factors were associated with increased risk of stomach cancer in blacks: consumption of smoked foods, relative risk (RR) = 1.7, and consumption of homemade sausage or home-cured meats, (RR) = 2.32. Fruits as a group and dietary vitamin C were found to exert strong protective effects for both blacks and whites, reducing the risk by more than half with high intake.

The relationship of diet to pancreatic cancer risk in Louisiana was examined in detail (21). Significant 50% elevations in risk were found with frequent consumption of breads and cereals, fresh and processed pork meats, and rice. Fruit consumption showed a significant protective effect (RR = 0.63), whereas vegetable consumption reduced risk only slightly and nonsignificantly (RR = 0.88). Analyses were conducted to test for dose-response effects in foods and nutrients. Consumption of fruits and of vitamin C was associated with significant decreasing gradients for both sexes. Interestingly, no excess risk for pork was found among persons who consumed a lot of fruit, but low-fruit consumers who were heavy pork consumers had a greater than twofold excess of risk of pancreatic cancer.

As part of the larger lung cancer study, a small case-control interview study of malignant mesothelioma was also conducted (48). Thirty-seven cases (32 with pleural tumors and 5 with peritoneal tumors) were compared with 37 matched controls. Cases and controls reported similar overall intake of the total of 59 food items. The only case-control difference related to vegetable intake. Cases reported less frequent consumption of home-grown produce, cruciferous vegetables (broccoli, turnips, cabbage, brussels sprouts, and greens), and all vegetables combined. An estimate of usual carotene intake was also significantly lower in cases. Significant reductions in risk were associated with increasing consumption of vegetables. The results of this small case-control study suggest that diet may be associated with risk of malignant mesothelioma. This hypothesis should be tested in larger studies.

Conclusion

The weight of the evidence from more than a decade of research throughout the world strongly supports the need for public health efforts to increase consumption of fruits and vegetables. Although there are nonnutrient compounds with cancer-chemoprevention potential in such food items, there seems to be little doubt that the antioxidant vitamins play a prominent role in their antineoplastic functions. This role is crosscultural and more prominent for the nonendocrine-related tumors. The magnitude of the risk-reducing potential of these antioxidants has been underestimated by the public health community. Even in the presence of such strong carcinogens as tobacco smoke, reductions of greater than 30% of the risk are expected.

In general, the risk-reducing effects are seen more consistently for fresh fruits and vegetables as a group than for each vitamin independently. Much research is needed on the mechanisms of action, but it seems reasonable to believe that these vitamins act in synergy. Their study in chemoprevention trials, given their practically nonexistent toxicity, should be encouraged. In addition to yields related to their efficacy in humans, the trials could throw new light onto the biology of the preneoplastic process.

REFERENCES

1. Slater TF, Block G, eds. Antioxidant vitamins and β Carotene in disease prevention. *Am J Clin Nutr.* 1991;53(suppl):1895–3965.

2. Tannenbaum A. Relationship of body weight to cancer incidence. *Arch Path.* 1940;30:509–517.
3. Armstrong B, Doll R. Environmental factors and cancer incidence in different countries, with special reference to dietary practices. *Int J Cancer.* 1975;15:617–631.
4. Correa P. Epidemiologic correlations between diet and cancer frequency. *Cancer Res.* 1981;41:3685–3690.
5. Winn DM, Ziegler RG, Pickle LW, *et al.* Diet in the etiology of oral and pharyngeal cancer among women from the southern United States. *Cancer Res.* 1984;44:1216–1222.
6. Ziegler R, Morris LE, Blot WJ, *et al.* Esophageal cancer among black men in Washington DC, II: role of nutrition. *J Natl Cancer Inst.* 1981;67:1199–1206.
7. Correa P, Fontham E, Pickle LW, *et al.* Dietary determinants of gastric cancer in south Louisiana inhabitants. *J Natl Cancer Inst.* 1985;75:645–654.
8. Negri E, La Vecchia C, Franceschi S, *et al.* Vegetable and fruit consumption and cancer risk. *Int J Cancer.* 1991;48:350–354.
9. Hirayama T. Lung cancer in Japan: effects of nutrition and passive smoking. In: Mizell M, Correa P, eds. *Lung Cancer Causes and Prevention.* Deerfield Beach: Verlag Chemie International; 1984: 175–195.
10. Wald N, Thompson SG, Densem JW, *et al.* Serum beta-carotene and subsequent risk of cancer: results from the BUPA study. *Br J Cancer.* 1988;57:428–453.
11. Willett WC. Diet and cancer: an overview. *New Engl J Med.* 1984; 310:697–703.
12. Ames B. Dietary carcinogens and anticarcinogens. *Science.* 1983; 221:1256–1264.
13. Wattenberg L. Inhibitors of chemical carcinogenesis. *Adv Cancer Res.* 1978;26:197–226.
14. Doll R, Peto R. The causes of cancer: quantitative estimates of avoidable risks of cancer in the United States today. *Nat Cancer Inst.* 1981;66:1191–1308.
15. McLaughlin JK, Gridley G, Block G, *et al.* Dietary factors in oral and pharyngeal cancer. *J Natl Cancer Inst.* 1988;80:1237–1243.
16. Gridley G, McLaughlin JK, Block G, *et al.* Diet and oral and pharyngeal cancer among blacks. *Nutr.* 1990;14:219–225.
17. La Vecchia C, Negri E, D Avanzo B, *et al.* Dietary indicators of laryngeal cancer risk. *Cancer Res.* 1990;50:4497–4500.

18. Mettlin C, Graham S, Priore R, *et al.* Diet and cancer of the esophagus. *Nutr Cancer.* 1981;2:143–147.
19. Decarli A, Liati P, Negri E, *et al.* Vitamin A and other dietary factors in the etiology of esophageal cancer. *Nutr Cancer.* 1987;10: 29–37.
20. Chyou P, Nomura A, Hankin J, Stemmermann G. A case-control study of diet and stomach cancer. *Cancer Res.* 1990;50:7501–7504.
21. Falk R, Pickle L, Fontham E, *et al.* Lifestyle risk factors for pancreatic cancer in Louisiana. *Am J Epidemiol.* 1988;128:324–336.
22. Olsen GW, Mandel JS, Gibson RW, *et al.* A case-control study of pancreatic cancer and cigarettes, alcohol, copper and diet. *Am J Public Health.* 1989;79:1016–1019.
23. LaVeccia C, Negri E, De Carli A, *et al.* Dietary factors in the risk of bladder cancer. *Nutr Cancer.* 1989;12:93–101.
24. Mills PK, Beeson WL, Phillips RL, Fraser GE. Bladder cancer in a low risk population: results from the Adventist Health Study. *Am J Epidemiol.* 1991;133:230–239.
25. Committee on Diet, Nutrition and Cancer, National Academy of Sciences. *Diet, Nutrition and Cancer.* Washington, DC: National Academy Press; 1982. National Research Council.
26. Pisani P, Berrino F, Maculuso M, *et al.* Carrots, green vegetables and lung cancer: a case-control study. *Int J Epidemiol.* 1986;15:463–468.
27. Ziegler RG, Mason TJ, Stemhagen A, *et al.* Carotenoid intake, vegetables and the risk of lung cancer among white men in New Jersey. *Am J Epidemiol.* 1986;123:1080–1093.
28. Koo LC. Dietary habits and lung cancer risk among Chinese females in Hong Kong who never smoked. *Nutr Cancer.* 1988;11: 155–172.
29. Fontham ETH, Pickle LW, Haenszel W, *et al.* Dietary vitamin A and C and lung cancer risk in Louisiana. *Cancer.* 1988;62:2267–2273.
30. LeMarchand L, Yashizawa CN, Kolonel LN, Hankin JR, Goodman MT. Vegetable consumption and lung cancer risk: a population based case control study in Hawaii. *J Natl Cancer Inst.* 1989;81: 1158–1164.
31. Hirayama T. Diet and cancer. *Nutr Cancer.* 1979;1:67–81.
32. Colditz GA, Branch LG, Lipnick RJ, *et al.* Increased green and yellow vegetable intake and lowered cancer deaths in an elderly population. *Am J Clin Nutr.* 1985;41:32–36.

33. Fraser GE, Beeson WL, Phillips RL. Diet and lung cancer in California Seventh-Day Adventists. *Am J Epidemiol.* 1991;133:683–693.
34. Bjelke E. Dietary vitamin A and human lung cancer. *Int J Cancer.* 1975;15:561–565.
35. Paganini-Hill A, Chao A, Ross RK, Henderson BE. Vitamin A, beta-carotene, and the risk of lung cancer: a prospective study. *J Natl Cancer Inst.* 1987;79:443–448.
36. Shekelle RB, Liu S, Raynor WJ, *et al.* Dietary vitamin A and the risk of cancer in the Western Electric study. *Lancet.* 1981;i: 1185–1190.
37. Zeigler RG. Vegetables, fruits and carotenoids and the risk of cancer. *Am J Clin Nutr.* 1991; 53:251S–259S.
38. Kark J, Smith AH, Switzer BR, Hames CG. Serum vitamin A (retinol) and cancer incidence in Evans County, Georgia. *J Natl Cancer Inst.* 1981;66:7–16.
39. Nomura AMY, Stemmermann GN, Heilbrun LK, *et al.* Serum vitamin levels and the risk of cancer of specific sites in men of Japanese ancestry in Hawaii. *Cancer Res.* 1985;45:2369–2372.
40. Salonen JT, Salonen R, Lappeteläinen R, *et al.* Risk of cancer in relation to serum concentrations of selenium and vitamin A and E: matched case-control analyses of prospective data. *Br Med J.* 1985;290:417–420.
41. Menkes MS, Comstock GW, Vuilleunier JP, *et al.* Serum beta-carotene, vitamin A and E, selenium and the risk of lung cancer. *N Engl J Med.* 1986;315:1250–1254.
42. Connett GW, Kuller LH, Kjelsberg MO, *et al.* Relationship between carotenoids and cancer: the multiple risk factor intervention trial (MRFIT) study. *Cancer.* 1989;64:126–134.
43. Knekt P, Aromaa A, Maatela J, *et al.* Vitamin E and cancer prevention. *Am J Clin Nutr.* 1991;53:2835–2865.
44. Stähelin HB, Gey KF, Eichholzer M, Ludin E. Beta-carotene and cancer prevention: the Basel study. *Am J Clin Nutr.* 1991;53 (suppl): 265S–269S.
45. Block G. Vitamin C and cancer prevention: the epidemiologic evidence. *Am J Clin Nutr.* 1991;53:270S–282S.
46. Knekt P, Aromaa A, Maatela J, *et al.* Serum micronutrients and risk of cancers of low incidence in Finland. *Am J Epidemiol.* 1991; 134:356–361.
47. Menkes MS, Comstock GW, Vuilleumier JP, Helsing KJ, Rider AA, Brookmeyer R. Serum beta-carotene, vitamins A and E, se-

lenium and the risk of lung cancer. *N Engl J Med.* 1986;315: 1250–1254.

48. Schiffmann MH, Pickle LW, Fontham E, *et al.* A case-control study of diet and mesothelioma. *Cancer Res.* 1988;48:2911–2915.

JoANN E. MANSON, MICHAEL A. JONAS, DAVID J. HUNTER, JULIE E. BURING, and CHARLES H. HENNEKENS

Prospective Cohort Studies of Vitamins and Cancer

ABSTRACT

Diet may play a major role in the etiology of cancer. Among the components of diet, several vitamins have been postulated to have chemopreventive properties, including beta-carotene, preformed vitamin A (retinol), vitamin C, and vitamin E.

Prospective cohort studies, both those analyzing dietary vitamin intake and serum levels, have contributed valuable information to the evidence on this subject. Studies of beta-carotene have been the most widely reported. The most convincing evidence to date suggesting a possible protective effect comes from prospective studies of epithelial cancer, especially lung cancer, most of which have found strong inverse relations of high intake of carotene-rich foods and subsequent risk. Prospective studies using baseline blood samples also tend to support a possible benefit. Vitamin A has also been extensively studied, but results have been conflicting. Vitamins C and E have been the focus of fewer investigations, with the results inconsistent with respect to an inverse association between dietary intake or prediagnostic serum levels and subsequent cancer. Large-scale randomized trials in men and women, which are ongoing or planned, are necessary to provide reliable data upon which to base rational clinical decision making and public policy.

Introduction

Diet has been hypothesized to play an important role in the etiology of human cancer. Doll and Peto (1) have suggested that dietary practices may cause as much as 35% of all malignancies. Evidence of a possible role of diet in cancer has included basic research, which has outlined plausible mechanisms by which certain nutrients may exert chemopreventive effects, as well as descriptive epidemiologic studies, which have raised the possibility that regional variations in dietary habits may explain, at least in part, the striking worldwide differences in cancer incidence.

Vitamins are a component of diet postulated to play a significant role in the etiology of cancer and have been the subject of a large number of analytic epidemiologic studies, using both case-control and prospective cohort designs (2). This paper reviews the evidence from prospective cohort studies of the four principal vitamins hypothesized to have cancer chemopreventive properties: beta-carotene (provitamin A), retinol (preformed vitamin A), vitamin C, and vitamin E. In contrast to case-control studies, in which exposure information is collected after the diagnosis of the outcome of interest, prospective cohort studies collect exposure data at baseline on a population free from disease and then follow subjects to track the subsequent occurrence of the outcomes of interest. Thus, prospective studies have the methodologic advantage of being less susceptible to the introduction of either selection bias or observation bias in the reporting of exposure data (3).

Prospective studies of vitamins and cancer generally can be divided into two categories: dietary intake investigations and blood-based investigations. In the former, dietary intake information is collected from a cancer-free population that is then followed over time to track the subsequent incidence of this disease. The incidence of cancer is then calculated according to levels of nutrient intake. In some dietary intake studies an estimate of individual vitamin consumption is calculated based on the vitamin content of foods consumed, whereas others simply categorize participants according to average intake of the principal vitamin-rich foods. The differing methods used to assess dietary intake in observational studies make direct comparisons more difficult. Nevertheless, all these studies provide information relevant to the totality of evidence.

In prospective blood-based studies, serum or plasma specimens are collected at base line from a population free from cancer that is then followed over time. In a few such studies, fresh specimens are assayed from all participants for levels of the nutrient under study, and these values are later compared between incident cancer cases and the remainder of the population. In most blood-based studies, however, because of the expense of conducting such a large number of assays, specimens are frozen until the end of the designated follow-up period, at which time samples are assayed from all incident cases and a sample of matched controls selected from the remainder of the population. Although such investigations are called nested case-control studies, they are methodologically more similar to prospective cohort studies because they collect exposure information at baseline before the occurrence of outcomes.

Beta-Carotene

Beta-carotene, or provitamin A, is principally found in green leafy or yellow vegetables, carrots, and certain fruits. Dietary beta-carotene is converted to preformed vitamin A, or retinol, in the intestines of individuals with retinol-deficiency. It could, therefore, indirectly play a role in cancer prevention if very low retinol levels are related to carcinogenesis (4). In well-nourished populations, however, most dietary carotene is absorbed directly from the intestine without undergoing transformation to retinol. Beta-carotene has potent antioxidant properties (4), which are postulated to inhibit later stages of carcinogenesis, perhaps by deactivating excited or singlet oxygen molecules, which may propagate malignant transformation of damaged DNA.

Dietary Intake Studies

A large number of dietary studies in different countries have assessed intake of carotene in relation to subsequent cancer (Table 1). In most locations, one or two foods are the source for most of the beta-carotene consumed by that population, such as carrots in the United States and dark green or leafy vegetables in Singapore. As a result, many epidemiologic studies have been able to address the beta-carotene hypothesis simply because their general dietary questionnaire collected information on the chief carotene-containing foods in that region. Most of these studies suggest an inverse relation of high carotene intake and risk of cancers of epithelial cell origin, with the most consistent evidence relating to lung cancer.

One of the largest dietary cohort studies that has been conducted involved 265 118 Japanese adults (5). In 1966, dietary information was collected from these participants, who were then followed over a 17-year period. During this time, 14 740 cancer deaths were recorded. Subjects were divided in quartiles according to intake of green and yellow vegetables. The relative risk of cancer death for men in the highest

Table 1. Dietary Studies of Beta-Carotene Intake and Cancer

Study	Site(s)	Cases	RR[a]	*P* Value[b]
Colditz *et al.* (6) Massachusetts	All	42	0.30	0.01
Heilbrun *et al.* (13) Hawaii	Colon	102 men	0.72	0.11
	Rectum	60 men	0.83	0.42
Hirayama (5) Japan	All	8794 men	0.76	0.02
		5946 women	0.87	0.03
Hsing *et al.* (9) U.S.	Prostate	149	0.90	NS[c]
Hunter *et al.* (12) U.S.	Breast	1439	0.89	0.08
Knekt *et al.* (8) Finland	Lung	24 male non-smokers	0.40	0.04
		93 male smokers	0.93	0.91
Kromhout (14) Holland	Lung	63 men	0.68	NS
Mills *et al.* (16) California	Pancreas	50	>1	NS
Paganini-Hill *et al.* (15) California	All	638	0.87	NS
Shekelle *et al.* (7) Chicago	All	208 men	0.77	0.11
	Lung	33 men	0.14	0.003
[d]Long-de and Hammond (11) U.S.	Lung	2952	0.56	<0.05
[d]Mills *et al.* (10) California	Prostate	180	0.60–0.88	0.02–0.31

[a]Relative risk estimates here and in the following tables report risk in highest category compared with lowest.
[b]Most values refer to test of trend.
[c]Not significant.
[d]Assessed intake of foods rich in beta-carotene and vitamin C.

quartile of intake compared with those in the lowest was 0.76 ($P = 0.02$). For women, the comparable risk estimate was 0.87 ($P = 0.03$). The strongest effect was seen for stomach cancer, for which men and women with the highest intake levels had a relative risk of 0.66 ($P = 0.03$ and 0.01, respectively). For lung cancer, men in the highest quartile were at significantly reduced risk, whereas no trend was apparent in women. The effect of beta-carotene on risk of cancer among smokers has received particular attention, since this group has significantly increased risks. Although the inverse relation of green and yellow vegetable intake and total cancer risk in this study seemed greater in smokers than in nonsmokers, there were no significant differences for lung cancer.

Six other studies have found statistically significant inverse associations between high dietary carotene intake and cancer risk (6–11). In a cohort of 1271 elderly residents of Massachusetts (6), high intake of carotene-containing vegetables was associated with a statistically significant 70% decreased risk in cancer mortality, after adjustment for cigarette smoking. In a 19-year follow-up in the Western Electric Study (7), strong and statistically significant inverse effects of high carotene intake on risks of lung cancer were observed among the total population (relative risk [RR] = 0.14) and among those with smoking histories of 30 or more years (RR = 0.12). When all other cancers were considered in aggregate, however, there was no apparent effect. In a study of 4538 Finnish men (8), high intake of carotene was not inversely associated with lung cancer risk overall, but there was a significant inverse trend in the subgroup of nonsmokers. Finally, in a study of fatal prostate cancer among 17 633 white men (9), there was no overall effect but statistically significant trends of an inverse relation of high carotene intake and fatal prostate cancer among older men (≥ 75) and a positive association in those under 75 years old.

In a cohort of approximately 14 000 Seventh-day Adventist men (10), there was a significant inverse relation of high intake of fruits and vegetables with prostate cancer. However, since the foods showing inverse associations were high in both beta-carotene and vitamin C, it was difficult to draw conclusions concerning the relative benefit of either vitamin. Similar difficulties exist in interpreting the findings of a large prospective study of the American Cancer Society (11). Dietary information was collected from 136 281 white men whose lung cancer mortality was tracked for 10 years. High fruit consumption was associated with a significantly reduced risk of lung cancer death (RR = 0.56), raising the possibility that the vitamin C content of the fruits may have an etiologic role. This effect was somewhat weaker among smokers (RR = 0.65). Intake of green salad was not as strongly associated with a reduced risk of fatal lung cancer in these data.

Five studies have reported either nonsignificant inverse associations or null findings regarding beta-carotene and cancer (12–16). A recent study of diet and breast cancer among 89 494 registered nurses found a nonsignificant trend of decreased risks of breast cancer with increasing carotene intake (12), and a study of Hawaiian men of Japanese ancestry found a nonsignificant inverse association between carotene intake and colon cancer (13). A 25-year follow-up study from the Netherlands (14) found a nonsignificant inverse relationship of beta-carotene intake with lung cancer mortality, but this relationship was no longer present after controlling for cigarette smoking. In other studies, beta-carotene intake was unrelated to total cancer incidence (15) and fatal pancreatic cancer (16).

Blood-Based Studies

The beta-carotene hypothesis has also been tested in a number of prospective studies in which blood samples were collected at baseline (Table 2). The results of such investigations have been inconsistent with respect to the relationship between prediagnostic beta-carotene levels and total cancer incidence. However, as with the studies of dietary carotene intake, the findings for lung cancer have more consistently demonstrated an inverse association.

Four of five blood-based studies of beta-carotene that have examined serum beta-carotene levels and subsequent lung cancer have reported statistically significant lower risks with increasing levels of beta-carotene (17–20), and the fifth (21) reported a strong inverse relation (RR = 0.43), but the trend test did not achieve statistical significance ($P = 0.08$). Specifically, in a cohort of British men (17), the RR of lung cancer in the highest quintile of serum beta-carotene was 0.41, with a statistically significant trend. A study of residents of Washington County, Maryland, reported significantly lower levels of beta-carotene in 99 subjects who later developed lung cancer than in 196 matched controls (18). This effect persisted after adjustment for smoking, with an RR of 0.45 for those in the highest serum quintile ($P = 0.008$). For squamous-cell lung cancer, the risk reduction was even greater (RR = 0.23). In case-control comparisons in the Prospective Basel Study (19), carotene levels were significantly lower among the total cancer group, as well as for lung and stomach cancers. However, in the risk estimates, significant protective trends of high carotene were seen only for lung and stomach malignancies. In a Hawaiian study in which 302 cases of cancer accrued (20), the lung was the only site for

Table 2. Blood-Based Studies of Beta-Carotene Levels and Cancer

Study	Site(s)	Cases	RR	*P* Value[a]
Burney *et al.* (44) Maryland	Pancreas	22	0.82	NS[b]
Comstock *et al.* (26) Maryland	Melanoma	20	0.53	0.16
	Rectum	34	1.25	0.26
	Basal cell	21	0.91	0.24
	Breast	30	1.11	0.43
Connett *et al.* (21) U.S.	Lung	66	0.43	0.08
Helzlsouer *et al.* (42) Maryland	Bladder	35	0.62	0.35
Hsing *et al.* (36) Maryland	Prostate	103	1.08	0.94
Knekt *et al.* (25) Finland	Sites of low incidence	115	0.86	NS
	Melanoma	10	0.03	<0.01
Knekt *et al.* (22) Finland	All	453 men	0.77	0.01
		313 women	1.0	0.26
Menkes *et al.* (18) Maryland	Lung	99	0.45	0.04
Nomura *et al.* (20) Hawaii	Lung	74	0.45	0.04
Schober *et al.* (43) Maryland	Colon	72	0.83	NS
Stahelin *et al.* (19) Basel	All	204	0.64	≤0.01
	Lung	68	0.54	≤0.05
	Stomach	20	0.29	≤0.01
	Gastrointestinal tract	37	0.60	NS
Wald *et al.* (17) U.K.	All	271	0.60	0.01
	Lung	50	0.41	0.008
Wald *et al.* (24) U.K.	Breast	39	0.36	NS
Willett *et al.* (23) U.S.	All	111	1.5[c]	0.49

[a]Most values refer to test of trend.

[b]Not significant.

[c]Measured total carotenoids, not beta-carotene specifically.

which there were significant differences in prediagnostic serum levels. After adjusting for cigarette smoking, there was a significant trend of lower risks with higher serum levels ($P = 0.04$), although the estimates for each quintile included unity.

In the Finnish Mobile Clinic Health Examination Survey (22), statistically significant lower base-line beta-carotene levels were reported in male, but not female, cancer patients. The differences were even greater for male lung cancer patients, but this benefit did not persist after adjusting for smoking. Only one study (23) has reported higher base-line carotene levels in those subsequently developing lung cancer. This analysis of blood specimens from the Hypertension Detection and Follow-up Program also found higher levels among subsequent cases of all cancer sites combined than in matched controls. In contrast to other studies, however, only total carotenoids were measured, not beta-carotene specifically. If beta-carotene is the truly protective component of carotenoids, it could be theorized that such an association may have been masked in this study. However, the Multiple Risk Factor Intervention Trial analyses (21), which measured both total carotenoids and beta-carotene, actually found lower levels of total carotenoids than beta-carotene among both all-cancer cases and lung cancer fatalities.

A serum study of breast cancer in Britain (24) found a strong trend toward decreased risks with greater levels of beta-carotene, but this did not reach statistical significance. The Finnish Mobile Clinic Health Examination Survey recently reported findings for 11 cancers of low incidence (25). There were lower levels for cases at several different sites, but the only significant trend was for melanoma ($P < 0.01$). In addition to lung cancer, the Washington County, Maryland, study also examined the relationship between serum beta-carotene and subsequent cancer at eight other sites (26). There were no statistically significant trends in the risk estimates, though the mean level in melanoma cases was 22% lower than that of controls.

Thus, several prospective blood-based studies have shown higher serum beta-carotene levels to be associated with decreased risks of cancer. There is more consistent evidence with respect to lung cancer, and in some studies the lung is the only site for which there are statistically significant trends. Although the chemopreventive effect of high serum beta-carotene may be specific to lung cancer, it is also possible that there were too few cases of other epithelial cell types to distinguish reliably between a true null and an uninformative null result.

Retinol

Retinol and other retinoids have been shown to have strong hormonelike effects on epithelial tissue cell growth and differentiation (27). Since carcinogenesis involves the disruption of normal cell differentiation, it has been hypothesized that retinol may have chemopreventive properties (28).

Dietary Intake Studies

Results of prospective cohort studies of dietary retinol intake and subsequent cancer risk are inconsistent (Table 3). A recent analysis of

Table 3. Dietary Studies of Retinol Intake and Cancer

Study	Site(s)	Cases	RR	*P* Value[a]
Heilbrun *et al.* (13) Hawaii	Colon	102 men	0.68	0.18
	Rectum	60 men	1.03	0.79
Hsing *et al.* (9) U.S.	Prostate	149	1.32	NS[b]
Hunter *et al.* (12) U.S.	Breast	1439 women	0.80	0.003
Knekt *et al.* (8) Finland	Lung	24 male non-smokers	0.68	0.72
		93 male smokers	1.37	0.08
Kromhout (14) Holland	Lung	63 men	NR[c]	NS
Paganini-Hill *et al.* (15) California	All	638	0.86	NS
Paganini-Hill *et al.* (29) California	All	445	1.0	NS
Shekelle *et al.* (7) Chicago	All	208	1.11	0.42
	Lung	33	2.0	0.38

[a]Most values refer to test of trend.
[b]Not significant.
[c]Not reported.

89 494 female registered nurses (12) found that high intake of preformed vitamin A from both diet and supplements was associated with a statistically significant decreased risk of breast cancer. Compared with those in the lowest quintile of intake, women in the highest had an RR of breast cancer of 0.80 (95% CL 0.69–0.95, $P = 0.003$). In contrast to these findings, however, six other prospective dietary studies have failed to find an inverse association between retinol intake and subsequent cancer risk (7–9, 13–15). The Western Electric Study (7), which found a very strong effect of beta-carotene intake on lung cancer risk, reported no effect of retinol, with cases actually consuming slightly higher amounts. Similarly, the Zutphen Study in Holland (14), which found a suggestive, though nonsignificant, effect of carotene intake on lung cancer, reported no apparent effect of retinol intake. A third study (8) also found no association of retinol intake with lung cancer, but information on liver intake, a principal source of dietary retinol, was unreliable in an assessment of short-term reproducibility ($r = 0.16$). One study (13) found lower retinol intake among both colon and rectal cancer patients than among controls, but the differences were not statistically significant and there was no trend in the risk estimates. A study of fatal prostate cancer (9) found no overall association, but elevated risks were associated with greater retinol intake in men under the age of 75 ($P < 0.05$), whereas older men had nonsignificantly lower risks. Finally, a study of residents of a California retirement community found no strong evidence of an association of dietary retinol (11) or vitamin A supplements (29) and subsequent prostate cancer risk.

Blood-Based Studies

More than twenty blood-based studies of serum retinol and subsequent cancer have been conducted (Tables 4–5), the vast majority of which have failed to demonstrate any significant relationship of prediagnostic retinol levels with risks of cancer. However, blood-based studies of retinol are more difficult to interpret, since blood retinol levels are only weakly correlated with dietary retinol intake in well-nourished populations (30).

Although three such studies initially suggested inverse associations between high serum retinol and overall cancer risk (22, 31, 32), in one (22), when cases from the first two years of follow-up were

Table 4. Blood-Based Studies of Retinol Level and Cancer at All Sites

Study	Sites	Cases	RR	*P* Value[a]
Coates *et al.* (38) Washington State	All	156	1.0	NS[b]
Connett *et al.* (21) U.S.	All	156	NR[c]	NS
Criqui *et al.* (41) U.S.	All	136	NR	NS
Fex *et al.* (46) Sweden	All	61	NR	NS
Kark *et al.* (48) Georgia	All	85	0.16	<0.05
Knekt *et al.* (22) Finland	All	453 men 313 women	0.71 0.67	0.02 0.08
Kok *et al.* (45) Holland	All	69	NR	NS
Nomura *et al.* (20) Hawaii	All	284	NR	NS
Peleg *et al.* (34) Georgia	All	135	0.83	NS
Salonen *et al.* (37) Finland	All	51	1.11	NS
Stahelin *et al.* (19) Basel	All	204	0.86	NS
Wald *et al.* (31) U.K.	All	86	0.48	0.025
Wald *et al.* (33) U.K.	All	227	1.10	NS
Willett *et al.* (23) U.S.	All	111	1.1	0.98

[a]Most values refer to test of trend.
[b]Not significant.
[c]Not reported.

excluded, the effects were markedly attenuated, and in another (31), continued follow-up showed that the apparent benefit was confined to the first three years of follow-up (33). These findings raise the possibility that low serum retinol may be a consequence, rather than a cause, of cancer. In the third study (32), conducted in Evans County, Georgia, the initial finding of a significant inverse relation of serum retinol and subsequent cancer was not confirmed in a second cohort study conducted in this community (34). Whereas the earlier study

Table 5. Blood-Based Studies of Retinol Levels and Cancer at Various Sites

Study	Site(s)	Cases	RR	*P* Value[a]
Burney *et al.* (44) Maryland	Pancreas	22	0.93	NS[b]
Friedman *et al.* (39) California	Lung	151	0.83	NS
Helzlsouer (42) Maryland	Bladder	35	1.3	NS
Hsing *et al.* (36) Maryland	Prostate	103	0.40	0.07
Knekt *et al.* (25) Finland	Sites of low incidence	115	0.90	NS
Menkes *et al.* (18) Maryland	Lung	99	0.88	0.68
Reichman *et al.* (35) U.S.	Prostate	84	0.45	0.02
Russell *et al.* (40) U.K.	Breast	30	NR[c]	NS
Schober *et al.* (43) Maryland	Colon	72	0.29	0.15
Wald *et al.* (24) U.K.	Breast	39	0.84	NS

[a] Most values refer to test of trend.
[b] Not significant.
[c] Not reported.

excluded cases diagnosed within 12 months of blood drawing, the later investigation eliminated cancer cases diagnosed in the first 24 months after blood collection, which would tend to further diminish the possible effect of preclinical disease on the study findings. Of perhaps greater relevance, the earlier study reported differential thawing and refreezing of study specimens.

Two studies (35, 36) found serum retinol to be associated with decreased prostate cancer risks, though in one study (36) overall median values in cases and controls were similar and the trend did not achieve statistical significance. Three studies that found no overall association reported inverse associations of high serum retinol and gastrointestinal cancer (23), stomach malignancies (19), and lung cancer (37). A large number of studies have reported no apparent effect of prediagnostic retinol levels of cancer at various sites (18, 20, 21, 38–46). Thus, as with studies of dietary intake, prospective blood-based investigations do not support any clear inverse association between serum retinol and subsequent cancer risk.

Total Vitamin A

Although most dietary intake studies distinguish between vitamin A intake from beta-carotene and retinol, one of the earliest analytic studies of diet and cancer related risk to total vitamin A intake from all sources (47). The initial five-year follow-up in this cohort of 8 278 Norwegian men reported a statistically significant inverse association of high vitamin A intake on subsequent lung cancer (RR = 0.31, $P < 0.01$). All but 4 of the 53 incident cases were smokers, so it was not possible to make an assessment concerning nonsmokers. A subsequent report from this cohort (48), which included an additional 5 480 men as well as 2 929 women, confirmed the earlier finding.

Vitamin C

Like beta-carotene, vitamin C has potent antioxidant properties, which form the basis for its hypothesized role in cancer prevention. Although it has been the subject of fewer prospective studies, available evidence is compatible with a possible role in cancer prevention (Table 6).

Dietary Intake Studies

Three dietary intake investigations have reported inverse relationships of vitamin C intake and risk of cancer (8, 13, 14). In a Finnish study of lung cancer (8), Knekt and colleagues reported a relative risk of 0.32 for nonsmokers in the upper tertile of vitamin C intake ($P < 0.01$), but no effect was apparent in smokers. Overall vitamin C intake in Finland was low in comparison with that in other countries, suggesting that a higher intake might be particularly beneficial in populations with relatively low overall vitamin C consumption. The Zutphen Study (14) also found an inverse association between vitamin C intake and lung cancer risk, with an RR of 0.36 for those in the highest quartile of intake. Somewhat surprisingly, adjustment for cigarette smoking did not materially alter the results. There was an inverse association with total cancer, but this was of borderline statis-

Table 6. Dietary Studies of Vitamin C Intake and Cancer

Study	Site(s)	Cases	RR	*P* Value[a]
Heilbrun *et al.* (13) Hawaii	Colon	102	0.53	0.01
	Rectum	60	1.25	0.71
Hunter *et al.* (12) U.S.	Breast	1439	1.03	0.67
Knekt *et al.* (8) Finland	Lung	24 nonsmokers	0.32	<0.01
		93 smokers	1.23	0.36
Kromhout (14) Holland	Lung	63	0.36	<0.01
Kvale *et al.* (48) Norway	Lung	168	0.88	0.65
Shekelle *et al.* (7) Chicago	All	208	NR[b]	NS[c]
	Lung	33	NR	NS
[d]Long-de and Hammond (11) U.S.	Lung	2952	0.56	<0.05
[d]Mills *et al.* (10) California	Prostate	180	0.60–0.88	0.02–0.31

[a]Most values refer to test of trend.
[b]Not reported.
[c]Not significant.
[d]Assessed intake of foods rich in vitamin C and beta-carotene.

tical significance ($P = 0.05$) and was attenuated further by control for smoking. As mentioned above, two studies (10, 11) have reported inverse relationships of high intake of fruits and vegetables rich in both vitamin C and beta-carotene.

The recent analyses from a cohort of female registered nurses (12) show no effect of dietary vitamin C, with or without supplements, on subsequent risks of breast cancer. Similarly, no effect of vitamin C was reported in two studies of lung cancer (7, 45).

Blood-Based Studies

Plasma vitamin C can be measured reliably only in fresh blood specimens or in those stored at very low temperatures (−70°C) after being chemically stabilized (49). For this reason, the Basel Study (19), which tested fresh specimens from all 2974 men taking part in the 1971–1973 follow-up examination, is the only large-scale prospective investigation that has assessed prediagnostic vitamin C levels and cancer risk (Table 7). There was a statistically significant difference in mean

Table 7. Blood-Based Studies of Vitamin C Levels and Cancer

Study	Site(s)	Cases	RR	*P* Value
Stahelin *et al.* (19) Basel	All	204	0.82	NS[a]
	Gastrointestinal tract	37	>60 yrs 0.45 ≤60 yrs 1.61	<0.05 NS
	Stomach	20	>60 yrs 0.35 ≤60 yrs 1.12	≤0.05 NS
	Lung	68	>60 yrs 0.71 ≤60 yrs 0.79	NS NS

[a]Not significant.

Mean Plasma Vitamin C (μmol/L)	
All cancers	
204 cases	47.61 ± 1.78
2421 controls	52.76 ± 0.44
$p < 0.01$	
Stomach cancer	
20 cases	42.86 ± 4.88
2421 controls	52.76 ± 0.44
$p < 0.05$	

plasma between cases and controls that achieved statistical significance overall as well as for stomach cancer fatalities. In addition, there were significant inverse associations between vitamin C levels and stomach and total gastrointestinal cancer among those patients over 60 years old.

Vitamin E

Vitamin E, which is also a dietary antioxidant, has been studied in a small number of cohort studies of dietary intake (Table 8) and more extensively in prospective blood-based investigations (Tables 9, 10).

Dietary Intake Studies

Knekt and colleagues (8) assessed vitamin E intake in relation to subsequent risk of lung cancer among 4538 Finnish men. Mean intake levels were identical in 117 subsequent cases and 4421 controls. Risk estimates were suggestive of an inverse association in nonsmokers,

Table 8. Dietary Studies of Vitamin E Intake and Cancer

Study	Site(s)	Cases	RR	*P* Value[a]
Heilbrun *et al.* (13) Hawaii	Colon	102	NR[b]	NS[c]
	Rectum	60	NR	NS
Hunter *et al.* (12) U.S.	Breast	1439	0.90	0.07
Knekt *et al.* (8) Finland	Lung	24 nonsmokers	0.33	0.12
		93 smokers	1.25	0.58

[a]Test of trend.
[b]Not reported.
[c]Not significant.

Table 9. Blood-Based Studies of Vitamin E Levels and Cancer

Study	Sites	Cases	RR	*P* Value[a]
Connett *et al.* (21) U.S.	All	156	NR[b]	NS[c]
Fex *et al.* (46) Sweden	All	61	NR	NS
Knekt *et al.* (50) Finland	All	453 men	0.79	0.026
Knekt (51) Finland	All	313 women	0.58	0.05
Kok *et al.* (45) Holland	All	69	0.23	<0.01
	Lung	18	NR	NS
Nomura *et al.* (20) Hawaii	All	284	NR	NS
Salonen *et al.* (37) Finland	All	51	0.62	NS
Stahelin *et al.* (19) Basel	All	204	1.15	NS
Wald *et al.* (53) U.K.	All	271	<1 yr 0.28 ≥1 yr 1.14	0.003 NS
Willett *et al.* (23) U.S.	All	111	1.2	0.87

[a]Most values refer to test of trend.
[b]Not reported.
[c]Not significant.

Table 10. Blood-Based Studies of Vitamin E Levels and Cancer at Various Sites

Study	Site(s)	Cases	RR	*P* Value[a]
Burney *et al.* (44) Maryland	Pancreas	22	1.96	NS[b]
Comstock *et al.* (26) Maryland	Melanoma	20	1.00	0.50
	Rectum	34	1.67	0.40
	Basal cell	21	2.50	0.15
	Skin	30	1.67	0.28
	Breast			
Helzlsouer *et al.* (42) Maryland	Bladder	35	0.57	0.18
Hsing *et al.* (36) Maryland	Prostate	103	1.0	0.90
Knekt *et al.* (25) Finland	Sites of low incidence	115	0.96	NS
	Melanoma	10	0.20	<0.01
Russell *et al.* (40) U.K.	Breast	30	NR[c]	NS
Schober *et al.* (42) Maryland	Colon	72	0.67	NS
Wald *et al.* (24) U.K.	Breast	39	0.19	<0.01

[a]Most values refer to test of trend.
[b]Not significant.
[c]Not reported.

where the RR in the highest intake tertile was 0.33 ($P = 0.12$). Two other dietary cohort studies (12, 13) have found no suggestion of an effect of vitamin E intake on cancer risk. In the Nurses' Health Study analysis of diet and breast cancer (12), the multivariate RR estimate was close to 1.0 for each quintile of intake. In a study of colon and rectal cancer in Hawaii (13), there were no significant differences in mean intake of vitamin E among cases and controls.

Blood-Based Studies

Most of the 19 blood-based studies of vitamin E have reported lower levels in prediagnostic specimens of those subsequently developing cancer than in controls; however, only in 5 were there statistically significant trends toward decreased risks with higher blood levels (18,

25, 45, 50–51). In separate reports from the large Finnish cohort study of Knekt and colleagues, lower baseline vitamin E levels were found in both male (50) and female (51) cancer patients. In the study in men (50), a protective RR estimate for high vitamin E levels persisted after control for cigarette smoking as well as after eliminating those cancers diagnosed within two years of blood drawing and subjects with signs suggestive of preclinical disease (*e.g.*, low serum cholesterol, low hematocrit). The possible beneficial effect appeared to be limited to cancers unrelated to smoking. In the study in women (51), significant trends were seen for an inverse association between higher vitamin E levels and risk of total cancer as well as all epithelial cancers, but there was no apparent effect on hormone-related malignancies (breast, endometrium, and ovary). These findings persisted after control for smoking and other possible confounding factors, as well as in analyses eliminating cancers diagnosed in the first two years of follow-up. A recent analysis of vitamin E in relation to cancers of low incidence in this cohort (25) found a statistically significant inverse relation of serum vitamin E and melanoma, but this was based on only 10 cases.

Vitamin E levels were significantly lower in lung cancer cases than in controls in the cohort study in Washington County, Maryland (18). The smoking-adjusted RR for the highest serum quintile was 0.40 ($P = 0.04$). A prospective Dutch cohort study involving 10 532 subjects (45) also found significantly lower mean vitamin E levels in cases than in controls. A study of breast cancer in England (24) reported lower levels in cases than in controls, but the authors later suggested that this may have been the result of differential degradation of vitamin E levels in specimens of cases (52). Seven studies of cancer at multiple sites found no clear association between vitamin E levels and cancer (19–21, 23, 46, 53), as was the case in studies of cancer of the colon (41), breast (38), pancreas (42), bladder (40), and prostate (9). In one prospective study in which vitamin E levels did not differ significantly between cases and controls (35), there was the suggestion of greater risk associated with low vitamin E levels in the presence of low selenium levels.

Conclusion

Prospective cohort studies, both dietary and blood-based, have contributed important information regarding the possible chemopreventive effects of vitamins on cancer incidence. The strongest evidence to emerge from prospective observational studies involves the possible role of beta-carotene in preventing cancer of epithelial cell origin, particularly lung cancer. There are also suggestive findings for two other antioxidant nutrients, vitamins C and E. In spite of the large number of studies of retinol, particularly blood-based investigations, evidence for its role in cancer prevention remains inconsistent.

All observational studies, whether case-control or prospective cohort, are limited in their ability to provide reliable data about whether vitamins decrease cancer risk. Other life-style factors associated with intake of vitamins may, in fact, be responsible for any decreased risks. Some dietary studies have found that intake of certain vegetables or fruits is more strongly protective than a high score on an index of the nutrient being studied. This raises the possibility that other components of fruits and vegetables, such as fiber, phenols, and indoles, lower cancer risks, either alone or in combination. Direct evidence can only come from randomized trials, which are able to control for both known and unknown confounding variables. Such trials must be of sufficient sample size and adequate duration of treatment and follow-up to allow for the emergence of any anticancer effect. A primary prevention trial of beta-carotene is already ongoing among male physicians (54), and a trial of beta-carotene and vitamin E in female nurses is beginning (55). Other randomized trials are testing these agents, as well as vitamin C and retinoids, in secondary prevention of cancer or among high-risk populations. Over the next several years, reliable data upon which to base rational clinical decision making and public health policy should emerge from these randomized trials assessing whether beta-carotene, retinol, vitamin C, and vitamin E materially reduce human cancer risks.

REFERENCES

1. Doll R, Peto R. The causes of cancer. *JNCI Monogr.* 1981;66: 1191–1308.
2. Hennekens CH, Mayrent SL, Willett W. Vitamin A, carotenoids and retinoids. *Cancer.* 1986;58:1837–1841.
3. Hennekens CH, Buring JE. *Epidemiology in Medicine.* Boston: Little, Brown and Co; 1987.
4. Peto R, Doll R, Buckley JD, Sporn MB. Can dietary beta-carotene materially reduce human cancer rates? *Nature.* 1981;290:201–209.
5. Hirayama T. A large-scale cohort study on cancer risks by diet—

with special reference to the risk-reducing effects of green-yellow vegetable consumption. In Hayashi Y., *et al.*, eds. *Diet, Nutrition and Cancer.* Tokyo: Japan Scientific Societies Press; 1986:41–53.

6. Colditz GA, Branch LG, Lipnick RJ, *et al.* Increased green and yellow vegetable intake and lowered cancer deaths in an elderly population. *Am J Clin Nutr.* 1985;41:32–36.
7. Shekelle RB, Lepper M, Liu S, *et al.* Dietary vitamin A and risk of cancer in the Western Electric Study. *Lancet.* 1981;2:1185–1190.
8. Knekt P, Jarvinen R, Seppanen R, *et al.* Dietary antioxidants and the risk of lung cancer. *Am J Epidemiol.* 1991;134:471–479.
9. Hsing AW, McLaughlin JK, Schuman LM, *et al.* Diet, tobacco use, and fatal prostate cancer: results from the Lutheran Brotherhood Cohort Study. *Cancer Res.* 1990;50:6836–6840.
10. Mills PK, Beeson L, Phillips RL, Fraser GE. Cohort study of diet, lifestyle, and prostate cancer in Adventist men. *Cancer.* 1989; 64:589–604.
11. Long-de W, Hammond EC. Lung cancer, fruit, green salad and vitamin pills. *Chin Med J.* 1985;98:206–210.
12. Hunter D, Stampfer MJ, Colditz G, *et al.* A prospective study of consumption of vitamins A, C, E and breast cancer risk. *Am J Epidemiol.* 1992. In press. Abstract.
13. Heilbrun LK, Nomura A, Hankin JH, Stemmermann GN. Diet and colorectal cancer with special reference to fiber intake. *Int J Cancer.* 1989;44:1–6.
14. Kromhout D. Essential micronutrients in relation to carcinogenesis. *Am J Clin Nutr.* 1987;45:1361–1367.
15. Paganini-Hill A, Chao A, Ross RK, Henderson BE. Vitamin A, beta-carotene, and the risk of cancer: a prospective study. *JNCI Monographs.* 1987; 79:443–448.
16. Mills PK, Beeson WL, Abbey DE, Fraser GE, Phillips RL. Dietary habits and past medical history as related to fatal pancreas cancer risk among Adventists. *Cancer.* 1988; 61:2578–2585.
17. Wald NJ, Thompson SG, Densem JW, Boreham J, Bailey A. Serum beta-carotene and subsequent risk of cancer: results from the BUPA Study. *Br J Cancer.* 1988; 57:428–433.
18. Menkes MS, Comstock GW, Vuilleumier JP, Helsing KJ, Rider AA, Brookmeyer R. Serum beta-carotene, vitamins A and E, selenium, and the risk of lung cancer. *N Engl J Med.* 1986;315: 1250–1254.

19. Stahelin HB, Gey KF, Eichholzer M, *et al.* Plasma antioxidant vitamins and subsequent cancer mortality in the 12-year follow-up of the Prospective Basel Study. *Am J Epidemiol.* 1991;133:766–775.
20. Nomura AMY, Stemmermann GN, Heilbrun LK, Salkeld RM, Vuilleumier JP. Serum vitamin levels and the risk of cancer of specific sites in men of Japanese ancestry in Hawaii. *Cancer Res.* 1985;45:2369–2372.
21. Connett JE, Kuller LH, Kjelsberg MO, *et al.* Relationship between carotenoids and cancer: the Multiple Risk Factor Intervention Trial (MRFIT) study. *Cancer.* 1989;64:126–134.
22. Knekt P, Aromaa A, Maatela J, *et al.* Serum vitamin A and subsequent risk of cancer: cancer incidence follow-up of the Finnish Mobile Clinic Health Examination Survey. *Am J Epidemiol.* 1990; 132:857–870.
23. Willett WC, Polk BF, Underwood BA, *et al.* Relation of serum vitamins A and E and carotenoids to the risk of cancer. *N Engl J Med.* 1984;310:430–434.
24. Wald NJ, Boreham J, Hayward JL, Bulbrook RD. Plasma retinol, beta-carotene and vitamin E levels in relation to the future risk of breast cancer. *Br J Cancer.* 1984;49:321–324.
25. Knekt P, Aromaa A, Maatela J, *et al.* Serum micronutrients and risks of cancers of low incidence in Finland. *Am J Epidemiol.* 1991;134:356–361.
26. Comstock GW, Helzlsouer KJ, Bush TL. Prediagnostic serum levels of carotenoids and vitamin E as related to subsequent cancer in Washington County, Maryland. *Am J Clin Nutr.* 1991;53: 260S–264S.
27. Wolback SB, Howe PR. Tissue changes following deprivation of fat soluble A vitamin. *J Exp Med.* 1925;42:753–777.
28. Lippman SM, Meyskens FL Jr. Vitamin A derivatives in the prevention and treatment of human cancer. *J Am Coll Nutr.* 1988; 7:269–284.
29. Paganini-Hill A, Ross RK, Gray GE, Henderson BE. Vitamin A and cancer incidence in a retirement community. *NCI Monogr.* 1985;69:133–135.
30. Willett WC, Stampfer MJ, Underwood BA, *et al.* Vitamin A supplementation and plasma retinol levels: a randomized trial among women. *JNCI Monogr.* 1984;73:1445–1448.
31. Wald N, Idle M, Boreham J, Bailey A. Low serum-vitamin-A and

subsequent risk of cancer: preliminary results of a prospective study. *Lancet.* 1980;2:813–815.
32. Kark JD, Smith AH, Switzer BR, Hames CG. Serum vitamin A (retinol) and cancer incidence. *JNCI Monogr.* 1981;66:7–16.
33. Wald N, Boreham J, Bailey A. Serum retinol and subsequent risk of cancer. *Br J Cancer.* 1986;54:957–961.
34. Peleg I, Heyden S, Knowles M, Hames CG. Serum retinol and risk of subsequent cancer: extension of the Evans County, Georgia, Study. *JNCI Monogr.* 1984;73:1455–1458.
35. Reichman ME, Hayes RB, Ziegler RG, *et al.* Serum vitamin A and subsequent development of prostate cancer in the first National Health and Nutrition Examination Survey Epidemiologic Follow-up Study. *Cancer Res.* 1990;50:2311–2315.
36. Hsing AW, Comstock GW, Abbey H, Polk BF. Serologic precursors of cancer: retinol, carotenoids, and tocopherol and risk of prostate cancer. *JNCI Monogr.* 1990;82:941–946.
37. Salonen JT, Salonen R, Lappetelainen R, Haenpaa PH, Alfthan G, Puska P. Risk of cancer in relation to serum concentrations of selenium and vitamins A and E: matched case-control analysis of prospective data. *BmJ.* 1985;290:417–420.
38. Coates RJ, Weiss NS, Daling JR, Morris JS, Labbe RF. Serum levels of selenium and retinol and the subsequent risk of cancer. *Am J Epidemiol.* 1988;128:515–523.
39. Friedman GD, Blaner WS, Goodman DS, *et al.* Serum retinol and retinol-binding protein levels do not predict subsequent lung cancer. *Am J Epidemiol.* 1986;123:781–789.
40. Russell MJ, Thomas BS, Bulbrook RD. A prospective study of the relationship between serum vitamins A and E and risk of breast cancer. *Br J Cancer.* 1988;57:213–215.
41. Criqui MH, Bangdiwala S, Goodman DS, *et al.* Selenium, retinol, retinol-binding protein, and uric acid: associations with cancer mortality in a population-based prospective case-control study. *Ann Epidemiol.* 1991;1:385–393.
42. Helzlsouer KJ, Comstock GW, Morris SJ. Selenium, lycopene, alpha-tocopherol, beta-carotene, retinol, and subsequent bladder cancer. *Cancer Res.* 1989;49:6144–6148.
43. Schober SE, Comstock GW, Hesling KJ, *et al.* Serologic precursors of cancer, I: prediagnostic serum nutrients and colon cancer risk. *Am J Epidemiol.* 1987;126:1033–1041.

44. Burney PGJ, Comstock GW, Morris JS. Serologic precursors of cancer: serum micronutrients and the subsequent risk of pancreatic cancer. *Am J Clin Nutr.* 1989;49:895–900.
45. Kok FJ, van Duijn CM, Hofman A, Vermeeren R, de Bruijn AM, Valkenburg HA. Micronutrients and the risk of lung cancer. *N Engl J Med.* 1987;316:1416. Letter.
46. Fex G, *et al.* Low plasma selenium as a risk factor for cancer death in middle-aged men. *Nutr Cancer.* 1987;10:221–229.
47. Bjelke E. Dietary vitamin A and human lung cancer. *Int J Cancer.* 1975;15:561–565.
48. Kvale G, Bjelke E, Gart JJ. Dietary habits and lung cancer risk. *Int J Cancer.* 1983;15:397–405.
49. Willett W. *Nutritional Epidemiology.* New York: Oxford University Press; 1990.
50. Knekt P, Aromaa A, Maatela J, *et al.* Serum vitamin E and risk of cancer among Finnish men during a 10-year follow-up. *Am J Epidemiol.* 1988;127:28–41.
51. Knekt P. Serum vitamin E level and risk of female cancer. *Int J Epidemiol.* 1988;17:281–288.
52. Wald NJ, Nicolaides-Bouman A, Hudson GA. Plasma retinol, beta-carotene and vitamin E levels in relation to the future risk of breast cancer. *Br J Cancer.* 1988;57:235. Letter.
53. Wald NJ, Thompson SG, Densem JW, Boreham J, Bailey A. Serum vitamin E and subsequent risk of cancer. *Br J Cancer.* 1987;56:69–72.
54. Steering Committee of the Physicians' Health Study Research Group. Final report on the aspirin component of the ongoing Physicians' Health Study. *N Engl J Med.* 1989;321:129–135.
55. Buring JE, Hennekens CH, for the Women's Health Study Research Group. The Women's Health Study: background and rationale. *J Myocardial Ischemia.* 1992;4:30–40.

LAURENCE N. KOLONEL, LOÏC LE MARCHAND, JEAN H. HANKIN, ABRAHAM M. Y. NOMURA, MARC T. GOODMAN, LYNNE R. WILKENS, and LUE PING ZHAO

Case-Control Studies on Vitamins and Cancer in a Multiethnic Population

ABSTRACT

Attempts to explain the remarkable differences in cancer rates among ethnic groups in Hawaii have centered on studies of environmental exposures, especially the diet. Risk factors, such as dietary fat, and possible protective factors, such as vitamins, have been investigated extensively.

Case-control studies that examined vitamin intake have been completed for several cancer sites, including the lung, prostate, bladder, and thyroid. Cancers currently under study, for which only preliminary data are available, include colorectal cancer, endometrial cancer, and malignant melanoma. Although the findings vary by cancer site, the results of the completed studies suggest that beta-carotene, other carotenoids, or vitamin C may be protective against lung and bladder cancer. However, because other constituents with potential anticancer properties are present in the fruits and vegetables that are the primary sources of these nutrients, the data have also been examined for the effects of specific foods and food groups. These analyses suggest that there may be interactions among various food constituents in their effects on cancer risk.

Data from the study of lung cancer were used to illustrate the potential impact of changes in food or nutrient-consumption levels on cancer incidence. Based on calculations of the attributable risk due to low intake of beta-carotene or vegetables as a group, it appeared that the incidence of lung cancer in our population could be lowered by 20% to 40% on the basis of diet, independent of changes in smoking behavior. These results support the value of public health measures that encourage greater intakes of vitamin A, vitamin C, and other substances with cancer-inhibiting properties.

Introduction

Remarkable differences in the incidence of common cancers, such as lung, breast, prostate, colon, and bladder, are seen in the ethnic populations of Hawaii (1). Since the various ethnic groups live and work in close proximity in a state with little heavy industry, it is natural to consider either genetic or cultural factors as explanations for these differences. Because several lines of evidence, including our own studies on migrant populations (2–5), argue against a primary genetic explanation for these common cancers, we have turned our attention to certain life-style factors, particularly the diet.

In the initial correlations of ethnic cancer incidence patterns with corresponding levels of exposure to dietary and other life-style factors in Hawaii, some striking discrepancies were apparent that could not readily be explained. For example, the usual diet of native Hawaiians contains much more fat than does that of the Hawaii Japanese (6), yet the incidence of colon cancer among the Japanese is nearly twice as high (Fig. 1). Again, native Hawaiian men smoke cigarettes to a similar extent as Japanese men (7), yet the incidence of lung cancer is more than twofolds higher in the Hawaiians (Fig. 2). Such observations suggested that other factors, possibly involving the diet, might protect against cancer. This was not inconsistent with the findings of some of the early epidemiologic studies of diet and cancer that, although emphasizing dietary components that *increased* cancer risk, also found that some foods and eating patterns were inversely associated with risk (8–11).

In this paper we describe the results of case-control studies on vitamins and other dietary constituents that may inhibit cancer formation. These studies were conducted over several years in the ethnic populations of Hawaii. We also discuss the potential impact that increased intake of these substances might have on future cancer incidence in our population.

The design and methods of data collection were similar for all studies. Briefly, cases were identified by a rapid-reporting system of the Hawaii Tumor Registry, a population-based registry covering the entire state of Hawaii and a participant in the Surveillance, Epidemiology and End Results (SEER) Program of the National Cancer Institute. Controls also were population based and, with few exceptions, were selected from households participating in the Health Surveil-

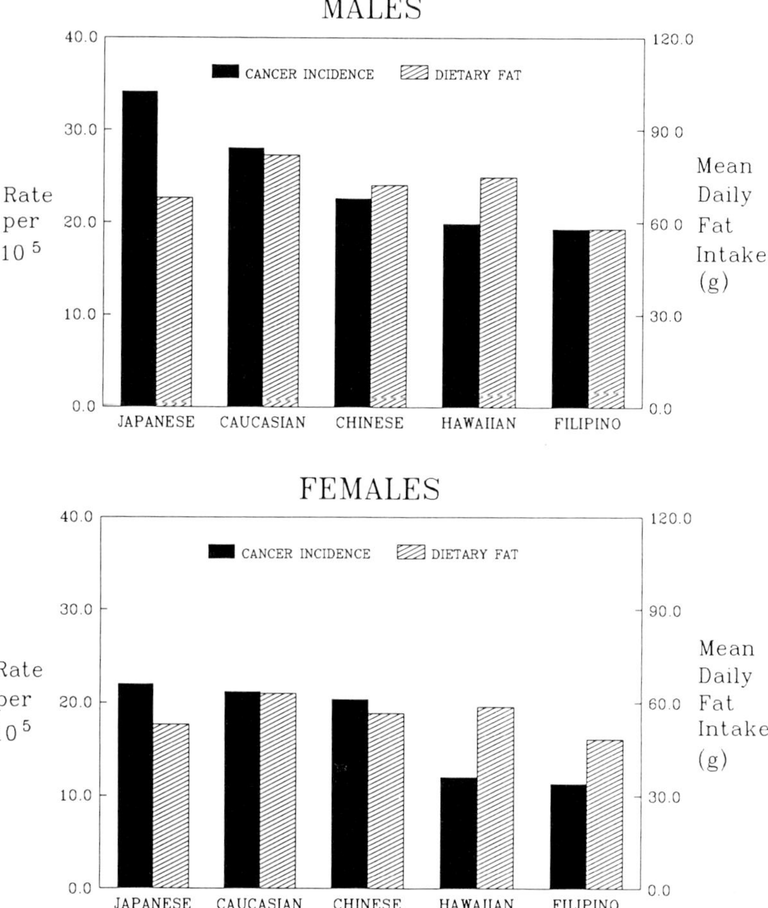

Figure 1. Fat intake and colon cancer incidence in Hawaii, 1978–1982, age-adjusted (world population standard).

lance Program of the Hawaii Department of Health (12). Controls were matched to the cases on age, sex, and, in some studies, ethnicity. The Health Surveillance Program surveys a randomly selected 2% of households throughout Hawaii each year to collect health-related data. Subjects for our studies were interviewed in person, at home, using a diet history method developed by one of us (13). We used a list of foods covering selected nutrients of interest, or the entire diet, to elicit information on frequency and amount of consumption. We used color photographs showing food items in three portion

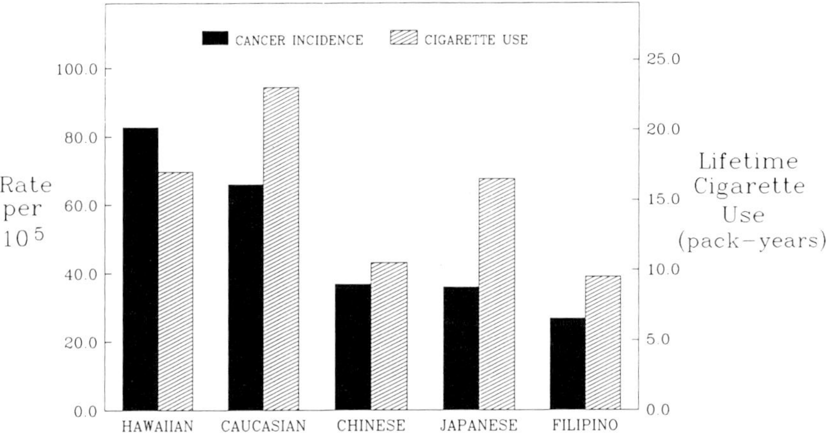

Figure 2. Lifetime cigarette use and lung cancer incidence in Hawaii (males), 1978–1982, age-adjusted (world population standard).

sizes to facilitate quantification. The analyses for these studies used multiple logistic regression to compute odds ratios associated with different levels of exposure to the risk factors of interest, with adjustment for appropriate confounding factors (14).

Studies of Selected Vitamin Intakes

Lung Cancer

Because of the poor correlation between cigarette smoking rates and the incidence of lung cancer among the ethnic populations of Hawaii, we decided to examine the role of vitamin A, beta-carotene, and vitamin C in the risk of this cancer.

In an initial case-control study conducted from 1979 through 1982 and involving 364 cases and 627 controls from the five main ethnic groups in Hawaii (15), we found no effect of dietary retinol or vitamin C on lung cancer risk, but a distinct protective effect, after controlling for cigarette smoking, or carotenoid intake in men but not women (Table 1). The odds ratio for the lowest quartile of intake relative to the highest in men was 2:2.

In a subsequent case-control study, conducted from 1983 through 1985, we used a similar design (with some modifications to the protocol for the dietary assessment) and interviewed 332 cases and 865 controls (16, 17). Again, we found a protective effect of beta-carotene

Table 1. Vitamin Intake[a] and Lung Cancer Risk, Study I

Intake Quartile	Odds Ratio[b] (95% C.I.)	
	Carotene	Vitamin C
	Males	
1 (High)	1.0	1.0
2	1.1 (0.7–1.9)	0.9 (0.6–1.5)
3	1.1 (0.7–1.9)	1.3 (0.7–2.2)
4 (Low)	2.2 (1.3–3.7)	1.6 (0.8–3.4)
	Females	
1 (High)	1.0	1.0
2	0.9 (0.4–2.0)	1.2 (0.6–2.4)
3	0.9 (0.4–2.1)	0.6 (0.2–1.5)
4 (Low)	0.6 (0.12–1.5)	0.7 (0.2–2.2)

Adapted, with permission, from reference 15.

[a] Includes supplements.

[b] Adjusted for age, ethnicity, pack-years of cigarette smoking, cholesterol intake, and occupational status.

and other carotenoids in men. In this study, a protective effect was seen in women as well (Table 2). These findings were consistent with the evidence from several other studies showing a protective effect of dietary beta-carotene on lung cancer risk (18, 19). Most of these reports were also based on case-control studies, though a few involved follow-up on cohorts. The findings from assays of beta-carotene in prediagnostic serum in some of these cohort studies (20–22) supported the results from the dietary intake assessments.

We also looked at the effect of vitamin C. In both studies, there was a protective effect in men. The effect was statistically significant in the second study, but there was no clear evidence of an effect in women (Table 2).

Bladder Cancer

We subsequently extended these studies to other cancer sites for which distinct ethnic differences in incidence existed in Hawaii. One such site was the bladder, where the incidence of cancer among Caucasian men and women in Hawaii is two to three times higher than among Japanese (1). During the period 1977–1986, we completed in-

Table 2. Vitamin Intake[a] and Lung Cancer Risk, Study II

Intake Quartile	Odds Ratio[b]			
	Retinol	Beta-Carotene	Other Carotenoids[c]	Vitamin C
		Males		
1 (High)	1.0	1.0	1.0	1.0
2	1.0	1.5	1.6	2.0
3	0.9	2.4	2.1	1.9
4 (Low)	0.9	1.9	2.0	1.9
P	.70	.001	.003	.01
		Females		
1 (High)	1.0	1.0	1.0	1.0
2	1.1	1.9	1.9	0.7
3	1.3	2.4	2.3	1.1
4 (Low)	1.0	2.7	2.9	1.4
P	.75	.01	.009	.42

Adapted, with permission, from reference 16.

[a]Food sources only.

[b]Adjusted for age, ethnicity, smoking status, pack-years of cigarette smoking, and cholesterol intake (males only).

[c]With vitamin A activity.

terviews with 195 men (87 Japanese and 108 Caucasian), and 66 women (37 Japanese and 29 Caucasian), each matched on age, sex, and ethnicity to two population controls (23).

The results showed no clear effect of carotenoids or retinol on bladder cancer in either sex, but an inverse association of vitamin C intake was seen in women (Table 3). These findings agree with most of the literature, which shows only weak evidence of dietary protective effects against this cancer (24).

Prostate Cancer

Prostate cancer rates in Hawaii are high among Caucasian men, somewhat lower among Hawaiian men, and much lower among Chinese, Japanese, and Filipino men (1). In a study of the relationship of diet to the risk of this cancer in Hawaii (25, 26), we interviewed 452 cases and 899 population controls from five ethnic groups from 1977 through 1983. We were surprised to find that the intake of retinol and carot-

Table 3. Carotene Intake[a] and Bladder Cancer Risk

Intake Quartile	Odds Ratio[b] (95% C.I.)		
	Retinol	Carotenoids[c]	Vitamin C
		Males	
1 (High)	1.0	1.0	1.0
2	1.2 (0.7–2.1)	0.7 (0.4–1.2)	1.1 (0.6–1.9)
3	1.1 (0.6–1.9)	1.0 (0.6–1.6)	1.3 (0.8–2.2)
4 (Low)	1.6 (0.9–2.7)	0.7 (0.4–1.2)	1.2 (0.8–2.1)
P	.10	.45	.41
		Females	
1 (Low)	1.0	1.0	1.0
2	1.1 (0.5–2.9)	0.6 (0.3–1.6)	1.0 (0.4–2.3)
3	1.0 (0.5–2.7)	1.3 (0.6–3.2)	0.9 (0.4–2.2)
4 (High)	1.0 (0.4–2.8)	0.5 (0.2–1.3)	0.4 (0.2–1.1)
P	.82	.31	.03

Adapted, with permission, from reference 23.

[a] Includes supplements.

[b] Adjusted for age, ethnicity, and pack-years of cigarette smoking.

[c] With vitamin A activity.

enoids (beta-carotene and others) was positively associated with risk among the older group of men (Table 4). Although such a finding was not inconsistent with certain laboratory findings on the potential for retinoids to enhance carcinogenesis (27) and with the results of other case-control studies (28, 29), it was disconcerting in terms of its implication for the potential contribution of these nutrients to cancer control intervention programs. Our further examination of this finding is discussed below.

For vitamin C, we also found elevated odds ratios in the older group of men for the upper two quartiles. However, these were not statistically significant and did not result in a significant trend.

Endometrial Cancer

Epidemiologic research on the relationship of diet to the risk of endometrial cancer is sparse (24). We are currently conducting a case-control study of this cancer in which dietary and other information is being collected. Preliminary data, based on interviews of 231 cases and 290 controls, do not suggest any effect of vitamin A, beta-

Table 4. Vitamin Intake[a] and Prostate Cancer Risk

Intake Quartile	Odds Ratio[b] (95% C.I.)			
	Retinol	Beta-Carotene	Other Carotenoids[c]	Vitamin C
		Age ≥70 Years		
1 (Low)	1.0	1.0	1.0	1.0
2	1.0 (0.6–1.5)	1.2 (0.8–1.9)	1.4 (0.9–2.1)	1.1 (0.7–1.7)
3	1.2 (0.8–1.9)	1.5 (0.9–2.3)	1.4 (0.9–2.2)	1.5 (0.9–2.3)
4 (High)	1.4 (0.9–2.1)	1.5 (0.9–2.3)	1.6 (1.0–2.5)	1.4 (0.9–2.3)
P	.10	.09	.08	.16
		Age <70 Years		
1 (Low)	1.0	1.0	1.0	1.0
2	0.8 (0.5–1.4)	1.5 (0.9–2.4)	1.4 (0.9–2.3)	0.8 (0.5–1.3)
3	1.1 (0.7–1.9)	1.1 (0.7–1.9)	1.1 (0.7–1.8)	1.0 (0.6–1.6)
4 (High)	0.9 (0.6–1.5)	1.0 (0.6–1.6)	0.9 (0.5–1.5)	0.7 (0.4–1.2)
P	.82	.55	.32	.27

Adapted, with permission, from reference 25.

[a]Includes supplements.

[b]Adjusted for age and ethnicity.

[c]With vitamin A activity.

carotene, other carotenoids, vitamin C, or vitamin E on the risk of this cancer (Table 5).

Malignant Melanoma

Although the etiology of malignant melanoma is clearly related to solar exposure and certain phenotypic characteristics, such as dysplastic nevus syndrome (30), it is plausible to consider that micronutrient constituents of the diet, including vitamin A, carotenoids, vitamin C, and vitamin E afford some protection (31).

In an ongoing study of this cancer, a variety of potential risk factors and their interactions are being examined. Preliminary data, based on 84 male and 58 female case-control pairs, do not show an independent effect of any of these micronutrients, however (Table 6).

Colorectal Cancer

An ongoing study by our group is examining the role of vitamins and other dietary constituents on colorectal cancer risk. Although a positive relationship to dietary fat and obesity has been reported in many

Table 5. Vitamin Intake[a] and Endometrial Cancer Risk (preliminary data)

Intake Quartile	Odds Ratio[b]				
	Vitamin A	Beta-Carotene	Other Carotenoids[c]	Vitamin C	Vitamin E
1 (High)	1.0	1.0	1.0	1.0	1.0
2	0.7	0.7	0.8	0.6	0.9
3	0.8	0.8	0.7	0.8	0.8
4 (Low)	1.0	1.0	0.9	1.0	1.6
P	.56	.64	.91	.53	.19

[a]Food sources only.
[b]Adjusted for age, ethnicity, age at menarche, age at menopause, history of diabetes, history of hypertension, and total calories.
[c]With vitamin A activity.

Table 6. Intake[a] of Selected Vitamins and Risk of Malignant Melanoma Among Whites (preliminary data)

Intake Tertile	Odds Ratio[b] (95% C.I.)			
	Retinol	Beta-Carotene	Vitamin C	Alpha-Tocopherol
		Males		
1 (Low)	1.0	1.0	1.0	1.0
2	1.1 (0.5–2.3)	1.1 (0.5–2.2)	1.2 (0.5–2.6)	1.0 (0.5–2.1)
3 (High)	1.0 (0.5–2.1)	1.1 (0.5–2.2)	0.9 (0.5–1.7)	0.8 (0.4–1.7)
P	0.94	0.82	0.63	0.53
		Females		
1 (Low)	1.0	1.0	1.0	1.0
2	1.2 (0.5–3.2)	1.3 (0.5–3.3)	0.6 (0.2–1.7)	0.7 (0.3–1.9)
3 (High)	1.8 (0.7–4.8)	1.2 (0.5–3.0)	2.5 (1.0–6.2)	1.1 (0.5–2.7)
P	0.26	0.72	0.04	0.73

[a]Food sources only.
[b]Subjects were matched by age.

studies of this cancer (32), there is less evidence regarding the possible protective effects of vitamins. Preliminary data based on interviews of 418 colon cancer patients, 174 rectal cancer patients, and 592 age-, sex-, and ethnicity-matched controls (Tables 7 and 8) do not show any association of vitamin intake with either colon or rectal can-

Table 7. Intake[a] of Selected Vitamins and Colon Cancer Risk (preliminary data)

Intake Tertile	Odds Ratio[b] (95% C.I.)			
	Retinol	Beta-Carotene	Vitamin C	Alpha-Tocopherol
		Males		
1 (Low)	1.0	1.0	1.0	1.0
2	1.3 (0.8–1.9)	0.9 (0.6–1.4)	1.0 (0.7–1.6)	0.8 (0.5–1.2)
3 (High)	1.6 (1.0–2.5)	0.9 (0.6–1.4)	0.8 (0.5–1.3)	1.1 (0.7–1.8)
P	0.08	0.61	0.32	0.43
		Females		
1 (Low)	1.0	1.0	1.0	1.0
2	1.4 (0.8–2.4)	0.9 (0.5–1.4)	1.4 (0.8–2.3)	1.1 (0.7–1.8)
3 (High)	1.2 (0.7–2.0)	1.0 (0.6–1.7)	1.3 (0.8–2.1)	1.1 (0.7–1.9)
P	0.73	0.92	0.34	0.73

[a]Food sources only.
[b]Subjects were matched by sex, age, and ethnicity.

Table 8. Intake[a] of Selected Vitamins and Rectal Cancer Risk (preliminary data)

Intake Tertile	Odds Ratio[b] (95% C.I.)			
	Retinol	Beta-Carotene	Vitamin C	Alpha-Tocopherol
		Males		
1 (Low)	1.0	1.0	1.0	1.0
2	1.3 (0.6–2.7)	0.5 (0.3–1.0)	0.8 (0.5–1.6)	1.0 (0.5–1.8)
3 (High)	1.3 (0.6–2.7)	0.7 (0.4–1.5)	0.5 (0.2–0.9)	0.7 (0.4–1.5)
P	0.64	0.67	0.03	0.36
		Females		
1 (Low)	1.0	1.0	1.0	1.0
2	0.6 (0.3–1.4)	1.7 (0.7–4.1)	1.1 (0.5–2.5)	0.7 (0.3–1.9)
3 (High)	0.7 (0.2–2.1)	0.9 (0.4–2.1)	1.4 (0.6–3.4)	1.6 (0.6–4.2)
P	0.64	0.86	0.50	0.21

[a]Food sources only.
[b]Subjects were matched by sex, age, and ethnicity.

cer, with the exception of a statistically significant inverse association between vitamin C intake and rectal cancer in males (Table 8).

Studies of Foods and Food Groups

Rationale

Most of the early studies of diet and cancer were based on simplified food-frequency questionnaires and did not assess nutrient intakes (8–11). Published reports from these studies referred to the consumption of high-fat foods or vegetables, often as generic food groups. Based on associations of these foods with cancer, effects of particular nutrient constituents, such as fat or vitamins, were inferred (33, 34). More comprehensive dietary assessments were obtained in subsequent studies, based on the use of frequency questionnaires and various means of estimating portion sizes, enabling investigators to compute nutrient intakes that could then be related to cancer risk. Naturally, this methodologic refinement was considered desirable.

As more information accumulated, including laboratory results on a variety of different carotenoids and nonnutritive food constituents with inhibitory properties against cancer (35, 36), we recognized that a focus on *nutrient* analyses could be misleading. Many different constituents with protective properties can be present in the same foods, and their interactive effects are not predictable at this time. Some of these components have not been quantified in foods, and others, no doubt, have not yet even been formally identified; thus, they are not included in current food composition data bases. There is also concern about the adequacy of the food composition data presently available for certain nutrients of interest (37). Consequently, we also examined foods and food groups in several of our studies.

Lung Cancer

As noted earlier, we have shown that quantitative estimates of the intake of beta-carotene, and of other carotenoids with vitamin A activity, supported a protective effect of these nutrients against lung cancer. We subsequently looked at foods and food groups that were especially rich in particular carotenoid constituents as a means of indirectly assessing their individual effects (16). For example, tomatoes

Table 9. Vegetable Intake and Lung Cancer Risk

Intake Quartile	Odds Ratio[a]				
	Carrots	Tomatoes	Dark Greens	Cruciferae	All Vegetables
			Males		
1 (High)	1.0	1.0	1.0	1.0	1.0
2	1.9	2.5	1.4	1.4	1.9
3	2.1	1.8	1.9	2.3	2.3
4 (Low)	2.8	2.3	2.0	2.2	2.7
P	<.001	.002	.003	.001	<.001
			Females		
1 (High)	1.0	1.0	1.0	1.0	1.0
2	2.2	1.5	3.7	3.2	3.2
3	3.7	3.1	3.4	4.6	3.0
4 (Low)	2.3	3.7	3.9	4.7	7.0
P	.01	<.001	.001	.001	<.001

Adapted, with permission, from reference 16.

[a] Adjusted for age, ethnicity, smoking status, pack-years of cigarette smoking, and cholesterol intake (males only).

were examined as an indicator of lycopene intake and dark green vegetables as a reflection of lutein.

This analysis showed that these vegetable sources were equally as strong as beta-carotene in their inverse association with lung cancer risk and that all vegetables as a group had an even greater effect, especially in women (Table 9). This suggests that several different constituents of vegetables may protect against lung cancer. Furthermore, these constituents may include protective components other than carotenoids and mechanisms of action other than antioxidation (35).

Bladder Cancer

In a similar analysis of the dietary data from the bladder cancer case-control study, the findings were more specific. Of the vegetables, only the dark greens, prominent sources of lutein as well as beta-carotene, showed a significant inverse association—in men (Table 10). The analysis of these data for all carotenoids with vitamin A activity

Table 10. Vegetable Intake and Bladder Cancer Risk

Intake Quartile	Odds Ratio[a]			
	Carrots	Papaya	Tomatoes	Dark Greens
		Males		
1 (Low)	1.0	1.0	1.0	1.0
2	1.1	1.2	0.8	1.2
3	0.7	1.3	0.8	0.9
4 (High)	1.0	1.2	0.7	0.6
P	.78	.62	.27	.02
		Females		
1 (Low)	1.0	1.0	1.0	1.0
2	0.5	1.0	1.0	1.4
3	0.6	0.9	1.2	0.9
4 (High)	0.5	1.3	0.9	0.8
P	.24	.59	.70	.41

Adapted, with permission, from reference 23.

[a] Adjusted for age, ethnicity, and pack-years of cigarette smoking.

(Table 3) did not show a protective effect. Thus, the specificity with regard to dark green vegetables is likely to reflect a particular carotenoid (*e.g.*, lutein) or some other constituent(s) of dark green vegetables.

Prostate Cancer

Having found a direct association of the intake of beta-carotene and other carotenes with prostate cancer risk in older men, we were prompted to examine the particular food sources of carotenoids that accounted for this observation (38). The result was unexpected (Table 11). Only one of the important sources of beta-carotene in our population, papaya, showed a significant relationship to prostate cancer risk and accounted for the overall association. Other carotenoid sources, such as dark green vegetables and tomatoes, showed no effect on risk.

Because papaya presumably contributes little to the diet of the other populations in whom a similar positive association with beta-carotene was reported (28, 29), the constituent responsible for the

Table 11. Vegetable and Fruit Intake and Prostate Cancer Risk

Intake Quartile	Odds Ratio[a] Carrots	Papaya	Tomatoes	Dark Greens	All Vegetables
		Age ≥70 Years			
1 (Low)	1.0	1.0	1.0	1.0	1.0
2	1.1	1.4	1.0	1.2	1.1
3	1.0	1.9	1.1	1.4	0.9
4 (High)	0.9	2.5	1.1	1.3	1.2
P	.46	.0001	.57	.39	.58
		Age <70 Years			
1 (Low)	1.0	1.0	1.0	1.0	1.0
2	1.1	1.0	1.4	0.9	1.3
3	1.0	0.8	1.3	1.2	1.0
4 (High)	0.8	1.3	0.9	0.7	0.8
P	.20	.43	.35	.21	.11

Adapted, with permission, from reference 38.

[a] Adjusted for age and ethnicity.

effect, if real, must occur in other foods. It appears that these foods are likely to be fruits. In a study in Japan (39), although beta-carotene showed a protective effect, fruits as a food group were positively associated with risk. In addition to beta-carotene, papaya contains significant amounts of the carotenoid beta-cryptoxanthin (G. R. Beecher, unpublished data).

Thyroid Cancer

In an attempt to explain not only the diversity of rates of thyroid cancer in Hawaii's ethnic groups but also the high rates compared with those for other populations of the world (1), we conducted a case-control study based on cases identified on Oahu between 1980 and 1987. The analysis included 191 cases and 441 age- and sex-matched population controls (41).

No effect was found for retinol, vitamin C, beta-carotene, or other carotenoids as assessed from the diet. Although vegetable sources of beta-carotene, lycopene, and lutein, as examined in our other studies,

Table 12. Vegetable and Seafood Intake and Thyroid Cancer Risk

	Odds Ratio[a] (95% C.I.)	
Intake Quartile	Goitrogenic Vegetables	Seafood
	Males	
1 (Low)	1.0	1.0
2	1.7 (0.6–4.8)	1.6 (0.5–4.6)
3	1.4 (0.5–3.8)	1.2 (0.4–3.6)
4 (High)	1.0 (0.3–3.0)	2.2 (0.7–7.0)
P	.63	.23
	Females	
1 (Low)	1.0	1.0
2	0.9 (0.5–1.6)	1.4 (0.7–2.5)
3	0.7 (0.4–1.3)	1.0 (0.5–1.8)
4 (High)	0.6 (0.3–1.2)	1.2 (0.6–2.2)
P	.10	.86

Adapted, with permission, from reference 41.

[a] Adjusted for age and ethnicity.

also showed no effect, goitrogenic vegetables were inversely associated with risk in women (Table 12). Goitrogenic vegetables have considerable overlap with vegetables in the cruciferous group, which are sources of several nonnutritive constituents with inhibitory effects against cancer (35). The inverse effect was strongest for broccoli, which does contain lutein, beta-carotene, and other carotenoids, as well as ascorbic acid.

Impact on Population

As a result of these studies, evidence is accumulating that consumption of certain foods reduces the risk of cancer. Although there is support for beta-carotene in particular, especially with regard to lung cancer, a role of other carotenoids, and possibly other nutritive and nonnutritive constituents in fruits and vegetables, is gaining support. This provides a rationale for an emphasis in public health programs on increasing the mean intake of these foods in the population.

With this in mind, we examined the data from the second and more comprehensive of our lung cancer studies in order to estimate the potential impact of changes in consumption levels. We chose this cancer because the lung is the site for which the inverse association with carotenoids and selected foods is best established. For the analysis, we computed the attributable risk of lung cancer due to low intake of beta-carotene and of vegetables as a group. Although five ethnic groups were included in the study, the attributable risk calculations were limited to the Japanese and Caucasians because the number of subjects in the other groups was too small to yield reliable estimates. Because the results were similar for the Japanese and the Caucasians, the two groups were combined for this analysis.

Since the lung cancer study was population based, the assumption for these computations that the controls for the study were a representative sample of the general population is reasonable. Quartiles of intake were determined separately for each sex group, based on the intake of the controls. Initially, relative risks, adjusted for ethnicity, smoking, and age, were computed by logistic regression. Then the attributable risk, defined as the ratio of the excess number of cancer cases due to a particular factor to the total number of cancer cases, was calculated using the following formula (14):

$$AR = (R-1)p/\,(Rp+(1-p))$$

where AR = attributable risk, R = relative risk, and p = percentage of the population in the exposed group (since quartiles were used, p = 0.25 for each intake level).

Table 13 shows the results of these calculations. These data suggest that the incidence of lung cancer in these ethnic groups could be lowered by 20% to 40% on the basis of diet, independent of changes in smoking behavior. For example, in the men with beta-carotene consumption in the lowest quartile of intake (<1984 mcg/day), 29% of lung cancer occurrence can be attributed to their low intake level.

Although these are crude estimates, they suggest that the contribution of these components of the diet to the incidence of lung cancer (and possibly other types of cancer) may be substantial. Thus, public health programs that encourage increased consumption of vegetables and vitamins may have an important cancer prevention potential.

Table 13. Attributable Risk of Lung Cancer with Beta-Carotene and Vegetable Intake

Beta-Carotene		Vegetables	
Intake Quartile (mcg/d)	AR[a] (%)	Intake Quartile (g/d)	AR[a] (%)
	Males		
1 (>5680)	0.0	1 (>192.9)	0.0
2 (3720–5680)	20.3	2 (127.2–192.9)	25.0
3 (1984–3719)	38.4	3 (76.0–127.1)	31.2
4 (<1984)	29.4	4 (<76.0)	34.0
	Females		
1 (>6600)	0.0	1 (>202.8)	0.0
2 (4221–6600)	27.5	2 (129.2–202.8)	10.2
3 (2500–4220)	31.4	3 (77.7–129.1)	32.9
4 (<2500)	40.6	4 (<77.7)	47.4

[a] Attributable risk, adjusted for age, ethnicity, pack-years of cigarette smoking, and intake of vitamin C, folic acid, and cholesterol (males only).

REFERENCES

1. Muir C, Waterhouse J, Mack T, Powell J, Whelan S. Cancer incidence in five continents, V. 1987;*IARC Sci. Pub.* 1987 (No. 88).
2. Doll R, Peto R. The causes of cancer: quantitative estimates of avoidable risks of cancer in the United States today. *J Natl Cancer Inst.* 1981;66:1191–1308.
3. Kolonel LN. Variability in diet and its relation to risk in ethnic and migrant groups. In: *Phenotypic Variation in Populations: Relevance to Risk Assessment.* New York: Plenum Press; 1988:129–135.
4. Kolonel LN, Hinds MW, Hankin JH. Cancer patterns among migrant and native-born Japanese in Hawaii in relation to smoking, drinking and dietary habits. In: Gelboin HV, *et al.*, ed. *Genetics and Environmental Factors in Experimental and Human Cancer.* Tokyo: Japan Sci. Soc. Press; 1980:27–40.
5. Kolonel LN, Nomura AMY, Hirohata T, Hankin JH, Hinds MW. Association of diet and place of birth with stomach cancer incidence in Hawaii Japanese and Caucasians. *Am J Clin Nutr.* 1981; 34:2478–2485.
6. Kolonel LN, Hankin JH, Nomura AMY, Hinds MW. Studies of

nutrients and their relationship to cancer in the multiethnic population of Hawaii. In: Poirier LA, Newberne P, Pariza M, eds. *The Role of Essential Nutrients in Carcinogenesis.* New York: Plenum Press: 1987;206:35–43.

7. Kolonel LN. Smoking and drinking patterns among five ethnic groups in Hawaii. In: Second Symposium on Epidemiology and Cancer Registries in the Pacific Basin, Maui, January 1978. *Natl Cancer Inst Monogr.* 1979;53:81–87.
8. Wynder EL, Kajitani T, Ishikawa S, Dodo H, Takano A. Environmental factors of cancer of the colon and rectum, II: Japanese epidemiological data. *Cancer.* 1969;23(5):1210–1220.
9. Graham S, Schotz M, Martino P. Alimentary factors in the epidemiology of gastric cancer. *Cancer.* 1972;30:927–938.
10. Haenszel W, Kurihara NM, Segi M, Lee R.K.C. Stomach cancer among Japanese in Hawaii. *J Natl Cancer Inst.* 1972;49:969–988.
11. Bjelke E. Dietary vitamin A and human lung cancer. *Int J. Cancer.* 1975;15:561–566.
12. Oyama N, Johnson DB. *Hawaii Health Surveillance Program: Survey Methods and Procedures.* Honolulu: Hawaii State Dept of Health; 1986. Research and Statistics Report No. 54.
13. Hankin JH. Twenty-third Lenna Frances Cooper Memorial Lecture: a diet history method for research, clinical and community use. *J Am Diet Assoc.* 1986;86:868–875.
14. Breslow NE, Day NE. Statistical methods for cancer epidemiology, 1: the analysis of case-control studies. *IARC Sci. Pub.* 1980 (No. 32).
15. Hinds MW, Kolonel LN, Hankin JH, Lee J. Dietary vitamin A, carotene, vitamin C and risk of lung cancer in Hawaii. *AM J Epidemiol.* 1984;119:227–237.
16. Le Marchand L, Yoshizawa CN, Kolonel LN, Hankin JH, Goodman MT. Vegetable consumption and lung cancer risk: a population-based case-control study in Hawaii. *J Natl Cancer Inst.* 1989; 81:1158–1164.
17. Goodman MT, Kolonel LN, Yoshizawa CN, Hankin JH. The effect of dietary cholesterol and fat on the risk of lung cancer in Hawaii. *Am J Epidemiol.* 1988;128:1241–1255.
18. Bertram JS, Kolonel LN, Meyskens FL, Jr. Rationale and strategies for chemoprevention of cancer in humans. *Cancer Res.* 1987; 47:3012–3031.

19. Willett WC. Vitamin A and lung cancer. *Nutr Rev.* 1990;48:201–211.
20. Peleg I, Heyden S, Knowles M, Hames CG. Serum retinol and risk of subsequent cancer: extension of the Evans County, Georgia, study. *J Natl Cancer Inst.* 1984;73:1455–1458.
21. Menkes MS, Comstock GW, Vuilleumier JP, Helsing KJ, Rider AA, Brookmeyer R. Serum beta-carotene, vitamins A and E, selenium, and the risk of lung cancer. *N Engl J Med.* 1986;315:1250–1254.
22. Nomura AM, Stemmermann GN, Heilbrun LK, Salkeld RM, Vuilleumier JP. Serum vitamin levels and the risk of cancer of specific sites in men of Japanese ancestry in Hawaii. *Cancer Res.* 1985; 45:2369–2372.
23. Nomura AMY, Kolonel LN, Hankin JH, Yoshizawa CN. Dietary factors in cancer of the lower urinary tract. *Int J Cancer.* 1991; 48:199–205.
24. Committee on Diet and Health. *Diet and Health.* Washington, DC: National Academy Press;1989.
25. Kolonel LN, Yoshizawa CN, Hankin JH. Diet and prostate cancer: a case-control study in Hawaii. *Am J Epidemiol.* 1988;127:999–1012.
26. Kolonel LN, Hankin JH, Yoshizawa CN. Vitamin A and prostate cancer in elderly men: enhancement of risk. *Cancer Res.* 1987; 47:2982–2985.
27. Welsch CW, Goodrich-Smith M, Brown CK, Crowe N. Enhancement by retinyl acetate of hormone-induced mammary tumorigenesis in female GR/A mice. *J Natl Cancer Inst.* 1981;67:935–938.
28. Graham S, Haughey B, Marshall J, *et al.* Diet in the epidemiology of carcinoma of the prostate. *J Natl Cancer Inst.* 1983;70:687–692.
29. Heshmat MY, Kaul L, Kovi J, *et al.* Nutrition and prostate cancer: a case-control study. *Prostate.* 1985;6:7–17.
30. Titus-Ernstoff L, Ernstoff MS, Duray PH, Barnhill RL, Holubkov R, Kirkwood JM. A relation between childhood sun exposure and dysplastic nevus syndrome among patients with nonfamilial melanoma. *Epidemiol.* 1991;2:210–214.
31. Le Marchand L. Dietary factors in the etiology of malignant melanoma. *Clin Dermatol.* In press.
32. Kolonel LN, Le Marchand L. The Epidemiology of Colon Cancer and Dietary Fat. In: Ip C, Rogers A, Birt D, Mettlin C, eds. *Progress in Clinical and Biological Research;* vol. 222: *Fat and Cancer.* New York: Alan R. Liss, Inc; 1986:69–91.
33. Phillips RL. Role of life-style and dietary habits in risk of cancer

among Seventh-Day Adventists. *Cancer Res.* 1975;35:3513–3522.

34. MacLennan R, Da Costa J, Day NE, Law CH, Ng YK, Shanmugaratnam K. Risk factors for lung cancer in Singapore Chinese, a population with high female incidence rates. *Int J Cancer.* 1977;20: 854–860.
35. Wattenberg LW. Inhibitors of chemical carcinogenesis. *Adv Cancer Res.* 1978;26:197–226.
36. Matthews-Roth MM, Krinsky NI. Effect of dietary fat level on UV-B induced skin tumors, and anti-tumor action of beta-carotene. *Photochem Photobiol.* 1984;40:671–673.
37. Beecher GR, Matthews RH. Nutrient composition of foods. In: Brown ML, ed. *Present Knowledge in Nutrition.* 6th ed. Washington, DC: International Life Sciences Institute, Nutrition Foundation; 1990:430–443.
38. Le Marchand L, Hankin JH, Kolonel LN, Wilkens LR. Vegetable and fruit consumption in relation to prostate cancer risk in Hawaii: a reevaluation of the effect of dietary beta-carotene. *Am J Epidemiol.* 1991;133:215–219.
39. Ohno Y, Yoshida O, Oishi K, Okada K, Yamabe H, Schroeder FH. Dietary beta-carotene and cancer of the prostate: a case-control study in Kyoto, Japan. *Cancer Res.* 1988;48:1331–1336.
40. Kolonel LN, Hankin JH, Wilkens, LR, Fukunaga FH, Hinds MW. An epidemiologic study of thyroid cancer in Hawaii. *Cancer Causes and Control.* 1990;1:223–234.

T. COLIN CAMPBELL, JUNSHI CHEN, BANOO PARPIA, and MING LI

Diets and Cancer Mortality Rates in Sixty-Five Counties in the People's Republic of China

ABSTRACT

We conducted a survey of dietary and other life-style characteristics of 130 villages located in 65 mostly rural counties in the People's Republic of China in 1983–1984 to investigate the chief correlates of disease mortality recorded earlier in 1973–1975. Fifty adults, half from each sex and 35 to 64 years of age, were included in each village. A total of 366 items of information eventually was collected, based on analyses of blood, urine, and food samples, a three-day household survey of food intakes, and completion of a questionnaire.

As reported in more depth elsewhere, vitamin status was recorded directly as the intakes of vitamin A, total carotenoids, thiamine, riboflavin, niacin, and vitamin C; by plasma activities of alpha- and beta-carotene, alpha- and gamma-tocopherol, retinol, retinol binding protein, and vitamin C; erythrocyte glutathione reductase (riboflavin); and urine excretion of and excess load of vitamin C and riboflavin. Plasma vitamin C was most consistently, and inversely, correlated with male cancer mortality rates, being statistically significant for esophageal cancer ($P < 0.001$), total aggregate cancers ($P < 0.001$), stomach cancer ($P < 0.01$), liver cancer ($P < 0.05$), and lung cancer ($P < 0.05$); although in the same direction, correlations of plasma vitamin C with female rates were not significant. Plasma beta-carotene also was quite consistent in the inverse direction for both sexes but was generally not statistically significant. Plasma retinol and tocopherol levels were not related to cancer mortality rates, both being influenced by blood lipid levels. Comparisons of Chinese vitamin status with Western-subject vitamin status revealed significant differences reflecting the much higher intake of plant foods in China. The implications of these findings are discussed in reference to the concept of chemoprevention as a means of cancer control.

In 1983 we conducted a comprehensive survey of dietary and other life-style characteristics on 6500 adults, one-half from each sex, 35 to 64 years of age, residing in 130 villages in 65 mostly rural counties in the People's Republic of China (1). The variables recorded in this survey then were compared with the widely varying rates of mortality for about four dozen different diseases, including about a dozen different cancers, recorded for the years 1973–1975 (2). Cancer of each organ site is highly localized geographically in China, as illustrated by the wide ranges of mortality rates for selected cancers in Table 1.

Included in the 1983 dietary/life-style survey were a number of indicators of vitamin status, which are summarized in Table 2. These indicators were obtained from analyses of blood, urine and food samples, individual questionnaire responses, and calculation of nutrient intakes from a three-day dietary survey of households. Further details on study design and other experimental procedures are available in the monograph of data published by Chen *et al.* (1).

Before reporting on the preliminary findings on vitamin intakes and cancer etiologies from this study, we will outline the framework within which we chose to interpret these data. These views are based

Table 1. Selected County-Level Cancer Mortality Rates in China[a]

Cancer	Sex	Mean	Minimum	Maximum
Esophageal	Male	31	<1	153
	Female	16	<1	100
Stomach	Male	31	2	133
	Female	14	<1	50
Liver	Male	24	2	96
	Female	8	1	23
Colorectal	Male	4	<1	24
	Female	3	<1	22
Lung	Male	7	<1	21
	Female	3	<1	9
Breast	Female	3	<1	9
Cervical	Female	10	1	34

From Chen *et al.* (1), by permission of Cornell University Press and Oxford University Press, and Li *et al.* (2).

[a]Cumulative sex- and rate-specific mortality rates per 1000 for ages 0–64 years.

Table 2. Variables Influencing Vitamin Status in the Survey of Chen *et al.*

Plasma factors
Alpha-carotene
Beta-carotene
Alpha-tocopherol
Gamma-tocopherol
Retinol
Vitamin C
Retinol bonding protein
Erythrocytes
Glutathione reductase (riboflavin)
Urine factors[a]
Vitamin C
Riboflavin
Nutrient Intakes[b]
Retinol
Total carotenoid
Thiamine
Niacin
Vitamin C
Questionnaire Responses
Frequencies of food intake[c]

[a]Excess excreted within 4 hours after administration of 500 mg of riboflavin or 5 mg of vitamin C.
[b]Mean intake of "reference man" (65 kg adult male doing light physical work), obtained from 3-day dietary survey (direct measurement) in each of 30 households per county.
[c]Frequency of consumption of major foods over the year was recorded as recalled by respondent to provide inferences on vitamin intake.

on the question of whether the cancer-modifying effects of individual nutrients should be considered within the context of the entire diet or in respect to individual nutrient supplements.

Among the many dietary factors reported to be involved in cancer development, several vitamins have been identified, including riboflavin, the retinoid/carotenoid group (vitamin A), the tocopherol group (vitamin E), and ascorbic acid (vitamin C), several of which are considered in this volume. These findings have generated considerable interest in the possible use of these micronutrients as food supplements to prevent cancer occurrence (3, 4), a concept generally referred to as chemoprevention. Interest in this concept was the original basis for the many studies that have been undertaken, particularly under the direction and/or funding of the National Cancer Institute (5), the American Cancer Society, and other agencies, to test in human intervention trials the ability of natural and synthetic vitamin analogues to prevent or reverse the development of various putatively preneoplastic lesions (3, 4). This relationship of micronutrient status and degenerative disease etiology has been the subject of numerous symposia and conferences, with one of the more recent and informative being held in 1989 in London (6).

The rationale for using nutrient supplements as a means of cancer control chiefly arises from the proposition that proscription of dietary change, that is, telling consumers what not to eat, is likely to be unaccepted by the consuming public. Thus, only modest dietary changes have been recommended (*e.g.*, reduce mean dietary fat intake to 30% or less of total calories and increase mean dietary fiber intake to 20–30 g/day), along with the hope that prescription of nutrient supplements and uniquely designed foods will be able to achieve what this modest dietary change cannot. However, although modest dietary change and prescription of nutrient supplements as means of cancer control receive most of the serious attention in public and investigative research communities, proscription of major dietary change should not be ignored.

Both empirical and theoretical considerations can be cited to question the reliability of using a public health strategy of chemoprevention as a primary means of cancer control. Virtually all empirical evidence implicating a role for vitamins and other micronutrients obtained in human studies suggests a comprehensive effect of entire diets, not of individual nutrient supplements. In fact, this conclusion was highlighted in the executive summary of the seminal 1982 report on diet, nutrition, and cancer by an expert committee of the National Academy of Sciences (NAS) (7) after reviewing the then-available literature. The recommendation of this committee to increase the consumption of vegetables, fruits, and whole cereal grains applied "only to foods as sources of nutrients—not to dietary supplements of individual nutrients." Thereafter, administrative court proceedings were undertaken by the United States Federal Trade Commission (8), with advice from the NAS, to bar the marketplace from making claims for cancer prevention by such nutrient supplements. It would appear that little, if any, new information has emerged to alter this view. For example, a perusal of the more recent reports on antioxidant vitamin status and cancer etiology presented at the 1989 London conference (6) generally affirms the findings of the 1982 NAS Diet, Nutrition and Cancer Committee (7). Thus, there appears to be distressingly little evidence to date to support the concept that chemoprevention should or could be a preferred strategy for cancer control by nutritional means, especially when compared with a strategy that forthrightly presents information showing the effects of the entire diet.

Even if individual nutrients are shown to alter tumor development in experimental animals—and indeed this has been the case—several almost insurmountable theoretical questions remain concerning the applicability of these findings to humans. For example, dose-response relationships for individual chemicals often are known to be vastly different between species, and when these differences are coupled with the virtually endless number and variety of interactions occurring between individual nutrients and other food constituents among free-living populations, the quantitative extrapolation of narrowly constrained experimental animal data to human use becomes severely limited.

Human intervention trials of individual nutrients do little to allay these concerns about the difficulty of extrapolating experimental animal data to human use. Favorable results obtained in these trials, if not resulting from chance alone, still must be constrained in their application to free-living populations by the experimental conditions used. A single nutrient shown to produce what appears to be a desirable effect of reducing the progression of a particular precursor preneoplastic lesion does virtually nothing to alter the underlying cause of the progression by the comprehensive effects of the entire diet. This scenario is analogous to a clinical trial that, for example, shows that beta-carotene reduces the progression of a preneoplastic precursor lesion in the lung among heavy smokers. Therefore, would it be appropriate to draw the conclusion that smoking might be continued if a beta-carotene tablet is also consumed? In arriving at the answer to this question, is it first necessary to question whether this tablet also would alleviate adverse effects in tissues other than the lung? If these are appropriate questions in the case of beta-carotene and tobacco use, then they should be even more apropos in the case of diets enriched in foods that yield, for example, high levels of fat, low levels of dietary fiber, and low levels of antioxidant nutrients. That is, the long-term consumption of such a diet conceivably exerts a much more comprehensive effect upon the body's myriad biochemical, physiological, and metabolic systems than does smoking. Therefore, if efficacy of nutrient supplements for free-living humans cannot be concluded, claims of health benefit become illusory, thereby diverting attention from alternative and possibly more effective means of cancer control, such as with the use of the comprehensive effects of the entire diet.

We believe that a strategy coupling only modest dietary changes with the use of nutrient supplements to reduce cancer risk suffers serious faults as a public health option—both empirically and theoretically. First, as already mentioned, present empirical evidence is not supportive of this approach. That the 1982 NAS report and two major 1989 reports—the NAS Diet and Health Report (9) and that of the London conference (6)—all have failed to demonstrate convincing evidence in human studies of the ability of antioxidant micronutrient supplements to prevent cancer (not precursor lesions), in spite of the huge effort expended during the seven years between the reports, makes us skeptical of the reasonableness of this approach. Admittedly, a casual reading of the vast literature on antioxidant micronutrients and disease etiology suggests that substantial evidence does exist for a chemopreventive effect of vitamin supplements on cancer development. However, a closer inspection of this literature reveals that many authors rather carelessly refer in their texts, perhaps even in their titles, to the singular effects of individual vitamins upon cancer etiology in their studies, often even discussing possible mechanisms of action, when in fact their experimental observations included only estimated intakes of foods and calculated intakes of nutrients, not the intakes of nutrient supplements. Often it is as if writers are overanxious to conclude positive effects for nutrient supplements.

On theoretical grounds, the incomprehensively dynamic biological interface between food input and disease outcome is far more complex than generally assumed by the prescription or chemoprevention strategy that oversimplifies biological and nutritional reality. It is puzzling to ponder, for example, the future form of a public health strategy of chemoprevention that undoubtedly will be able to draw upon a virtually unlimited variety of potentially active compounds. Already there are more than a thousand empirically documented compounds known to "chemoprevent" cancer under experimental conditions (4), and surely this list is a mere sampling of possible chemopreventive compounds present in foods. And this list includes only a few of the more than six hundred carotenoids, just to name one class of food constituents (10). Digressing for a moment, let us note that virtually all of these carotenoids surely are capable of inhibiting to varying degrees the development of one or more experimental tumors. For example, we have evidence that beta-carotene, though the most ubiquitous carotenoid, is not the most active chemopreventive analogue of this group of compounds (11, 12).

There are many substantial questions that cannot be ignored in research efforts used to justify chemoprevention as a means of cancer control. Which one (or group) of the seemingly unlimited number of chemopreventive compounds will be chosen—and regulated—for consumer use? And what will be the dosage levels to be recommended for the average citizen? Will these recommendations be for all individuals or just for selected people? Will there be a recommended upper limit of intake, and if so, how will limits be monitored or controlled? (Upper limits of intake are of particular concern for the more toxic fat-soluble "vitamins."*) This latter question is potentially serious, since some individuals who perceive a high risk of cancer may overdose. Will higher than normal levels of intake sustained over a long period of time alter the body's natural abilities to absorb, metabolize, and distribute normal intakes of these substances? For example, once the body becomes physiologically adapted to higher-than-normal levels of intake of a particular nutrient supplement, would sudden withdrawal precipitate a disease outcome opposite from that which is desired?

We find the emphasis given to chemoprevention as a primary means of cancer control, especially in the absence of forthright information on the benefits of changing the entire diet, to be consistent with the philosophy of Western medicine that emphasizes curative rather than preventive practices and that is based on the proposition that disease prevalence is best controlled through the use of "magic

*According to classical definition, a vitamin is an essential nutrient; thus "vitamins" A and D are not vitamins.

bullet" interventions such as routine pharmaceuticals, surgery, and tissue-targeted cytoxic agents. Unfortunately, the more comprehensive effects of broadly based dietary habits upon disease occurrence too often are acknowledged and promoted only rather begrudgingly by primary health care workers. A strategy that promotes the use of a broadly based diet, particularly a diet constituted mostly or entirely of a variety of good-quality plant foods, would allow the intakes of nutrients and other constituents involved in degenerative disease inhibition to be well within ranges commonly found in nature, where unfavorable toxicities, interactions, and time-dependent adaptations to individual nutrients are controlled homeostatically. It is the more comprehensive effect of total diets and broad food groups, rather than the isolated contributions of individual nutrients or even individual foods, that is likely to exert the broadest range of disease interventions. In the final analysis, the goal of an ideal public health policy on cancer control by dietary means should be to prevent the largest proportion of all cancers for the largest number of people while minimizing undesirable toxicities and unsuspected increases in other chronic degenerative diseases.

Thus, we believe that the following brief summary of our findings on vitamin status and cancer etiology in our cross-sectional study in China (1) should be regarded primarily as an indication of the broader effects of dietary habits upon cancer mortality rates, not the effects of single nutrients. Vitamin status among the Chinese when compared with comparable Western subjects is shown in Table 3. Some of these comparisons indicate that tissue levels and activities for these vitamins are determined by more than vitamin intake levels alone. For example, mean total carotenoid intake among the Chinese is double that of Westerners, yet plasma levels are somewhat lower. Similarly, mean vitamin C intake among the Chinese is twice that of Westerners, but plasma levels are comparable.

The intake of retinol, only found in animal foods, is far higher among Westerners, but circulating plasma levels essentially are identical. Homeostatic control appears to be exceedingly impressive considering the exceptionally wide range of intakes. On the question of riboflavin (1, 13), mean intake is about 2.5 times higher among Westerners, undoubtedly owing to the very high consumption of riboflavin-rich dairy products (14). Similarly in China, riboflavin intake was highly dependent on dairy food consumption as measured in the

Table 3. Comparison of Vitamin Status Among Chinese and Western Subjects

Vitamin Indicator	Range of Chinese Village Means	Range of Western Individuals' Means
Plasma beta-carotene (μg/dL)	2.3–32.2	2.5–69.0
Plasma alpha-tocopherol (μg/dL)	460–1040	500–2000
Plasma retinol (μg/dL)	25–68	30–65
Plasma vitamin C (mg/dL)	0.3–3.2	0.6–2.0
Plasma retinol binding protein (mg/dL)	1.9–4.4	4.0–5.0
Erythrocyte EGR (activity coefficient)	1.07–1.82	0.87–1.21
Dietary retinol (RE/d)	0–280[a] (mean = 27.8)	990
Dietary total carotenoid (mg/d)	0–3000 (mean = 836)	429
Dietary riboflavin (mg/d)	0.4–2.7 (mean = 0.8)	0.7–4.7 (mean = 1.9)
Dietary vitamin C (mg/d)	6–429 (mean = 140)	7–315 (mean = 73)

From Chen *et al.* (1), by permission of Cornell University Press and Oxford University Press. See (1) for further details on characteristics of Western subjects.

[a] Excludes one ethnic minority county of mostly herdspeople of 1550 RE/d.

three-day dietary survey ($r = 0.81$, $P < 0.001$), although this survey involved only a few northern counties of nomadic herdspeople where dairy foods are consumed (1). Erythrocyte glutathione reductase activity, a biomarker of riboflavin status, was associated with riboflavin intake ($P < 0.01$).

Within the data set, several indicators suggest that greater intakes of foods rich in antioxidant micronutrients are protective against cancer mortality rates. A summary of these observations, with the detailed analysis to be published elsewhere, is as follows.

Relationships between vitamin status indicators and cancer mortality rates first were explored by comparison of univariate correlation coefficients (Table 4). Plasma ascorbic acid levels were most consistently protective, exhibiting statistically significant inverse associations for several cancers among males, with the strongest and most

Table 4. Univariate Correlation Coefficients for Plasma Levels of Vitamin Status Indicators and Various Cancer Mortality Rates

Mortality Rate	Sex	Vitamin C	Beta-Carotene	Alpha-Tocopherol	Retinol
Esophagus	M	−.45[a]	−.14	.22	−.12
	F	−.18	−.11	−.02	.03
Stomach	M	−.27[b]	−.24	.11	−.21
	F	−.06	−.20	.15	.02
Liver	M	−.28[c]	.04	.23	−.15
	F	−.02	−.08	.05	−.17
Colorectal	M	−.16	−.04	.26[c]	.10
	F	.01	−.17	.09	−.07
Lung	M	−.29[c]	−.03	.09	−.11
	F	−.12	.04	.11	−.01
Breast	F	−.22	−.09	.24	.15
Cervix	F	−.16	−.11	.15	.01
All Cancers	M	−.43[a]	−.12	.25[c]	−.07
	F	−.14	−.12	.09	.02

From Chen *et al.* (1), by permission of Cornell University Press and Oxford University Press.

[a] $2P < 0.001$.
[b] $2P < 0.01$.
[c] $2P < 0.05$.

significant correlations being those for total cancer ($P < 0.001$) and esophageal cancer ($P < 0.001$). Although inverse associations also were found for seven of the eight mortality rates for females, none was statistically significant.

Most associations for beta-carotene also were inverse, though none was statistically significant. Plasma alpha-tocopherol exhibited a tendency to be positively correlated with cancer mortality rates. This is undoubtedly due to the influence of blood lipid levels upon circulating levels of alpha-tocopherol that were correlated, for example, with plasma total cholesterol ($P < 0.01$), apolipoprotein A1 ($P < 0.001$), and triglyceride ($P < 0.05$) (1). Beta-carotene also had a tendency to be positively correlated with various plasma cholesterol fractions, though none was significant.

We used multiple regression analysis to investigate the relative importance of each variable adjusting for potential confounding factors for each cancer site. This analysis confirmed the impressions gained from examination of the univariate correlations noted above. Antioxidant factors including vitamin C and beta-carotene were most significant for cancers of the esophagus and stomach for both sexes. After adjustment for other variables in the model (*e.g.*, plasma levels of total cholesterol, beta-carotene, and selenium), plasma vitamin C exhibited the strongest associations, being significant for cancers of the esophagus, liver, and lung in males; no significant associations were observed for females. Similarly, a significant independent effect for beta-carotene only was observed for stomach cancer in both sexes. Plasma selenium was inversely associated with cancers of the esophagus and stomach in both sexes. The joint effects of these variables, that is, plasma total cholesterol, vitamin C, beta-carotene, and selenium, plus specific factors for each cancer, account for a relatively large proportion of the variation in the cancer mortality rates, ranging from 29% to 37% for cancers of the esophagus, stomach, and colorectum for males. For females the antioxidant factors, excepting the effect of plasma beta-carotene upon stomach cancer, did not contribute significantly to the explanatory power of the model; specific factors accounted for most of the variation in these cancer mortality rates.

Although riboflavin status is beyond the scope of this paper, our findings (13) on this vitamin may illustrate an issue often overlooked in investigations of this kind. A few years ago it was hypothesized that riboflavin deficiency is associated with the prevalence of esophageal cancer (16, 17, 18), and on this basis, intervention trials were mounted to investigate the ability of a riboflavin supplement, along with other nutrients, to inhibit esophagitis (18, 19, 20), a putative precursor lesion of esophageal cancer. Similar to the impressions of other investigators of riboflavin status in China (17, 21), we observed that as many as 90% of individuals might be deficient in riboflavin, thus superficially supporting the hypothesis that the high rate of esophageal cancer in China is partially attributable to a deficiency in this vitamin. Given the strength of our data showing a widespread deficiency and given the odd fact that riboflavin sufficiency is generally related to foods that mostly enhance rather than reduce cancer risk, we undertook a more careful review of the previous literature said to support the currently recommended levels of riboflavin intake. These levels, if inappropriately high, would lead to the false impression of widespread deficiency. Our literature analysis suggested that these recommendations very likely were set much too high, thus substantially reducing the alleged deficiency of this vitamin in China. Investigation of a particular vitamin deficiency therefore must take full account of the basis for the presumed deficiency. If riboflavin intakes in China are not deficient, then riboflavin supplementation perhaps would not affect cancer or its precursor lesions, an observation that has been borne out in intervention trials in China (20).

Our final observation concerns the data on the type of diet likely to yield maximum prevention of cancer development. We have begun analysis of this question. One of the more significant observations from our studies is that the range of plasma cholesterol in China is very low by Western standards, being only about 100–190 mg/dL (range of village means). Moreover, the principal dietary correlates of plasma cholesterol in China generally are similar to those observed for Western subjects, that is, increased meat ($P < 0.05$), animal protein ($P = 0.06$), and fat intake ($P < 0.05$), and decreased intake of dietary complex carbohydrates (approximately 0.10 to < 0.01 for various fiber fractions). Such a dietary relationship is quite remarkable since these dietary factors are, by Western standards, already hypocholesterolemic (with averages of fat intake at 14.5% of calories, dietary fiber at 33 g per day, and animal protein [mammalian and avian] at 7% of total protein [compared with 70% in the United States]). Thus, within this range of dietary and metabolic experience in China, one easily could surmise that diseases common in the West should be relatively sparse. However, interpretations of these data have shown that breast cancer, after adjustment for known risk factors, is positively associated ($P \sim 0.05$) with fat intake (range is 6% to 24% of calories) (22), colon and rectal cancers are positively associated with low dietary fiber intake ($P \sim 0.05$) (23), and of most interest, aggregate rates of degenerative diseases (cancers, heart diseases, diabetes) ($P < 0.01$) (24) are positively associated with plasma cholesterol ($P < 0.01$).

Thus, it would appear that diets containing even small amounts of foods that elevate fat levels much above about 10% of calories and reduce fiber intakes much below 50 to 60 g per day are associated with an increased prevalence of these diseases. In this analysis, we cannot rule out the possibility that the life-style conditions associated with industrialization and urbanization help account for the significant increases in the mortality rates for these diseases, because it is within such settings that diets usually become richer in foods tending to encourage these diseases.

ACKNOWLEDGMENTS

This paper was supported in part by National Institutes of Health grant 5RO1CA33638, the Chinese Academy of Preventive Medicine, the United Kingdom Imperial Cancer Research Fund, the United States Food and Drug Administration, the American Institute for Cancer Research, and several American industry groups, notably Shell Oil Company, Mobil Oil Company, Hoffman-LaRoche, and CPC International.

REFERENCES

1. Chen J, Campbell TC, Li J, Peto R, eds. *Diet, Life-style and Mortality in China: A Study of the Characteristics of 65 Chinese Counties.* New York: Cornell University Press; 1990.
2. Li J-Y, Liu B-Q, Li G-Y, Chen Z-J, Sun X-D, Rong S-D. Atlas of cancer mortality in the People's Republic of China: an aid for cancer control and research. *Int J Epidemiol.* 1981;10:127–133.
3. Bertram J, Kolonel LN, Meyskens FL Jr. Rationale and strategies for chemoprevention of cancer in humans. *Cancer Res.* 1987;47: 3012–3031.
4. Malone WF, Kelloff GJ, Boone C, Nixon DW. Chemoprevention and modern cancer prevention. *Prev Med.* 1989;18:553–561.
5. Greenwald P. Manipulation of nutrients to prevent cancer. *Hosp Pract.* 1984;19:119–134, 124–126, 131–134.
6. Slater TF, Block G. Antioxidant vitamins and β-carotene in disease prevention: proceedings of a conference held in London, UK. *Am J Clin Nutr.* 1989;53:189S–396S.
7. National Research Council. *Diet, Nutrition and Cancer.* Washington, DC: National Academy Press; 1982.
8. FTC judge sets one human trial as standard for supplement claims. *Abbrev.* 46–49.
9. National Research Council. *Diet and Health: Implications for Reducing Chronic Disease Risk.* Washington, DC: National Academy Press; 1989.

10. Bendich A, Olson JA. Biological actions of carotenoids. *FASEB J.* 1989;3:1927–1932.
11. He Y. *Effects of Carotenoids and Dietary Carotenoid Extracts on Aflatoxin B_1-Induced Mutagenesis and Hepatocarcinogenesis.* Ithaca, NY: Cornell University; 1990. PhD dissertation.
12. He Y, Campbell TC. Effects of carotenoids on aflatoxin B_1-induced mutagenesis in *S. typhimurium* TA 100 and TA 98. *Nutr Cancer.* 1990;13:243–253.
13. Campbell TC, Brun T, Chen J, Feng Z, Parpia B. Questioning riboflavin recommendations on the basis of a survey in China. *Am J Clin Nutr.* 1990;51:436–445.
14. Adams CF. *Nutritive Value of American Foods, in Common Units.* Washington, DC: US Department of Agriculture; 1975.
15. Chen J, Geisler C, Pampla B, Li J, Campbell TC. Antioxidant-status and cancer mortality in China. *Int J Epidemiol.* 1992;21. In press.
16. Yang CS, Miao J, Yang W, *et al.* Diet and vitamin nutrition of the high esophageal cancer risk population in Linxian, China. *Nutr Cancer.* 1982;4:154–164.
17. Ershow AG, Zheng SF, Li G, Li J, Yang CS, Blot WJ. Compliance and nutritional status during feasibility study for an intervention trial in China. *J Natl Cancer Inst.* 1984;73:1477–1481.
18. Munoz N, Hayashi M, Lu JB, Wahrendorf J, Crespi M, Bosch F. Effect of riboflavin, retinol and zinc on micronuclei of buccal mucosa and of esophagus: a randomized double-blind intervention study in China. *J Natl Cancer Inst.* 1987;79:687–691.
19. Zheng S, Ershow AG, Yang CS, *et al.* Nutritional status in Linxian, China: effects of season and supplementation. *Int J Vitam Nutr Res.* 1989;59:190–199.
20. Munoz N, Wahrendorf J, Lu LB, *et al.* No effect of riboflavin, retinol and zinc on prevalence of precancerous lesions of oesophagus: randomized double-blind intervention study in high-risk population of China. *Lancet.* July 20, 1985;2(ii):111–114.
21. Yang CS, Sun Y, Yang Q. Vitamin A and other deficiencies in Linxian, a high esophageal cancer incidence area in northern China. *J Natl Cancer Inst.* 1984;73:1449–1453.
22. Marshall JR, Qu Y, Chen J, Parpia B, Campbell TC. Additional ecologic evidence: lipids and breast cancer mortality among women age 55 and over in China. *Eur J Cancer.* 1991. In press.

23. Campbell TC, Wang G, Chen J, Robertson J, Chao Z, Parpia B. Dietary fiber intake and colon cancer mortality in The People's Republic of China. In: Kritchevsky D, Bonfield C, Anderson JW, eds. *Dietary Fiber.* New York, NY: Plenum Publishing Corporation; 1990:473–480.
24. Campbell TC, Chen J, Brun T, *et al.* China: from diseases of poverty to diseases of affluence: policy implications of the epidemiological transition. *Ecol Food Nutr.* 1991. In press.

PART III

The Use of Vitamins in Precancerous Lesions

DONNA H. RYAN and BARRY STARR

Vitamins as Chemotherapeutic and Chemopreventive Agents

ABSTRACT

Therapy with retinoids has produced objective responses in patients with some types of skin cancer, and tretinoin is effective in producing terminal differentiation and complete remission in acute promyelocytic leukemia. Cancer chemoprevention trials are under way evaluating the activity of multiple vitamin preparations, beta-carotene, retinoids, vitamin C, vitamin E, vitamin B_{12}, vitamin B_6, and folate. Since carcinogenesis is a multistage process that can occur over decades in humans, efficient evaluation of chemopreventive agents requires research strategies utilizing intermediate biologic end points. Preneoplasia, classically defined histologic cellular change, is being redefined by advances in molecular and cell biology. Vitamins have been exploited as unproven remedies to vulnerable cancer patients, but now vitamins and their derivations have an emerging role in cancer chemotherapy and chemoprevention.

Introduction

Of the nearly thirty chemoprevention trials currently under way with National Cancer Institute sponsorship, over half employ vitamins or vitamin derivatives. The first cancer chemoprevention trial, begun in 1981, employs beta-carotene or a placebo in 22 071 male physicians and evaluates cancer development at all sites. Although we are over ten years into that study, it is still too early to draw conclusions. Carcinogenesis is a multistep process and can occur over decades. Chemopreventives can be evaluated on a faster track when the target population has already developed histologic change that predictably leads to cancer. In this volume five papers discuss vitamin chemoprevention in patients with preneoplasia.

Genetic change can continue to occur within cells classified as cancer cells. Genomic instability of malignant cells results in progressive abnormalities of chromosome structure and number and gene expression, and worsening clinical prognosis. Since the changes from preneoplasia to frank neoplasia to further altered neoplastic cells are a continuum, a review of the published clinical evidence of chemopreventive and chemotherapeutic activity of vitamins seems in order.

No discussion of vitamins and cancer is complete without a mention of the unfortunate exploitation of vitamins as cures for cancer. In a famous instance of quackery, laetrile and pangamic acid were promoted as "vitamins" B_{17} and B_{15} (1). These toxic and ineffective compounds are not, and have never been, considered vitamins. "Mega-vitamin therapy" (massive doses of vitamins) and "metabolic therapy" (a combination of vitamins, enemas, and diet) are two currently fashionable, unproven cancer remedies (2). Vitamin C has also been the center of a controversy in cancer treatment. Touted by Linus Pauling, a Nobel prize–winning chemist, as a cure-all (3), the use of vitamin C in patients with terminal cancer has been shown to be ineffective cancer therapy (4).

The Vitamin A Family

Most of the existing clinical data supporting chemotherapeutic or chemopreventive activity of vitamins centers on evaluation of the 2000 natural and synthetic chemical compounds that constitute the vitamin A family. Beta-carotene is a precursor of vitamin A; its analogues are called carotenoids. Retinol analogues and derivatives are called retinoids. The first-generation derivatives of retinol, tretinoin (transretinoic acid) and isotretinoin (13-*cis*-retinoic acid), were developed as acne remedies. The second-generation etretinate was developed as a treatment for psoriasis. Toxicity (hepatocellular abnormalities, mucocutaneous dryness, increased intracranial pressure, teratogenesis) has driven the search for derivatives, and the third-generation arotenoid and its ethyl ester appear to be highly potent and less toxic. A first-generation retinoid, 4-hydroxyphenyl retinamide (4-HPR), appears relatively nontoxic in early trials. There is some concern about potential for UV-induced skin cancer in patients taking carotenoids and retinoids based upon data from animal models, and monitoring for this complication is recommended. Table 1 lists the vitamin A family members discussed in this review.

Table 1. The Vitamin A Family

Carotenoids	Retinoids
Beta-carotene	Retinol
	Tretinoin (transretinoic acid)
	Isotretinoin (13-*cis*-retinoic acid)
	Etretinate
	Arotinoid-ethyl ester
	4-Hydroxyphenyl retinamide

Beta-Carotene

Because of its minimal toxicity, beta-carotene is favored for large chemoprevention trials. The preclinical evidence for beta-carotene is strong, but the jury is still out on its efficacy. In a study of 1805 patients judged at risk for nonmelanoma skin cancer by virtue of prior skin cancer, there was no benefit in terms of reduced skin cancer incidence from treatment with beta-carotene when given at a dose of 50 mg per day over a five-year period. There was essentially no toxicity with beta-carotene in that trial (5).

Beta-carotene does show activity in regression of oral leukoplakia. In a study that began as a randomized trial of beta-carotene versus 13-*cis*-retinoic acid (6), 11 of the first 16 patients refused to participate unless guaranteed the less toxic agent. In that study, beta-carotene at 30 mg per day produced 2 complete and 15 partial regressions of oral leukoplakia out of 24 patients with no significant toxicity. Beta-carotene and vitamin A both show activity in a study of oral leukoplakia using intermediate biologic end points (7). Indian fishermen who chew tobacco-containing betel quids were studied for frequency of oral leukoplakia, micronuclei in oral mucosa cells, and alterations in nuclear textures as end points. Whereas vitamin A produced remission of leukoplakia in 57% and reduction of micronuclei in 96% of the patients, beta-carotene resulted in remission of leukoplakia in 14.8% and reduction of micronuclei in 98%.

Retinoids in Oral Leukoplakia

Retinoids have been investigated in at least four studies of leukoplakia, detailed in Table 2. Since many leukoplakia chemoprevention trials indicate that the effect is dependent on taking the drug and that

Table 2. Retinoids in Oral Leukoplakia

Agent	Response	Reference
13-*cis*-retinoic acid, topical	9/11	8
13-*cis*-retinoic acid, topical	1/5	9
13-*cis*-retinoic acid	19/24	
vs		
Transretinoic acid	16/24	10, 11
vs		
Etretinate	22/24	
13-*cis*-retinoic acid	16/24	
vs		12
Placebo	2/20	

Table 3. Retinoids in Actinic Keratoses

	Response[a]	Reference
Transretinoic acid, topical	24 CR, 27 PR/60	13
Transretinoic acid, topical	46 CR, 47 PR/93	14
Etretinate, po	35 CR, 8 PR/46	15
Etretinate, po	10 CR, 27 PR/44	
vs		16
Placebo	1 CR, 1 PR/42	

[a]CR = complete response; PR = partial response.

when the retinoid is stopped leukoplakia returns, toxicity will be a major consideration in chemoprevention. Further research is needed to demonstrate the validity of reversal of leukoplakia and reduction of micronuclei as valid biologic end points in prevention of oral cancer with retinoids of beta-carotene.

Retinoids in Preneoplastic Skin Disorders

Preneoplastic skin disorders include actinic keratoses and dysplastic nevi. Table 3 describes clinical trials of retinoids in active keratoses. One of those listed by Moriarty and colleagues (16) reported a double-blind crossover study of 25 mg of oral etretinate given three times daily in 17 patients. The complete response and partial response in 44 patients compare favorably with the placebo group's one complete response and one partial response out of 42 patients. Toxicity, chiefly mucocutaneous dryness, was reversed when the dose was lowered, and the regimen was considered well tolerated.

Response of dysplastic nevi to topical transretinoic acid applied by occlusion was documented clinically in three of five patients in a randomized double-blind study (17). Seven of the 15 biopsies of nevi in those five patients showed disappearance or reversion to benign nevi. There was no clinical or histologic response in the placebo-treated group.

Retinoids in Established Skin Cancer

For established basal-cell carcinoma and malignant melanoma, responses to higher doses of retinoids have been demonstrated and are reviewed elsewhere (18). In advanced squamous-cell carcinoma of the skin, 13-*cis*-retinoic acid given at 1 mg/kg per day for 4 days has produced well-documented, impressive regression in 4 patients (19). Reports of 6 additional responses in 10 similarly treated patients are documented. Although most patients with squamous-cell carcinoma of the skin are cured with surgery or radiotherapy, for refractory disease retinoids appear to hold more promise than conventional cytotoxic chemotherapy. A preliminary report of 22 patients treated with 13-*cis*-retinoic acid at 1 mg/kg per day and alpha-interferon at 3 MU per day describes 6 complete and 10 partial responses. Only 3 of the 9 patients with metastasis responded, but response occurred in all patients with locally advanced disease (20).

Retinoids in Skin Cancer Prevention

In patients with xeroderma pigmentosum (XP), 13-*cis*-retinoic acid has shown activity in prevention of skin cancer. DiGiovanna and colleagues, whose paper is included in this volume, have worked with XP patients whose risk of developing skin cancer is 1000 times that of the general population. In five XP patients treated with 13-*cis*-retinoic acid at 2 mg/kg per day for two years, there was a 63% reduction in the incidence of basal-cell and squamous-cell skin cancer during treatment (21). The study demonstrated a rapid decrease in the rate of development of skin cancer after starting the retinoid treatment and rapid return to skin cancer risk on stopping the retinoid treatment.

Retinoids in Laryngeal Papillomatosis

Laryngeal papillomatosis is a disorder that may progress to squamous-cell carcinoma. The disorder responds to alpha-interferon in roughly 50% of patients. In one report of 6 patients with recurrent, progressive disease, 13-*cis*-retinoic acid at a dose of 1–2 mg/kg per day produced a complete response in 3 patients (22). In another report, 28 (67%) of 42 patients taking etretinate at a dose of 1 mg/kg per day showed a complete regression of laryngeal papillomatosis (23).

Retinoids in Head and Neck Cancer Prevention

For patients who have been treated for squamous-cell carcinoma of the head and neck, 10% to 40% will develop a second primary cancer. Results from a recent study have generated enthusiasm for the use of retinoids in prevention of second primary head and neck cancers. In a randomized trial of 103 patients who had been treated with surgery and/or radiotherapy for head and neck cancer, there was no significant difference in the number of recurrences of the primary cancers between a group taking 13-*cis*-retinoic acid (50–100 mg/m^2 per day orally for 12 months) and a group taking a placebo. Yet, when evaluated at 32 months, of the 13-*cis*-retinoic acid group, only 4% had developed a second primary tumor compared with 24% of the placebo group. The risk of second primary cancer in this clinical setting makes some toxicity acceptable, and in the study, toxicity (predominantly mucocutaneous dryness and hypertriglyceridemia) was mild or moderate. Nine of the 47 patients in the 13-*cis*-retinoic acid group discontinued therapy because of toxic effects compared with 3 of the 51 patients in the placebo group (24).

Retinoids in Mycosis Fungoides

The activity of 13-*cis*-retinoic acid and arotinoid ethyl ester in mycosis fungoides has been reviewed by Lippman (18). Table 4 summarizes the larger trials of retinoids in mycosis fungoides. Although these retinoids have demonstrated activity in mycosis fungoides with responses that can last months, further study is needed to define the optimal retinoid and its role in relation to other therapeutic options that are available in mycosis fungoides. Trials are under way to evaluate transretinoic acid in this disease.

Table 4. Retinoids in Mycosis Fungoides

Agent	Response[a]	Duration	Reference
13-*cis*-retinoic acid 1–2 mg/kg/day	3 CR, 8 PR/25	>8 mo, median	25
13-*cis*-retinoic acid 0.1–2.0 mg/kg/day	6 CR, 13 PR/28		26
13-*cis*-retinoic acid 1–2 mg/kg/day	6/6 symptomatic relief	>9 mo, median	27
Etretinate 1 mg/kg/day	1 CR, 7 PR/11		28
Arotinoid-ethylester .05 mg/wk–.3 mg/day, po	1 CR, 2 PR/6	102+ (CR) PR>10 mo, mean CR>23 mo	29

[a]CR = complete response; PR = partial response.

Retinoids in Hematologic Malignancy

The induction of remission in patients with acute promyelocytic leukemia (APL) using transretinoic acid is an exciting advance and represents a new treatment approach in this disease. Unlike the traditional cytoreduction approach to remission induction, transretinoic acid induces differentiation of promyelocytic leukemia cells. There is a characteristic (t15, 17) translocation in APL cells, and the breakpoint cluster region on chromosome 17 has been shown to involve the retinoic acid receptor alpha (RAR-α) (30). The APL cells express a mutant for RAR-α. Treatment of patients with transretinoic acid results in striking hyperleukocytosis that resolves despite continued drug treatment and high rates of complete remission. Observations of morphology, cell-surface immunophenotype, and fluorescent in situ hybridization with chromosome 17 probes demonstrate maturation of the leukemic cells (31). In one series of 11 APL patients treated with transretinoic acid, 9 entered remission (31). In another, 47 of 50 APL patients treated with transretinoic acid achieved remission (32). The mechanism whereby transretinoic acid effects differentiation in cells with mutated RAR-α-receptor is unknown. The clinical observations of activity are exciting; this agent may be superior to conventional chemotherapy for remission induction of APL, and trials are under way to define its optimal use in this disorder.

Although there are reports of improvement in myelodysplastic syndrome with 13-*cis*-retinoic acid, a double-blind, placebo-controlled randomized trial failed to demonstrate its efficacy in a study of 68 patients with this disorder (33). There was also failure to demonstrate response to 13-*cis*-retinoic acid in a small (12 evaluable subjects) trial of elderly patients with acute myeloid leukemia (34).

Retinoids in Cervical Dysplasia

Topical application of transretinoic acid via a cervical cap resulted in complete regression in 10 of 18 patients with cervical dysplasia (35).

Retinoids in Bladder Cancer

European studies (Table 5) have investigated the effectiveness of oral etretinate at 50 mg daily in preventing new bladder papilloma in patients who, following surgery for bladder papilloma, were disease free. Two randomized, placebo-controlled trials showed a positive effect (36, 37), whereas another showed no benefit (38) in a subject population with higher average histologic grade and larger numbers of recurrences prior to study entry. There are few studies and small numbers of cases describing the activity of retinol, transretinoic acid, and 4-hydroxyphenyl retinamide in bladder papilloma therapy and prevention reviewed by Malone (39).

Table 5. Etretinate in Bladder Cancer

		Response	Reference
Etretinate	11/15	papilloma prevention	36
vs			
Placebo	4/15		
Etretinate	19/23	<3 papillomas recurring	37
vs		at ≥ 12 mo	
Placebo	15/29		
Etretinate	20/33	papilloma recurrence	38
vs		reduced or absent	
Placebo	26/40		

Retinoids in Bronchial Metaplasia

Etretinate at 25 mg per day was given to 34 smokers who had bronchial metaplasia demonstrated at bronchial biopsy. Upon rebiopsy at six months, 10 of 11 subjects who completed the therapy showed improvement in bronchial metaplasia.

Vitamin C and Vitamin E

There is interest in vitamins C and E as potential chemopreventives in bowel cancers. They may be effective in the prevention of recurrence of colorectal polyps. A double-blind randomized trial (40) involving 200 patients who had prior polypectomies evaluated the results of a dosage of 400 mg each of vitamins C and E daily versus a placebo. After two years of supplementation, 41.7% of the vitamin-supplement group had polyps on colonoscopy, compared with 50.7% of the placebo-treated subjects. This study sample size is too small for statistical significance; larger trials are needed to evaluate the role of vitamins C and E in chemoprevention of colon cancer. In another randomized, double-blind study of 36 evaluable patients, a dosage of 3 g daily of vitamin C or a placebo was given for two years to patients with familial polyposis coli. There was a statistically significant reduction in polyp area in the vitamin-treated group (41). In a study of 5 patients with familial polyposis after ileorectal anastomosis, a dosage of 3 g of ascorbic acid daily for 4–13 months was associated with polyp disappearance in 2 patients, partial polyps regression in 2 patients, and increased polyps in 1 patient (42).

Vitamin D

Although vitamin D has not been used as a chemopreventive, preclinical data support its role in calcium regulation as a potential for colon cancer chemoprevention. In high-risk individuals, that is, familial colon cancer kindred with a high colon cell turnover rate, calcium supplementation was shown to reduce the turnover rate (43). That study used [3H]thymidine labeling of epithelial cells in colonic mucosa crypts and measured rates and patterns of labeling in subjects on calcium supplementation. Half of the subjects demonstrated a decrease in crypt hyperproliferation. In the half that did not demonstrate the overall decrease in crypt proliferation, there was a decrease in the size of the proliferative compartment at the crypt base, a pattern typical of individuals at decreased risk of colon cancer. This demonstrates the need to assess the efficacy of calcium in prevention of colonic adenomatous polyps.

Vitamin B_{12} and Folate

Vitamin B_{12} and folate play key roles in cellular proliferation and differentiation. In an early evaluation of women taking oral contraceptives, folate was found to improve cervical dysplasia (44). In the preliminary report of a randomized trial comparing vitamin B_{12} (0.5 mg/day) and folate (10 mg/day) for four months versus a placebo, 73 heavy-smoking men with bronchial squamous atypia were evaluated by sputum cytology. The B_{12} and folate–treated group had significantly greater reduction in cellular atypia. The limitations of the study—small sample size and short duration of study—require cautious interpretation (45).

Conclusion

The data from the several dozen clinical trials reviewed herein support activity of vitamins as both chemotherapeutic and chemopreventive agents. The retinoids show activity in established cancers as well as premalignant disorders. The activity of retinoids extends beyond epithelial tumors; lymphoid and myeloid malignancies respond. There are positive indications regarding the use of transretinoic acid in acute promyelocytic leukemia. Newer retinoids such as 4-HPR and arotinoid may have greater therapeutic efficacy and less toxicity. Clinical evaluation of the retinoids is an exciting and interesting area as oncologists seek the proper role for these therapeutic agents. The jury is out on the role of beta-carotene as an effective chemopreventive, but time and the results of ongoing chemoprevention trials will resolve this question. There may also be a place for vitamins C, E, and B_{12} and folate in our cancer-prevention armamentarium. The next decade holds the prospect of our beginning to understand the role of the diverse group of chemicals known as vitamins in cancer prevention.

REFERENCES

1. Herbert V. *Nutrition Cultism Facts and Fictions.* Philadelphia: George F. Stickley Company; 1980.
2. Cassileth BR. Unorthodox cancer medicine. *Cancer Invest.* 1986;4: 591–598.
3. Pauling L. *How to Live Longer and Feel Better.* New York: W A Freeman; 1986.
4. Moertel CG, Fleming TR, Creagan ET, *et al.* High dose vitamin C versus placebo in the treatment of patients with advanced cancer who have had no prior chemotherapy. *N Engl J Med.* 1985;311: 137–141.
5. Greenberg ER, Baron JA, Stuket TA, *et al.* A clinical trial of beta carotene to prevent basal-cell and squamous cell cancers of the skin. *N Eng J Med.* 1990;323:789–794.
6. Garewal HS, Meyskens FL, Killen D, *et al.* Response of oral leukoplakia to beta-carotene. *J Clin Oncol* 1990;8:1715–1720.
7. Stich HF, Mathew B, Sankaranarayanan R, Nair MK. Remission of precancerous lesions in the oral cavity of tobacco chewers and maintenance of the protective effect of beta-carotene or vitamin A. *Am J Clin Nutr.* 1991;53:2985–3045.
8. Shah JP, Strong EW, DeCosse JJ, Itri L, Sellers P. Effect of retinoids on oral leukoplakia. *Am J Surg.* 1983;146:466–469.
9. Pindborg JJ, Jolst O, Renstrup G, Roed-Petersen B. Studies in oral leukoplakia. *J Am Dent Assoc.* 1968;76:767–771.
10. Koch HF. Biochemical treatment of precancerous oral lesions: the effectiveness of various analogues of retinoic acid. *J Maxillofac Surg.* 1978;6:59–63.
11. Koch HF. Effect of retinoids on precancerous lesions in oral mucosa. In: Orfanos CE, Braun-Falco O, Farber EM, *et al.*, eds. *Retinoids: Advances in Basic Research and Therapy.* Berlin: Springer-Verlag; 1981:307–312.
12. Hong WK, Endicott J, Itri LM, *et al.* 13-*cis*-retinoic acid in the treatment of oral leukoplakia. *N Engl J Med.* 1986;315:1501–1505.
13. Bollag W, Ott F. Vitamin A acid in benign and malignant epithe-

lial tumors of the skin. *Acta Derm Venereol Suppl (Stockh)*. 1975; 74:163–166.

14. Belisario JC. Recent advances in topical cytotoxic therapy of skin cancer and pre-cancer. In: *Melanoma and Skin Cancer.* Sydney, Australia: 1972:349–365. Proceedings of the International Cancer Conference.
15. Grupper C, Beretli B. Cutaneous neoplasia and etretinate. In: Spitzy KH, Karrer K, eds. *Retinoids: A New Approach to Prevention and Therapy of Cancer.* Vienna: B H Egarmann; 1983:24–27. Proceedings of the 13th International Congress of Chemotherapy Symposium.
16. Moriarty M, Dunn J, Derregu A, *et al.* Etretinate in treatment of actinic keratoses: a double-blind crossover study. *Lancet.* 1982: 364–365.
17. Edwards L, Jaffe P. The effect of topical tretinoin on dysplastic nevi: a preliminary trial. *Arch Dermatol.* 1990;126:494–499.
18. Lippman SN, Meyskens FL. Results of the use of vitamin A and retinoids in cutaneous malignancies. *Pharmacol Ther.* 1989;40: 107–122.
19. Lippman SM, Meyskens FL. Treatment of advanced squamous cell carcinoma of the skin with isotretinoin. *Ann Intern Med.* 1987;107:499–501.
20. Lippman SM, Parkinson DR, Weber RS, *et al.* Isotretinoin plus-interferon: effective therapy of advanced squamous cell carcinoma (SCC) of the skin. *Proc Am Soc Clin Oncol.* 1991;10:197.
21. Kraemer KH, DiGiovanna JJ, Moshell AN, *et al.* Prevention of skin cancer in xeroderma pigmentosum with the use of oral isotretinoin. *N Engl J Med.* 1988;318:1633–1637.
22. Alberts DS, Coulthard SW, Meyskens FL. Regression of aggressive laryngeal papillomatosis with 13-cis retinoic acid. *J Biol Response Mod.* 1984;5:124–128.
23. Bickler E. The role of aromatic retinoid in the treatment of laryngeal keratinizing disorders and dysplasias. In: Spitzy KH, Karrer K, eds. *Retinoids: A New Approach to Prevention and Therapy of Cancer.* Vienna: B H Egarmann; 1983:36–37. Proceedings of the 13th International Congress of Chemotherapy Symposium.
24. Hong WK, Lippman SM, Itri LM, *et al.* Prevention of second primary tumors with isotretinoin in squamous-cell carcinoma of the head and neck. *N Engl J Med.* 1990;323:795–801.

25. Kessler JF, Jones SE, Levine N, *et al.* Isotretinoin and cutaneous helper T-cell lymphoma (mycosis fungoides). *Arch Dermatol.* 1987; 123:201–204.
26. Molin L, Thomsen K, Volden G, *et al.* 13-*cis*-retinoic acid in mycosis fungoides: a report from the Scandinavian Mycosis Fungoides Group. In: Saurat JH, ed. *Retinoids: New Trends in Research and Therapy.* Basel: Karger; 1985:341–344.
27. Neely SM, Mehlmauer M, Feinstin DI. The effect of isotretinoin in six patients with cutaneous T-cell lymphoma. *Arch Intern Med.* 1987;147:529–531.
28. Claudy AL, Rouchouse B. Treatment of cutaneous T-cell lymphomas with retinoid. In: Saurat JH, ed. *Retinoids: New Trends in Research and Therapy.* Basel: Karger; 1985:335–340.
29. Hoting E, Meissner K. Arotenoid-ethylester: effectiveness in refractory cutaneous T-cell lymphoma. *Cancer.* 1988;62:1044–1048.
30. deThe H, Chomienne C, Lanotte M, *et al.* The t (15;17) translocation of acute promyelocytic leukemia fuses the retinoic acid receptor gene to a novel transcribed locus. *Nature.* 1990;347:558–561.
31. Warrell RP, Frankel SR, Miller, WH, *et al.* Differentiation therapy of acute promyelocytic leukemia with tretinoin (all-trans-retinoic acid). *N Engl J Med.* 1991;324:1385–1393.
32. Chen Z-X, Xue Y-Q, Zhang R, *et al.* A clinical and experimental study on all-transretinoic acid-treated acute promyelocytic leukemia patients. *Blood.* 1991;78:1413–1419.
33. Koeffler HP, Heitjan D, Mertelsmann R, *et al.* Randomized study of 13-*cis*-retinoic acid or placebo in the myelodysplastic disorders. *Blood.* 1988;71:703–708.
34. Kramer ZB, Boros L, Wiernik PH, *et al.* 13-*cis*-retinoic acid in the treatment of elderly patients with acute myeloid leukemia. *Cancer.* 1991;67:1484–1486.
35. Surwit EA, Graham V, Droegenmueller W, *et al.* Evaluation of topically applied transretinoic acid in the treatment of cervical intraepithelial lesions. *Am J Obstet Gynecol.* 1982;143:821–823.
36. Alfthan O, Tarkkanen J, Grohn P, *et al.* Tigason (etretinate) in prevention of recurrence of superficial bladder tumors. *Eur Urol.* 1983;9:6–9.
37. Studer VE, Biedermann D, Chollet P, *et al.* Prevention of recurrent superficial bladder tumors by oral etretinate; preliminary re-

sults of a randomized, double-blind multicenter trial in Switzerland. *J Urol.* 1984;131:47–49.

38. Pederson H, Wolf H, Jensen SK, *et al.* Administration of a retinoid as prophylasis of recurrent non-invasive bladder tumors. *Scand J Urol Nephrol.* 1984;18:121–123.
39. Malone WF, Kelloff GJ, Pierson H, Greenwald P. Chemoprevention of bladder cancer. *Cancer.* 1987;60:650–657.
40. McKeown-Eyssen G, Holloway C, Jazmaji V, *et al.* A randomized trial of vitamins C and E in the prevention and recurrence of colorectal polyps. *Cancer Res.* 1988;48:4701–4705.
41. Bussey HJ, DeCosse JJ, Descaner EE, *et al.* A randomized trial of ascorbic acid in polyposis coli. *Cancer.* 1982;50:1434–1439.
42. DeCosse JJ, Adams MB, Kuzma JF, *et al.* Effect of ascorbic acid on rectal polyps of patients with familial polyposis. *Surgery.* 1975;78: 608–612.
43. Lipkin M, Friedman E, Winnver, Newmark H. Colonic epithelial cell proliferation in responders and non-responders to dietary calcium. *Cancer Res.* 1989;49:248–254.
44. Butterworth CE, Hatch KD, Gore H, *et al.* Improvement in cervical dysplasia associated with folic acid therapy in users of oral contraceptives. *Am J Clin Nutr.* 1982;35:73–82.
45. Heimburger DG, Alexander CB, Birch R, *et al.* Improvement in bronchial squamous metaplasia in smokers treated with folate and vitamin B_{12}. *JAMA.* 1988;259:1525–1530.

HARINDER S. GAREWAL

The Role of Vitamins and Nutrients in Oral Leukoplakia

ABSTRACT

The reversal or suppression of premalignant lesions is an important strategy for the prevention of cancer. Oral cavity cancer is a common neoplasm whose frequency varies markedly from one region of the world to another. Oral leukoplakia is a premalignant lesion for oral cancer. Epidemiologic, laboratory, and animal studies strongly suggest that antioxidant vitamins and nutrients, such as beta-carotene and alpha-tocopherol, are inhibitors of oral cancer formation. Hence, there is increasing interest in studying these nontoxic substances as chemopreventive agents. Early clinical studies suggest that beta-carotene, alone or in combination with low doses of vitamin A, can reverse oral leukoplakia in short-term trials lasting three to six months. Our pilot study using beta-carotene at a dosage of 30 mg per day for three to six months resulted in a 70% response rate without toxicity. We are now conducting a longer (18-month), placebo-controlled, randomized study to test whether these remissions produced by beta-carotene are durable. Trials using alpha-tocopherol, either alone or in combination with other nutrients, are also ongoing. Such studies will help define a chemopreventive role for these nontoxic agents in oral cavity cancer.

Introduction

Oral and pharyngeal cancers are common malignancies, the head and neck area being the sixth most frequent cancer site overall (1). Their incidence varies from one part of the world to another with some of the highest rates occurring in developing countries, where often as many as 25% to 30% of all cancers occur in the oral cavity (2, 3). In the United States approximately 42 000 new cases of head and neck cancer occur annually, resulting in about 12 000 deaths (4). Despite the introduction of new strategies for the management of advanced oral cancer, there has been no demonstrable improvement in the survival rate of patients afflicted with this disease. In fact, five-year survival rates in the early 1970s and those achieved in the 1980s are essentially identical.

Perhaps the most promising approach to reducing the morbidity and mortality from oral cancer lies in its prevention. This statement is based on the well-defined etiologic associations with respect to tobacco use, betel quid chewing, and alcohol consumption (5, 6). Tobacco, either smoked or chewed, causes in excess of 70% of head and neck cancers (5). Thus, elimination or reduction of the use of this noxious agent will have a significant impact on the incidence of this disease. Additionally, a large body of evidence suggests a role for nutritional agents, particularly those related to vitamin A (retinoids and carotenoids), in inhibiting oral carcinogenesis. As described elsewhere in this volume, substantial epidemiologic and laboratory evidence exists for a protective role for these nutrients in a variety of malignancies, including oral cavity cancer. More recently, this finding has been corroborated by clinical trials demonstrating the ability of these agents to reverse premalignant changes in the oral cavity.

Why Target Premalignant Lesions?

Although it may seem obvious why premalignant lesions are targeted in clinical trials, the reasons vary considerably from one setting to another. It is therefore important to keep the overall objective of a treatment program in perspective if we are to design clinically meaningful studies, the results of which will have the potential to make a real impact on cancer morbidity and mortality.

It is widely believed that cancer develops through a series of steps called initiation, promotion, and progression. Premalignant lesions are the first clinically identifiable lesions along this pathway. In one sense, therefore, they are intermediate markers that allow recognition of an organ or tissue as having been affected by the carcinogenesis process. Therefore, the search for interventions that lead to reversal or suppression of these lesions constitutes an important strategy for cancer prevention, for example, reduction in colon polyps as a preventive approach to colon cancer.

Premalignant lesions or conditions have been characterized for the vast majority of human cancers. However, the word *premalignant* signifies a wide range of cancer risk, depending on the particular lesion in question. Some precancerous conditions are associated with an overwhelming cancer risk during an individual's lifetime, for example, familial polyposis of the colon, Bloom's syndrome. Close monitoring is mandatory for patients afflicted with such conditions. Furthermore, any interventions that can lead to a significant decrease in cancer risk would be highly desirable, even if associated with some side effects and morbidity of their own. Overall, however, such very high-risk syndromes account for only a minority of human cancers. The vast majority of precancerous lesions, as a rule, will not become manifest as cancer during an individual's lifetime. For example, people with sporadic adenomatous polyps of the colon, particularly if they are small, have a very low frequency of development of colon cancer. Furthermore, the incidence and prevalence of such premalignant lesions usually far exceed the incidence and prevalence of the corresponding malignancy. Hence, in developing interventions to prevent or reverse these lesions, the associated treatment toxicities and side effects become of paramount importance, since most subjects receiving the treatment are not destined to develop cancer. In other words, the ultimate goal of chemopreventive strategies directed at the reversal of common premalignant lesions is to develop interventions for the prevention of cancer and not merely treatment of the premalignant lesions. It is important to keep this objective in mind when designing such studies to avoid subjecting patients at little risk of actually developing cancer to agents with significant side effects.

The majority of oral cavity premalignant lesions fall into the category of leukoplakia, defined as a white patch or plaque on the mucosa that cannot be rubbed off and is not attributable to a specific disease entity (7). In general, the simple form of this condition has a rather low malignant potential, in the range of 1% or less per year (8). Certain clinical features are associated with a greater risk of transformation. Grossly, the presence of a reddish component (erythroplakia), speckled leukoplakia, or a proliferative verrucous type of lesion are associated with a higher transformation rate (8, 9). Overall, however, these high-risk varieties are relatively uncommon in the United States. At the microscopic level, the presence of severe dysplasia is associated with greater cancer risk (8).

Oral leukoplakia is an excellent model for chemoprevention studies looking for reversal of the condition, mainly because of its well-known association with oral cancer and the ease with which it can be repeatedly accessed. Nevertheless, as with other premalignant lesions, the ultimate objective of any intervention trial conducted in leukoplakia must be kept in mind when selecting modalities to be tested. If the objective is to develop a treatment applicable to the small minority of patients with high-risk lesions, as defined earlier, that are not amenable to standard treatments such as removal of local irritants, surgical excision or cryosurgery, then some degree of toxicity of the treatment may be acceptable. In this category would be studies that have tested such agents as topical bleomycin, which has shown efficacy (10, 11). However, if the objective is to test strategies for the prevention of oral cancer, then clearly such toxic agents will never be useful, even if found to be active. Such trials must therefore involve use of nontoxic agents that can be safely supplemented. It is in this context that interest has intensified recently in the potential role of vitamins and other nutrients in reversing oral leukoplakia. The majority of clinical trials have thus far been done with vitamin A and related compounds. Therefore, this paper focuses on trials using these agents.

Vitamin A, Beta-Carotene, and Related Compounds in Oral Cancer Prevention

Vitamin A plays an important role in the normal differentiation of epithelial tissues (12). Carotenoids, a group of over three hundred different compounds that form the red, orange, and yellow pigments in plants, can serve as vitamin A precursors and have antioxidant and anticarcinogenic activities of their own. Beta-carotene is biologically one of the most important carotenoids, since it can be converted in mammalian tissues to yield two molecules of vitamin A. In the developing world, carotenoids serve as the dietary source of approximately 80% to 90% of vitamin A as compared with only 50% in the United States. Carotenoids that are not converted to vitamin A circulate with fats and are deposited in many tissues throughout the body. These deposited carotenoids may have a direct protective role.

As discussed elsewhere in this volume, there is considerable epidemiologic evidence linking an increased risk of cancer of the aerodigestive tract, including oropharyngeal cancer, with a low intake of foods containing carotenoids, that is, vegetables and fruits. Similarly, in laboratory studies carotenoids have been shown to have antimutagenic activity in bacterial and cell culture systems (13, 14). Particularly relevant to oral cancer prevention is the demonstration that beta-carotene can block genotoxic damage induced in Chinese hamster ovary cells by tumor promoters that include extracts of areca nut, which is an integral part of betel quid and has been linked to oral cancer causation (15). In animal experiments, it has been shown that vitamin A, beta-carotene, and vitamin E (alpha-tocopherol) are inhibitors of oral carcinogenesis in the hamster cheek pouch model in which lesions are induced by applying a carcinogen to the hamster cheek pouch (16–22). These laboratory and epidemiologic observations have led to clinical trials directed toward the reversal of oral leukoplakia in humans as the next step in determining a potential role for these compounds in oral cancer prevention.

Clinical Studies in Oral Leukoplakia

Retinoids

It has been known for nearly three decades that very high doses of vitamin A can reverse the hyperkeratosis associated with oral leukoplakia (23). However, the significant toxicity associated with a high dose of vitamin A precluded use of this modality as a cancer prevention approach. Since then, several trials have been conducted demonstrating the efficacy of various retinoids, both natural and synthetic, in reversing leukoplakia. The retinoids 13-*cis*-retinoic acid, transretinoic acid, and etretinate are all effective, leading to response rates in the range of 50% to 90% (24–27). However, all these treatments are associated with significant toxicity. Furthermore, relapses occur in the majority of patients after therapy is discontinued, most often within one to two months of treatment cessation, thereby pointing to a need for long-term interventions if cancer prevention is to be the goal.

The clinical toxicity of the retinoids at the doses used in the above trials essentially precludes their use for the primary prevention of oral cancer, despite their effectiveness. The agent in this class that has attracted the greatest interest is 13-*cis*-retinoic acid, which has been used at a dose of 1–2 mg/kg per day. Studies presently under way plan to use lower doses with the hope of reducing toxicity (.25–.50 mg/kg per day). However, since the lesions relapse soon after drug discontinuation, it is anticipated that prolonged use, probably over several years, will be necessary. Although lower doses of 13-*cis*-retinoic acid are less toxic than the high doses, extensive clinical use of this agent for dermatologic indications has shown that even a very low dosage of 13-*cis*-retinoic acid (0.1–0.2 mg/kg per day) can produce significant toxicities, particularly with prolonged use (28, 29). In this regard, recent use of this drug in a trial for skin cancer prevention involved approximately 10 mg per day total dosage (*i.e.*, 0.1–0.15 mg/kg per day). This was ineffective in the prevention of recurrent skin cancer, but perhaps more important from our standpoint, it was associated with significant toxicity (30). Therefore, it is unlikely that 13-*cis*-retinoic acid will serve as a useful agent for the primary prevention of oral cancer. It may, however, play a role in the treatment of the occasional severely dysplastic, high-risk oral premalignant lesion that is not amenable to presently available standard treatments.

Beta-Carotene and Beta-Carotene–Containing Combinations

Because of its lack of toxicity and ready availability, beta-carotene is an attractive agent to test for potential use in oral cancer prevention (Table 1). Stich and colleagues have reported a series of studies showing that beta-carotene, alone or in combination with vitamin A, can decrease the incidence of micronucleated cells in exfoliated oral mucosal cells from populations considered to be at high risk for oral cancer (31). Increased frequency of micronucleated cells is thought to reflect genotoxic damage produced by carcinogens.

Stich *et al.* have also reported clinical results of a series of trials in India using vitamin A alone or in combination with beta-carotene (31, 32). This study differs from the other trials discussed in this paper in that the lesion studied is associated primarily with the chewing of betel nuts and other substances. Furthermore, the study population may have had some degree of pre-existing vitamin A deficiency. In one study, treatment consisted of beta-carotene (180 mg/week, group I), beta-carotene plus vitamin A (100 000 IU/week, group II), or a placebo (group III) given twice weekly for six months. At six

Table 1. Oral Leukoplakia Trials Using Beta-Carotene

Investigator	Agent(s)	CR[a] (%)	PR[b] (%)	OR[c] (%)	Country
Stich	Beta-carotene	15	NS[d]	NS	India
Stich	Beta-carotene + vitamin A	27	NS	NS	India
Garewal	Beta-carotene	8	63	71	U.S.
Garewal	Beta-carotene vs Placebo (18 months)	Ongoing study			U.S.
Kaugars	Beta-carotene + vitamin E + vitamin C	Ongoing study			U.S.
Winn	vitamin E	Ongoing study			U.S.

[a]CR = complete response.
[b]PR = partial response.
[c]OR = overall response.
[d]NS = not stated.

months, 15% of the patients in group I, 27.5% in group II, and only 3% in group III had complete remission of their lesions (31). The appearance of new lesions was strongly inhibited in the treatment groups. In a more recent trial using 200 000 IU of vitamin A alone per week for six months, Stich *et al.* have reported a 57% complete response rate with complete suppression of new lesions (32).

Studies with beta-carotene in Western populations have also been conducted recently. We have reported a pilot trial of beta-carotene alone given at a dosage of 30 mg daily for three to six months (33). We observed a response rate of 71% in 24 evaluable patients. Of particular importance was the fact that no clinically significant toxicity was observed through the duration of this trial that could be attributed to beta-carotene. Since beta-carotene has been shown to produce changes in the cellular immune system in animal models and in in vitro studies, we measured the percentage of various immune cells in a subset of our study patients taking beta-carotene. An increase in the percentage of natural killer cells was found, accompanied by a smaller increase in helper T-cell numbers (34). These changes were qualitatively similar to those reported previously in vitro.

We have followed this pilot experience by initiating a larger trial of longer duration. In this study all subjects are treated with beta-carotene at a dosage of 60 mg per day for six months. At six months, all responding patients are randomized to continue beta-carotene or a placebo for an additional twelve months. This blinded, randomized trial is designed to determine whether responses can be maintained by continuation of the chemopreventive agent, an important point that needs to be established. Present experience from all the short-term trials discussed earlier is that a majority of lesions will recur after discontinuation of the test agent. However, the converse, that continued use of the agent will prevent recurrence, is not necessarily true and needs to be proved.

Another study involving a combination of antioxidant agents, including beta-carotene, is being conducted by Kaugars *et al.* (35). In this trial, patients receive a combination of beta-carotene, alpha-tocopherol, and vitamin C. Once again, this is essentially a nontoxic combination, and preliminary results appear encouraging. Although alpha-tocopherol alone is very active in the animal model system, there are no published trials of its use as a single agent in oral leukoplakia.

Future Directions

In summary, current data suggest that both vitamin A and beta-carotene play a role in the reversal and suppression of oral leukoplakia. Although beta-carotene has an effect on its own, the trials conducted by Stich *et al.* in India suggest that combining this agent with low doses of vitamin A may result in a greater complete response rate. Owing to the known toxicities of vitamin A, however, especially when used over a long period of time at dosages in excess of about 25 000 IU per day, caution must be exercised when using this agent for primary cancer prevention. Trials with other agents and combinations are in progress. Particularly interesting are studies using a combination of antioxidant, anticarcinogenic agents such as beta-carotene and alpha-tocopherol.

In this paper we have focused on one study population, that is, subjects with oral leukoplakia. Another important group of subjects to target for chemopreventive approaches are those who have had an early primary head and neck cancer that is considered cured. These patients are known to be at high risk for developing a second primary cancer of the aerodigestive tract (36–39). It is reasonable to speculate that agents active in reversing preneoplastic lesions might be active in reversing the "field cancerization" defect thought to underlie this increased incidence of second cancers (40). A recent report of an adjuvant trial using high-dose 13-*cis*-retinoic acid in patients with all stages of head and neck cancer showed a remarkable reduction in the incidence of second primary tumors, although it failed to show a significant adjuvant effect, that is, a reduction in recurrence of the original tumors (41). Toxicity was again a major problem, leading to premature discontinuation of therapy in a third of the patients. Trials using lower doses of 13-*cis*-retinoic acid are ongoing. Based on recent results showing activity in oral leukoplakia, trials using beta-carotene or beta-carotene plus low-dose vitamin A to prevent second cancers have also been initiated.

These early exciting results on the ability of nontoxic nutrients with antioxidant and anticarcinogenic activity to reverse established precancerous lesions have generated considerable optimism and enthusiasm for the likelihood of preventing oral cavity cancers. It is also possible that similar results may hold for other malignancies, particularly those involving the upper aerodigestive tract, which have closely linked etiologies to oral cavity cancer and are involved in a common "field cancerization" phenomenon. This possibility of an effective chemoprevention approach has led to the design of several studies using vitamin and nutrient supplementation in aerodigestive tract cancer prevention, the results of which should become available in the near future.

ACKNOWLEDGMENTS

The research for this paper was supported in part by United States Public Health Service grant CA25702.

REFERENCES

1. Parkin SM, Laara E, Muir CS. Estimates of the worldwide frequency of sixteen major cancers. *Indian J Cancer.* 1988;41:184–197.
2. Dunham LJ. A geographic study of a relationship between oral cancer and plants. *Cancer Res.* 1968;28:2369–2371.
3. Baden E. Tabac et cancers de la region oropharyngee et des

bronches: donnees actuelles. *Rev Med Joulouse.* 1978;14:549–560.

4. Silverberg E, Boring CC, Squires TS. Cancer statistics. *CA.* 1990; 40:9–26.
5. United States Department of Health and Human Services. *The Health Consequences of Smoking and Cancer:* A Report of the Surgeon General. Washington, DC: US Government Printing Office; 1982. DDHS publication (PSII) 82-5107.
6. Muir CS, Kirk R. Betel, tobacco and cancer of the mouth. *Br J Cancer.* 1990;14:597–608.
7. Kramer IRH, Luers RB, Pindborg JJ, Sobin LH. Definition of leukoplakia and related lesions: an aid to studies on oral precancer. *Oral Surg Oral Med Oral Pathol.* 1978;46:518–539.
8. Silverman S, Shillitoe EJ; S. Silverman, ed. *Etiology and predisposing factors in oral cancer.* 3rd ed., American Cancer Society;1990: 7–39.
9. Hansen LS, Olson JA, Silverman S. Proliferative verrucous leukoplakia: a long-term study of thirty patients. *Oral Surg Oral Med Oral Pathol.* 1985;60:285–298.
10. Wong F, Epstein J, Millner A. Treatment of oral leukoplakia with topical bleomycin: a pilot study. *Cancer.* 1989;64:361–365.
11. Hammersley N, Ferguson MM, Rennie JS. Topical bleomycin in the treatment of oral leukoplakia: a pilot study. *Br J Oral Maxillofac Surg.* 1985;23:251–258.
12. Hicks RM. The scientific basis for regarding vitamin A and its analogues as anticarcinogenic agents. *Proc Nutr Soc.* 1983;42: 83–93.
13. Som S, Chatterjee M, Bannerjee MR. Beta-carotene inhibition of 7,12-dimethylbenz(a)anthracene-induced transformation of murine mammary cells *in vitro. Carcinogenesis.* 1984;5:937–940.
14. Bertram JS, Peng A, Rundhaug JE. Carotenoids have intrinsic cancer preventive action. *FASEB J.* 1988;2:1413A. Abstract.
15. Stich HF, Dunn BP. Relationship between cellular levels of beta-carotene and sensitivity to genotoxic agents. *Int J Cancer.* 1987; 38:713–717.
16. Burge-Bottenbley A, Shklar G. Retardation of experimental oral cancer development by retinol acetate. *Nutr Cancer.* 1983;5:121–129.
17. Schwartz J, Suda D, Light G. Beta-carotene is associated with the regression of hamster buccal pouch carcinoma and induction of

tumor necrosis factor in macrophages. *Biochem Biophys Res Commun.* 1987;136:1130–1135.

18. Shklar G, Schwartz J, Grau D, *et al.* Inhibition of hamster buccal pouch carcinogenesis by 13-*cis*-retinoic acid. *Oral Surg.* 1980;50: 45–52.
19. Shklar G, Marefat P, Kornhauser A, *et al.* Retinoid inhibition of lingual carcinogenesis. *Oral Surg.* 1980;49:325–332.
20. Shklar G. Oral mucosal carcinogenesis in hamsters: inhibition by vitamin E. *J Natl Cancer Inst.* 1982;68:791–797.
21. Odukoya O, Hawach F, Shklar G. Retardation of experimental oral cancer by topical vitamin E. *Nutr Cancer.* 1984;6:98–104.
22. Suda D, Schwartz J, Shklar G. Inhibition of experimental oral carcinogenesis by topical beta-carotene. *Carcinogenesis.* 1986;7: 711–715.
23. Silverman S, Eisenberg E, Renstrap G. A study of the effects of high doses of vitamin A on oral leukoplakia (hyperkeratosis) including toxicity, liver function and skeletal metabolism. *J Oral Ther Pharmacol.* 1965;2:9.
24. Koch HF. Biochemical treatment of precancerous oral lesions: the effectiveness of various analogues of retinoic acid. *J Maxillofac Surg.* 1978;6:59–63.
25. Koch HF. Effect of retinoids on precancerous lesions of oral mucosa. In: Orfanos CE, Braun-Falco O, Farber EM, *et al.*, eds. *Retinoids: Advances in Basic Research and Therapy.* Berlin: Springer; 1981:307–312.
26. Shah JP, Strong EW, DeCosse JJ, *et al.* Effect of retinoids on oral leukoplakia. *Am J Surg.* 1983;146:466–470.
27. Hong WK, Endicott J, Itri LM, *et al.* 13-*cis*-retinoic acid in the treatment of oral leukoplakia. *N Engl J Med.* 1986;315:1501–1505.
28. Strauss JS, Rapini RP, Shalita AR, *et al.* Isotretinoin therapy for acne: results of a multicenter dose-response study. *J Am Acad Dermatol.* 1984;10:490–496.
29. Jones DH, King K, Miller AJ, Cunliffe WJ. A dose-response study of 13-*cis*-retinoic acid in acne vulgaris. *Br J Dermatol.* 1983;108: 333–343.
30. Tangrea JA. The isotretinoic-basal cell carcinoma prevention trial: results of the three year intervention phase. In: Proceedings of the 15th annual meeting of the American Society of Preventive Oncology; 1991; Seattle.

31. Stich HF, Rosin MP, Hornby AP, *et al.* Remission of oral leukoplakias and micronuclei in tobacco/betel quid chewers treated with beta-carotene and with beta-carotene plus vitamin A. *Int J Cancer.* 1988;42:195–199.
32. Stich HF, Hornby AP, Mathew B, *et al.* Response of oral leukoplakias to the administration of vitamin A. *Cancer Lett.* 1988;40: 93–101.
33. Garewal HS, Meyskens FL, Killen D, *et al.* Response of oral leukoplakia to beta-carotene. *J Clin Oncol.* 1990;8:1715–1720.
34. Prabhala RH, Garewal HS, Hicks MJ, Sampliner RE, Watson RR. The effects of 13-*cis*-retinoic acid and beta-carotene on cellular immunity in humans. *Cancer.* 1991;67:1556–1560.
35. Kaugars G, Brandt R, Carcaise-Edinboro P, Strauss R, Kilpatrick J. Beta-carotene supplementation in the treatment of oral lesions. *Oral Surg Oral Med Oral Pathol.* 1990;70:607–608.
36. McGuirt WF, Mathews B, Kaufman JA. Multiple simultaneous tumors in patients with head and neck cancer. *Cancer.* 1982;50: 1195–1199.
37. Karp DD, Guralnik E, Guidice LA, *et al.* Multiple primary cancers: a prevalent and increasing problem. *Proc Am Soc Clin Oncol.* 1985;4:13. Abstract.
38. Shapshay S, Hong WK, Fried M, *et al.* Simultaneous carcinomas of the esophagus and upper aerodigestive tract. *Otolaryngol Head Neck Surg.* 1980;88:373–377.
39. Kotwall C, Razack MS, Sako K, Roa U. Multiple primary cancers in squamous cell cancer of the head and neck. *J Surg Oncol.* 1989;40:97–99.
40. Slaughter DP, Southwick HW, Smejkal W. Field cancerization in oral stratified squamous epithelium clinical implications of multicentric origin. *Cancer.* 1953;5:963–968.
41. Hong WK, Lippman SM, Itri LM, *et al.* Prevention of second primary tumors with isotretinoin in squamous-cell carcinoma of the head and neck. *N Engl J Med.* 1990;323:795–801.

DOUGLAS C. HEIMBURGER

Premalignant Lesions of the Lung

ABSTRACT

Associations have been described between foods (especially vegetables and fruits) and a number of micronutrients and lung cancer. Principal among the potentially protective nutrients is beta-carotene, but there is also evidence that folic acid, vitamins C and E, and selenium may play a role in impeding bronchial carcinogenesis.

Human and animal studies have documented a graded progression from normal bronchial mucosa to cancer, involving squamous metaplasia with mild, moderate, and severe atypia as intermediate stages. These classic cytopathologic features are the best established premalignant lesions of the lung and have been used as intermediate end points in most completed and ongoing human lung cancer chemoprevention trials. Attempts have been made to quantify them through computerized measurements and statistical constructs such as the Atypia Status Index.

However, these morphologic changes are preceded by genetic and molecular events that could represent more sensitive, earlier markers. Measurements proposed for use in chemoprevention trials include genetic alterations expressed as ploidy (cellular DNA content), micronuclei, and DNA adducts, and cellular hormones, gene products, and enzymes such as epidermal growth factor, cytokeratins, involucrin, and transglutaminase.

In using any of these putative intermediate end points and biomarkers in chemoprevention trials, investigators must be careful to avoid confounding due to regression to the mean. This is the phenomenon whereby persons selected for extreme values of a variable will tend to have less extreme values, closer to the population mean, on subsequent measurements. Several methods can be used to eliminate the regression effect in the design of clinical trials.

Two chemoprevention trials completed to date (one published) have tested whether the retinoid etretinate can reduce the severity of bronchial squamous metaplasia and atypia. Although one trial suggested a chemopreventive effect of etretinate and the other did not, both were probably confounded by regression to the mean, leaving the effect of the treatment unclear. A third completed trial, using a combination of folic acid and vitamin B_{12}, showed a reduction in the severity of atypia after four months. Ongoing trials are using isotretinoin or beta-carotene alone or combined with retinol or alpha-tocopherol in smokers and/or asbestos workers. Some studies require the presence of premalignant lesions in sputum samples or bronchial brushings or biopsies. Most are using one or more of the intermediate end points described above, although some are using cancer itself as the end point.

Introduction

As discussed elsewhere in this volume, a number of foods and micronutrients are thought to protect against lung cancer. Epidemiologic studies show especially strong, and repeatedly confirmed, associations between dietary intake of vegetables and fruits and lower risks of lung cancer. Investigations of the particular protective nutrients in these foods and their mechanisms of action have mostly been directed toward retinoids because of strong evidence, both epidemiologic and experimental, that beta-carotene confers a reduced risk for lung cancer. However, although the evidence favoring them is weaker, other nutrients such as folic acid, selenium, and vitamins C and E, as well as nonnutritive substances, may share some of the credit for the beneficial effects of vegetables and fruits. Although animal studies show a protective effect for vitamin A, epidemiologic studies do not well support this role in humans.

Because these dietary covariates prevent the isolation of single-nutrient effects in epidemiologic studies, the effort to elucidate them in humans requires randomized, controlled trials with specific interventions. However, as with other malignancies, the lengthy gap between tumor initiation and clinical lung cancer renders the use of cancer incidence as the end point costly, slow, and potentially risky in terms of return on research dollars invested. Issues of long-term compliance in intervention groups, treatment contamination in control groups, comingling of incident with preexisting subclinical cases, and the possibility that, in secondary prevention trials, intervention will be applied too late to show an effect threaten the feasibility of such trials (1). Additionally, single-nutrient trials may miss important nutrient interactions, which one would not want to discover only after a decade or more of study. For these reasons, the use of premalignant lesions and biological markers as intermediate end points is gaining increasing prominence.

In the lung the principal challenge in pursuing these end points is in sampling them. In contrast to the skin, oral cavity, and cervix, the bronchial mucosa, from which most lung cancers arise, is relatively inaccessible. To obtain pure samples of bronchial cells requires bronchoscopically obtained bronchial brushings or biopsies, a procedure that is somewhat cumbersome and costly. Sputum samples, which are easier to obtain, have been used in several of the human chemoprevention trials to date. However, they have significant limitations that make the probability of missing mucosal lesions substantial. Among these are differential abilities among subjects to produce sputum from deep in the lungs and possible differential shedding of cells among areas of the lung and among sampling times. All of the premalignant lesions and biological markers to be discussed in this paper, if monitoried with sputum samples, are subject to these limitations.

Classic Bronchial Premalignant Lesions

It is well established that during carcinogenesis bronchial mucosal cells pass through progressively abnormal stages that culminate in squamous-cell carcinoma. Normal columnar epithelial cells are replaced by cells that have undergone squamous differentiation, to produce squamous metaplasia. These cells initially look like normal squamous cells, then exhibit progressive atypia that is labeled mild, moderate, or severe according to classic cytopathological criteria, before frank cancer cells appear. Although all stages of this process are rarely observed in humans, leaving the possibility that some of them may be skipped, animal studies have documented this progression in detail (2). The process is reversible up to the final stage (3), even spontaneously, leaving both the prospect that it can be used to monitor preventive efforts and the possibility that spontaneous regression may confound interpretation (4). Until proved otherwise, the same must be assumed to be true for all putative intermediate end points.

Among candidate intermediate end points for human chemoprevention trials, the substantial clinical and experimental experience with these cytophatologic changes makes them the most clearly linked with cancer. They have been used in nearly all of the current chemoprevention trials. However, even if the sampling problems can be resolved, at least two significant limitations remain. First, there is substantial subjectivity involved in assigning a score to a cell, producing both intra- and interobserver variation (5). Pathologists and cytotechnologists normally make qualitative judgments (is cancer present or not?) rather than quantitative ones (how far along a continuum is this cell?), and are often not practiced in making the sorts of assessments required in chemoprevention trials. Greenberg and Swank and their colleagues have attempted to solve this problem by quantitating morphologic features in sputum cells using computerized image analysis (3, 6). They have documented that composites of these features are related to the degree of atypia and have distilled some of them statistically into an Atypia Status Index.

But even this does not address the second limitation, which is that morphologic changes themselves may be relatively late phenomena. They are necessarily preceded by genetic and molecular events, and these events may be much more sensitive in charting the progression or reversal of carcinogenesis.

Genetic and Molecular Markers

Malignancy begins with genetic mutations that are preserved, leading to abnormalities in gene expression and loss of control over cell growth and reproduction. Many of these mutations result in cells that are aneuploid, containing abnormal, usually elevated, amounts of DNA. In their canine model of carcinogenesis, Benfield *et al.* have documented a progressive increase in nuclear DNA content and in the prevalence of aneuploidy as the bronchial mucosa approaches malignancy (2). Ono *et al.* noted that even severely atypical, aneuploid changes are reversible in this model if the carcinogen is removed (7). Auer and colleagues observed a correlation between DNA content and classic atypical features in human sputum cells across the entire spectrum from normal to invasive carcinoma (8). Further, among established malignancies, aneuploid tumors are generally more aggressive than euploid ones, making aneuploidy a marker both of malignant potential and of prognosis (9).

Although ploidy is often measured with flow cytometry, which requires very large cell numbers and results in discarding of cells, slide-based computer image analysis systems allow for measurement of DNA content in individual cells and small groups of cells, with simultaneous morphologic assessment if desired. Traditionally, Feulgen staining is utilized, but vital dyes such as acridine orange and Hoechst stains are applicable as well (10). This technique renders repetitive DNA measurements, such as would be required in chemoprevention trials, feasible.

When genetic damage occurs in epithelial tissues as a result of exposure to carcinogens or other genotoxic agents, chromosomal fragments called micronuclei are often observed (11). After Feulgen staining of cells, these can be counted. Their prevalence is increased in both premalignant and malignant lesions from a variety of tissues and in the bronchial mucosa of current cigarette smokers (12). Their presence in normal cells adjacent to premalignant lesions suggests that they appear before the morphologic expression of atypia.

The successful use of micronuclei as an intermediate end point in chemoprevention trials in persons with leukoplakia, a premalignant lesion of the oral cavity, suggests that they may be useful in the lung as well (13). Their use, however, may be limited by the following: their quantitation is labor intensive (though this may be improved with image analysis); sputum samples are probably not suitable for their assessment; and in the human lung, they are as yet linked conclusively only with cigarette smoking and not with bronchial metaplasia or lung cancer.

Adducts of DNA represent another index of genetic damage induced by cigarette smoke. Their levels are increased in virtually all body tissues in cigarette smokers, in a dose- and time-related fashion (14). Dunn *et al.* recently reported that DNA adduct levels in bronchial biopsies are correlated positively with intensity of current smoking and alcohol intake and negatively with number of years since quitting smoking and fruit and juice intake (using a crude measure of dietary intake) (15). However, they also noted substantial overlap between smokers and nonsmokers in the ranges of adduct levels, a problem that probably pertains to most of the proposed intermediate end points. In addition, the persistence of elevated levels of DNA adducts in tissues for years after smoking cessation may compromise their use in chemoprevention trials, and they are also subject to the drawbacks noted for micronuclei.

Another group of potential markers of premalignancy are the mediators of the squamous differentiation that results in metaplasia in injured epithelial tissues. This has been described as a two-step process. The first step is recruitment of quiescent (G_0) cells into the cell cycle, producing hyperplasia (16). This step is stimulated by vitamin A deficiency, epidermal growth factor, and transforming growth factor-α. The second step involves terminal cell division and subsequent expression of the squamous phenotype. This step is attended by changes in the elaboration of certain cytokeratins and in the activity of the enzyme transglutaminase and the level of its substrate, involucrin, which are responsible for formation of a cross-linked protein envelope in squamous-cell differentiation. Although transglutaminase and involucrin are codistributed in the superficial layers of normal epithelial cells, in premalignant tissues their synthesis is uncoupled, and they appear in cell layers in which they are not normally found (17).

Cytokeratins are intermediate-sized filaments present in epithelial cells. Many different types of keratins characteristic of particular cell types can be distinguished by monoclonal antibodies. Studies in a wide variety of human and animal tissues have noted that during step 2 of abnormal squamous differentiation, the types of keratins expressed, and their distribution among cell layers, change. Lippman and colleagues are examining their utility as biomarkers of carcinogenesis (18).

A final potential molecular marker derives from the expression of specific antigens on the surfaces of cells in various states of premalignancy. Antigens such as glycolipids and proteins have been described that are characteristic of particular cancer cell types. Using immunostaining of sputum specimens from the Johns Hopkins Lung Project, which evaluated the efficacy of sputum cytology screening for early detection of lung cancer, Tockman *et al.* reported that two monoclonal antibodies together predicted subsequent malignancy with 91% sensitivity and 88% specificity if the specimens were obtained within two years prior to the diagnosis of cancer (19). However, as they acknowledged, because normal sputum samples were discarded in the Johns Hopkins project, the specimens they studied were preselected for atypia, so the sensitivity of their antigens has not yet been compared directly with classic cytopathology. In fact, in some specimens, morphologic atypia preceded antigen expression by as much as two years. Nevertheless, antigens expressed early in the process of carcinogenesis, if reversible, may prove to be useful markers.

Many of the studies describing patterns of the newer markers in various tissues are subject to the limitations of the morphologic gold standards (metaplasia, atypia, leukoplakia, etc.). Many markers do not yet have data indicating whether they will be more sensitive, expressed earlier, or more specific than the gold standards. Possibly the studies with the most promise of overcoming these limitations are cell-culture studies and animal studies monitoring the markers throughout carcinogenesis. But before any of them can receive widespread use in human chemoprevention trials, they must be validated in humans.

Regression to the Mean—Biological and Methodological Sources

Whenever persons are screened for extreme values of a biological marker and that marker is subsequently used as an end point in a clinical trial, a risk exists for confounding due to regression to the mean. Regression to the mean is the phenomenon whereby persons with an extreme observed value of a variable tend to have less extreme values, closer to the population mean, on subsequent measurements (20). Any group selected for values deviating more than a given amount from the population mean at a point in time will contain some persons whose values appear extreme only because of random fluctuation or errors in measurement (21)—biological and methodological sources of error, respectively. Although best described in relation to trials of treatment for hypertension and hypercholesterolemia, regression to the mean will occur when any continuous biological variable is similarly measured in a select group.

Therefore, if a researcher screens a group of persons at elevated risk for lung cancer, such as smokers, selects a subgroup with a level of a putative intermediate end point deviating from the mean, and then remeasures the end point, the subgroup will almost certainly appear to have improved. If a placebo group is included, the change may be misinterpreted as placebo effect. This subtle but serious issue will potentially confound every intermediate end point trial that does not address it. There are several ways to reduce or eliminate regression to the mean.

If a subgroup must be selected for study, the most straightforward approach is to use separate screening and base-line data points. The researcher screens a population (such as smokers) that is expected to have a high prevalence of abnormal values of the end point (such as sputum samples for bronchial metaplasia and/or atypia). If a purer sample of persons with especially extreme values is needed, the screening can be extended to two separate measurements at varying intervals, with truncation of the group occurring both times, below the same or different thresholds (20, 22). In the case of bronchial intermediate end points this will generally be too cumbersome. In either case, when the desired subgroup is identified, the end point is remeasured at the time of entry to the trial; only the final measurement is used as the base line, and its results do not influence randomization.

The regression effect can be reduced, but not eliminated, by using an average of several measurements of the end point both to select the study group and to establish the base line for subsequent comparison. This approach, however, is not appropriate for some of the bronchial intermediate end points such as atypia, in which the researcher is interested in the appearance of the worst few cells rather than the average. It may be feasible for other end points such as micronuclei or DNA adducts.

A third way to minimize regression is to reduce methodological sources of error as much as possible. This will have a substantial effect if the great majority of measurement error is methodological and not biological, as is probably the case with sputum samples. Many smokers do not produce sputum consistently, and many samples actually contain no material from the lungs. Further, even "adequate" specimens have a high probability of failing to reveal lesions that are present. In preparing for a chemoprevention trial, we screened smokers for bronchial metaplasia and atypia, using two sputum specimens (23). We found that, in persons with metaplasia and/or atypia present in one of two specimens, 47% of the duplicate specimens contained no abnormalities, and 33% were unsatisfactory (containing no alveolar macrophages); only 20% of duplicate samples were also abnormal. In the actual trial recruitment we used three specimens for screening and, to control for regression to the mean, obtained five additional sputum samples in the metaplastic study group at the time of enrollment (24). Only 54% of these specimens contained metaplastic cells—a marked regression.

In our preliminary screening with two sputum specimens we detected an apparent 32% prevalence of metaplasia. With three specimens, the prevalence rate was 43%. In a trial with similar design, the Concerned Smoker Study, Arnold *et al.* used even more intensive screening with three pooled samples, each of which contained three sputum specimens (a total of nine), and detected atypia (not just metaplasia) in 77% (A. Arnold, personal communication). These results suggest that if the researcher sampled exhaustively, all persons with a history of smoking 15 or more pack-years might prove to have some metaplasia and/or atypia, and that its failure to appear in sputum specimens is primarily due to sampling limitations. It is not certain that screening with sputum samples really yields a group with a higher prevalence of metaplasia than the general population of heavy smokers. If this is the case, regression to the mean could be substantially reduced by more quantitative sampling, such as with bronchial brushings obtained through a bronchoscope.

Fourth, the regression effect can be removed if a study group is selected for a characteristic other than the end point to be measured. Subjects could be chosen according to their smoking history alone and then randomized. Levels of metaplasia and/or atypia in bronchial brushings could be measured before and after an intervention is applied. If metaplasia is virtually ubiquitous in heavy smokers, this approach has merit; the same would be true for any intermediate end point that is found in virtually all smokers.

Finally, even if the base-line mean and background variance of the end point have been definitely established through multiple measurements, it is critical to use a concurrent control group as the final means of separating treatment effect from regression to the mean.

Human Chemoprevention Trials

Only two completed human chemoprevention trials in persons at high risk for lung cancer have been reported in the literature, but a third has been completed and several others are in various stages of progress. Nearly all have used retinoids and/or beta-carotene. These trials will be summarized here, with emphasis on the populations being studied, the agents and end points used, and their status as of October, 1991.

Completed Trials

The first reported trial was conducted by Misset and colleagues in France (25). The population comprised 40 volunteers, each smoking a minimum of 15 pack-years and having an "index of metaplasia" greater than 15%. This index is the proportion of bronchoscopically obtained bronchial biopsies containing metaplasia out of a total of 10 predetermined biopsy sites. The investigators obtained biopsies before and after a 6-month treatment with the synthetic retinoid etretinate. They noted both a significant reduction in the index of metaplasia after treatment in most subjects and a complete resolution of metaplasia in four subjects who ceased smoking during the trial. The investigators mention only the prevalence of metaplasia; atypia, which may be a more important morphologic feature, is not mentioned.

The major limitation of this trial is that it cannot be purged of the effect of regression to the mean. The initial bronchoscopy was used to select a group with the desired degree of metaplasia, and the screening data were used as the base-line data. Although bronchoscopy probably removed most of the methodological measurement error, there was no placebo group to control for biological variability, which Band *et al.* noted to be substantial (4). All subjects were treated and served as their own controls.

The relevance of this unknown factor is underscored by the results of the Concerned Smoker Study, which has already reported recruitment methods and progress (26), compliance (using blood etretinate levels, pill counts, and sputum specimen delivery) (27, 28), and interobserver variation in sputum scoring (5). Arnold and his colleagues in Hamilton, Ontario, treated smokers with bronchial atypia with the same dose of etretinate used in the French trial and for the same length of time. Similarly, they did intensive screening for the desired abnormality and used the screening results as base-line data. By contrast, they used sputum samples rather than bronchoscopy, focused on atypia, and used a concurrent placebo group. Their results can be viewed as either the same as or as strikingly different from those of Misset *et al.* As in the latter trial, atypia in the treatment group improved significantly; in contrast, the placebo group, absent in the latter trial, improved equally (A. Arnold, personal communication). In actual fact, the Concerned Smoker Study may be no more "negative" than the French trial was "positive," because in neither can the effect of regression to the mean be removed in order to estimate a treatment effect. It may be possible for Arnold *et al.* to reanalyze their data in order to reduce the regression effect, but the best maneuver would have been to resample the subjects' sputum at the time of randomization to establish a more accurate base line for the selected group.

The final completed trial was conducted by our group in Birmingham (24). After detecting regression to the mean in a pilot trial, we changed the design and screened smokers for bronchial metaplasia and atypia (requiring only the former) using three sputum specimens, resampled their sputum at the time of randomization, and treated half of the enrolled group with folic acid and vitamin B_{12}. After four months, sputum samples in the treatment group showed significantly greater reduction in atypia score than did those in the placebo group. Although we attempted to refine the results by retrospectively measuring bronchial cell DNA content with image analysis, we experienced too much cell loss during destaining and restaining to produce evaluable results. Although this study was limited by its small sample size (n = 73) and the inherent problems of sputum sampling and scoring, it was probably not compromised by regression to the mean. The results suggest that folic acid, found in high quantities in many of the vegetables that protect against lung cancer, may reduce the severity of smoking injury and perhaps inhibit carcinogenesis.

Ongoing Trials

I am aware of four ongoing chemoprevention trials specifically addressing lung cancer. McLarty *et al.* in Tyler, Texas, are treating a group of asbestos workers with bronchial metaplasia and atypia, based on sputum samples, with retinol plus beta-carotene. The principal end point is improvement in atypia, although a reduction in the incidence of lung cancer may be seen. They have randomized 758 subjects and will follow each for a minimum of three years; those randomized earliest will have been observed for up to seven years (J. McLarty, personal communication). Follow-up should be completed in 1993.

A trial using beta-carotene and/or alpha-tocopherol for an average of six years in Finnish smokers, supported by the United States National Cancer Institute, is near completion. To be eligible to participate in this trial, subjects were required only to have a history of smoking five or more cigarettes per day. The trial is using the incidence of lung cancer and all cancers as the end point. The treatments or placebos are applied in a 2 × 2 factorial design, in an attempt to evaluate the effects of beta-carotene and alpha-tocopherol both independently and in combination. The study's recruitment and compliance results during a feasibility pilot phase have been published (29). The initial goal was to randomize 19 500 subjects.

Omenn and colleagues in Seattle are conducting a trial of supplementation with retinol and beta-carotene or a placebo in 14 000 smokers and in 4000 smokers with additional histories of significant asbestos exposure (30). Titled the Carotenoid and Retinoid Efficacy Trial, it will use the incidences of bronchogenic carcinoma and mesothelioma over a five-year period as end points. Substantial recruitment has been completed and is continuing.

In the only trial specifically designed both to test a chemopreventive agent and to validate multiple putative biomarkers, Lippman *et al.* in Houston are treating smokers who have an index of metaplasia greater than 16%, detected in bronchial biopsies from six standard sites, with isotretinoin (13-*cis*-retinoic acid) or a placebo (18). In addition to monitoring metaplasia, they are measuring the prevalence of micronuclei and mitotic figures, as well as levels of epidermal growth factor, involucrin, cytokeratins, proliferating cell nuclear antigen, and DNA polymerase-α. They have reported an association of micronuclei with smoking (12).

Conclusions

Future chemoprevention trials, particularly those using agents having less than substantial data behind them, will require the use of intermediate end points. All putative end points, particularly the newly proposed ones, must be validated in some way. In this regard it seems that bronchoscopy will be the preferred method for ensuring adequate and specific bronchial cell yields. Through this means, and by appropriate study design, regression to the mean must be eliminated in each study. Once other agents have substantial data bases favoring protective roles against lung cancer, as retinoids do now, longer-term trials using cancer as the principal end point will be appropriate. Even then, intermediate end points will be useful, and bronchoscopy may still be the preferred means of obtaining bronchial samples.

Once trials produce consistent answers, the knowledge gained will need to be applied. All involved uniformly agree that cessation of smoking will remain the best and most reliable means of preventing lung cancer. Beyond that, pharmacological and/or dietary means—and for the latter, either natural or technological methods—may be used to expose persons at varying levels of risk for cancer to the most effective agents. In the meantime, we should not lose sight of the consistently beneficial role shown for a high intake of vegetables and fruits.

REFERENCES

1. Zelen M. Are primary cancer prevention trials feasible? *J Natl Cancer Inst.* 1988;80:1442–1444.
2. Benfield JR, Hammond WG, Paladugu RR, Pak HY, Azumi N, Teplitz RL. Endobronchial carcinogenesis in dogs. *J Thorac Cardiovasc Surg.* 1986;92:880–889.
3. Greenberg SD, Spjut HJ, Estrada RG, Hunter NR, Greinia C. Morphometric markers for the evaluation of preneoplastic lesions in the lung: diagnostic evaluation by high-resolution image analysis of atypical cells in sputum specimens. *Anal Quant Cytol Histol.* 1987;9:49–54.
4. Band PR, Feldstein M, Saccomanno G. Reversibility of bronchial marked atypia: implication for chemoprevention. *Cancer Detect Prev.* 1986;9:157–160.
5. Browman GP, Arnold A, Levine MN, *et al.* Use of screening phase data to evaluate observer variation of sputum cytodiagnosis as an outcome measure in a chemoprevention trial. *Cancer Res.* 1990;50: 1216–1219.
6. Swank PR, Greenberg SD, Winkler DG, *et al.* Cell atypia profiles for monitoring preneoplastic changes in pulmonary squamous cell carcinogenesis. *Pathol Immunopathol Res.* 1986;5:47–53.
7. Ono J, Auer G, Caspersson T, *et al.* Reversibility of 20-methylcholanthrene-induced bronchial cell atypia in dogs. *Cancer.* 1984; 54:1030–1037.
8. Auer G, Kato H, Nasiell M, Roger V, Zetterberg A, Karlen L. Cy-

tophotometric DNA-analysis of atypical squamous metaplastic cells, carcinoma *in situ,* and bronchogenic carcinoma. In: Nieburgs HE, ed. *Cancer Detection in Specific Sites: Prevention and Detection of Cancer. Part II: Detection.* New York: Marcel Dekker; 1980:2;1465–1476.

9. Merkel DE, Dressler LG, McGuire WL. Flow cytometry, cellular DNA content, and prognosis in human malignancy. *J Clin Oncol.* 1987;5:1690–1703.
10. Aufferman W, Bocking A. Early detection of precancerous lesions in dysplasias of the lung by rapid DNA image cytometry. *Anal Quant Cytol Histol.* 1985;7:218–226.
11. Rosin MP, Dunn BP, Stich HF. Use of intermediate endpoints in quantitating the response of precancerous lesions to chemopreventive agents. *Can J Physiol Pharmacol.* 1987;65:483–487.
12. Lippman SM, Peters EJ, Wargovich MY, *et al.* Bronchial micronuclei as a marker of an early stage of carcinogenesis in the human tracheobronchial epithelium. *Int J Cancer.* 1990;45:811–815.
13. Stich HF, Rosin MP, Hornby AP, Mathew B, Sankaranarayanan R, Nair MK. Remission of oral leukoplakias and micronuclei in tobacco/betel quid chewers treated with beta-carotene and with beta-carotene plus vitamin A. *Int J Cancer.* 1988;42:195–199.
14. Randerath E, Miller RH, Mittal D, Avitts TA, Dunsford HA, Randerath K. Covalent DNA damage in tissues of cigarette smokers as determined by ^{32}P-postlabeling assay. *J Natl Cancer Inst.* 1989;81:341–347.
15. Dunn BP, Vedal S, San RHC, *et al.* DNA adducts in bronchial biopsies. *Int J Cancer.* 1991;48:485–492.
16. Jetten AM. Multistep process of squamous differentiation of tracheobronchial epithelial cells: role of retinoids. *Dermatologica.* 1987;175(S1):37–44.
17. Rice RH, Chakravarty R, Chen J, O'Callahan W, Rubin AL. Keratinocyte transglutaminase: regulation and release. *Adv Exp Med Biol.* 1988;231:51–61.
18. Lippman SM, Lee JS, Lotan R, Hittelman W, Wargovich MJ, Hong WK. Biomarkers as intermediate end points in chemoprevention trials. *J Natl Cancer Inst.* 1990;82:555–560.
19. Tockman MS, Gupta PK, Myers JD, *et al.* Sensitive and specific monoclonal antibody recognition of human lung cancer antigen on preserved sputum cells: a new approach to early lung cancer detection. *J Clin Oncol.* 1988;6:1685–1693.

20. McMahan CA. Regression toward the mean in a two-stage selection program. *Am J Epidemiol.* 1982;116:394–401.
21. Curnow RN. Correcting for regression in assessing the response to treatment in a selected population. *Stat Med.* 1987;6:113–117.
22. McMahan CA. Regression toward the mean in a two-stage selection program, II: correlated within-subject observations. *Am J Epidemiol.* 1987;125:912–916.
23. Heimburger DC, Krumdieck CL, Alexander CB, Birch R, Dill SR, Bailey WC. Localized folic acid deficiency and bronchial metaplasia in smokers: hypothesis and preliminary report. *Nutr Int.* 1987; 3:54–60.
24. Heimburger DC, Alexander CB, Birch R, Butterworth CE, Bailey WC, Krumdieck CL. Improvement in bronchial squamous metaplasia in smokers treated with folate and vitamin B_{12}: report of a preliminary randomized double-blind intervention trial. *JAMA.* 1988;259:1525–1530.
25. Misset JL, Mathe G, Santelli G, *et al.* Regression of bronchial epidermoid metaplasia in heavy smokers with etretinate treatment. *Cancer Detect Prev.* 1986;9:167–170.
26. Arnold A, Johnstone B, Stoskopf B, *et al.* Recruitment for an efficacy study in chemoprevention: the Concerned Smokers Study. *Prev Med.* 1989;18:700–710.
27. Browman GP, Arnold A, Booker L, Johnstone B, Skingley P, Levine MN. Etretinate blood levels in monitoring of compliance and contamination in a chemoprevention trial. *J Natl Cancer Inst.* 1989;81:795–798.
28. Arnold AM, Browman GP, Johnstone B, Skingley P, Booker L, Levine MN. Chemoprevention for lung cancer: evidence for a high degree of compliance. *Cancer Detect Prev.* 1990;14:521–525.
29. Albanes D, Virtamo J, Rautalahti M, *et al.* Pilot study: the US-Finland lung cancer prevention trial. *J Nutr Growth Cancer.* 1986; 3:207–214.
30. Omenn GS, Goodman GE, Kleinman GD, *et al.* The role of intervention studies in ascertaining the contribution of dietary factors in lung cancer. *Ann N Y Acad Sci.* 1988;534:575–583.

JOHN J. DiGIOVANNA, KENNETH H. KRAEMER, GARY L. PECK, and DONITA L. ABANGAN

Oral Isotretinoin Is Effective in the Prevention of Skin Cancer in Patients with Xeroderma Pigmentosum

ABSTRACT

Xeroderma pigmentosum is a rare, autosomal recessive disorder manifested by sun sensitivity, increased freckling, and defective DNA repair. Typically, patients with xeroderma pigmentosum develop large numbers of skin cancers, often starting at an early age. Five patients with xeroderma pigmentosum were cleared of existing cancers, then treated for two years with a high dosage (2.0 mg/kg per day) of isotretinoin, a derivative of vitamin A. These patients had a significant decrease in the number of new basal- and squamous-cell carcinomas compared to the two-year interval before treatment. After the drug was discontinued, the incidences of new skin cancers returned to pretreatment levels. To determine if chemoprevention could be attained with less toxicity, seven xeroderma pigmentosum patients were treated with a low dose (0.5 mg/kg per day) of isotretinoin. In most of the patients, during low-dose treatment, the frequency of skin cancers decreased in comparison to the interval without treatment. Mucocutaneous and laboratory toxicities were less frequent with the low-dosage treatment. We found that oral isotretinoin is effective in the prevention of skin cancer in patients with xeroderma pigmentosum; the lowest effective, least toxic dosage varies among patients.

Introduction

Skin cancer is the most common malignancy occurring in the United States, with approximately 600 000 new cases each year (1). Moreover, the incidence of skin cancer is increasing at an alarming rate.

The most common types of skin cancers are basal-cell carcinomas and squamous-cell carcinomas. Although these tumors only rarely metastasize, they have the capacity to be locally invasive and destructive and to cause significant morbidity.

The term *retinoid* refers to a group of compounds that includes vitamin A and its synthetic derivatives. Several naturally occurring vitamin A compounds exist. Some of these compounds have been shown to have specific biologic functions. Retinol is a common form of vitamin A that can be metabolized into the compounds that are necessary to fulfill all of the organism's functions that require vitamin A activity. Retinol can be metabolized to all-transretinoic acid. All-transretinoic acid has been studied for the treatment of a variety of disorders. The 13-*cis* isomer of all-transretinoic acid, 13-*cis*-retinoic acid (isotretinoin, Hoffman LaRoche), is a synthetic derivative that also occurs naturally in the human body in small quantities. When given systemically, 13-*cis*-retinoic acid has less clinical toxicity than all-transretinoic acid. Over two thousand synthetic derivatives have been synthesized in an effort to find active metabolites.

Vitamin A was initially related to cancer in 1926 when rats fed a diet deficient in vitamin A were found to develop carcinomas of the stomach (2). A main impetus for the development of the synthetic retinoids was their potential as anticancer agents. Some of them have been studied for cancer treatment and prevention. Early studies used isotretinoin systemically at high doses, and assessed its effect as a treatment for skin cancer (3, 4). Although in these studies isotretinoin was effective in causing resolution of some basal-cell carcinomas, the cure rates were low and the toxicities were significant. While systemic isotretinoin therapy did not appear to be useful as a treatment for most basal-cell carcinomas, some patients appeared to have a decrease in the development of new skin cancers while on isotretinoin therapy (5).

Xeroderma pigmentosum (XP) is an extremely rare autosomal recessive genodermatosis. This disorder is characterized by sun sensitivity and a deficiency in the repair of ultraviolet-damaged DNA (6). Consequently, patients with XP develop skin cancers at a frequency of more than 1000 times that of the general population (7). In addition these individuals begin to develop skin cancers at a very early age. Because of the high rate of new skin cancer formation in patients with XP, they are good candidates for studies of cancer prevention in humans.

In an effort to determine whether isotretinoin would be effective in the prevention of new skin cancers in patients who were developing large numbers of tumors, a study was undertaken in the Clinical Center at the National Institutes of Health to evaluate the ability of systemic isotretinoin to prevent skin cancer in patients with XP.

Study Design

Patients were chosen who had typical clinical features of XP and a high frequency of skin cancers. Clinical features included photosensitivity, xerosis, large numbers of freckles, lentigines, and irregular pigmented lesions in sun-exposed areas. All patients had a history of two or more skin cancers per year for the previous two years. Records were obtained from referring physicians to determine the number of histologically diagnosed skin cancers. Before treatment began, photographs were obtained of the entire skin surface with many close-ups. Routine blood tests including liver function tests, fasting triglycerides and cholesterol levels, urinalysis, and x-rays of the spine were obtained. A complete physical and an ophthalmologic examination were also performed. Before treatment all existing skin cancers were removed. Patients were seen at intervals of two weeks, one month, two months, and then at least every three months. At each visit the patient's skin was examined by at least two dermatologists, and all unusual lesions were photographed. A biopsy was done on any lesion suspected of being a skin cancer to obtain histological verification. The lesion was then treated appropriately. Patients were treated with isotretinoin (Accutane, Hoffman LaRoche) at 2 mg/kg per day in two equal doses. At each clinic visit, blood and urine tests were repeated. After two years of treatment isotretinoin was discontinued, and patients were observed for at least one year off isotretinoin.

Patients who continued to develop new tumors off treatment were enrolled in phase II of the study. For these patients, isotretinoin was restarted at the low dosage of 0.5 mg/kg per day, and patients were observed for the development of new skin cancers for at least one year. Patients who did not have an adequate response to this dosage would subsequently be treated (phase III) with the intermediate dosage of 1.0 mg/kg per day of isotretinoin.

Results

Phase I: High-Dosage Trial of Oral Isotretinoin

Seven patients with XP were enrolled in phase I (high-dosage—2.0 mg/kg per day). The results of this study have been published (8). Five patients from 10 to 39 years old were able to tolerate the high dosage for two years and completed the study. These patients had 8 to 43 histologically confirmed basal-cell or squamous-cell carcinomas in the two-year interval before treatment. Two additional patients (a 5-year-old girl and a 16-year-old boy) were unable to complete the protocol because of persistent laboratory abnormalities.

Response to Treatment

In the five patients studied, the total number of tumors decreased from 121 (mean, 24; range 8 to 43) in the two years before treatment to 25 (mean, 5; range 3 to 9) in the two years of treatment. This was a mean reduction of the tumor rate of 63% ($P = 0.019$). The results of the study for each patient are summarized in Table 1. Four of these five patients had a reduction in the number of tumors during treatment compared with the number of tumors that occurred before treatment. This improvement was noted quickly, within two months of the start of treatment. After a two-year treatment interval, isotretinoin was stopped. During the posttreatment period there was an increase in the frequency of skin cancers in all five patients. This increase oc-

Table 1. Number of Skin Cancers in Patients with Xeroderma Pigmentosum Treated with Oral Isotretinoin (2 mg/kg/day)

Patient (Age, Sex)	Before Treatment (2 yrs)	During High-Dose Treatment (2 yrs)	After Treatment (12–14 mos)
1 (19, F)	43 (21.5)	3 (1.5)	18 (18.0)
2 (12, F)	37 (18.5)	4 (2.0)	29 (38.7)[a]
3 (17, M)	23 (11.5)	6 (3.0)	20 (20.0)
4 (39, M)	10 (5.0)	3 (1.5)	4 (3.4)
5 (10, M)	8 (4.0)	9 (4.5)	10 (10.0)

Adapted with permission from Kraemer *et al.* (8).

[a] Treatment was resumed after nine months because of the large number of tumors that appeared after the drug was discontinued.

curred rapidly and was apparent within three months of stopping treatment. There was an 8.5-fold increase in the annual rate of occurrence of tumors (range, 2- to 19-fold) in the posttreatment period as compared with the treatment period ($P = 0.007$). The best response to treatment was seen in those patients who had the highest frequency of tumors before treatment.

SIDE EFFECTS

All patients treated experienced cheilitis and xerosis of the skin, especially on the face. These conditions were usually relieved with topical lubricants. Patients with XP have chronic eye problems even without retinoid therapy. These patients often develop conjunctivitis and have eyelid deformity from surgical procedures. After chronic ophthalmologic problems they may develop ectropion. Blepharitis and conjunctivitis were increased by isotretinoin therapy. Some elevations in serum triglyceride levels and abnormalities in liver function tests occurred while patients were on isotretinoin. Some patients had increased peak levels of triglyceride, ranging from 1.5 to 8 times their normal levels. Dietary adjustment usually lowered triglyceride levels to the normal range. Occasional abnormalities in liver function tests occurred in three patients, but in these patients results of tests became normal with continued treatment. One patient had persistent liver function test abnormalities. That patient was unable to continue treatment for the entire two-year period at the high dosage and therefore was withdrawn from the protocol. Mild arthralgias of the spine and peripheral joints occurred in some patients.

Phase II: Low-Dosage Trial of Oral Isotretinoin

We can conclude from phase I of this study that isotretinoin is effective in the prevention of new skin cancers in patients with XP. Because of the severity of the mucocutaneous and laboratory toxicities, we considered the high dosage too toxic for long-term therapy. We were therefore interested in continuing this study for a second phase to determine whether a low dosage (0.5 mg/kg per day) of isotretinoin, also given orally, would be effective in the chemoprevention of skin cancers in patients with XP.

All seven patients who were enrolled in the phase I trial were included in phase II of the study—the five patients who were able to tolerate isotretinoin at 2 mg/kg per day for two years and the two patients whose dosage had to be lowered because of toxicity. Patients were treated with oral isotretinoin at 0.5 mg/kg per day for one year and followed for the incidence of new tumors and toxicity. In comparison to the interval without treatment, the frequency of skin cancers occurring during the low-dosage treatment decreased in most patients. In some patients, there was an apparent dose response. Furthermore, mucocutaneous toxicity and laboratory abnormalities were less severe with the low-dosage treatment. This study is continuing in an effort to better define the therapeutic effect and toxicities of isotretinoin in this condition.

Summary

The first phase of this study was a high-dosage trial of oral isotretinoin in the chemoprevention of skin cancer in patients with XP. That part of the study demonstrated that oral isotretinoin was effective in the prevention of skin cancer in XP patients actively developing large numbers of new tumors. In this study all tumors were removed before beginning oral isotretinoin therapy. We did not assess whether isotretinoin would be effective in the treatment of existing tumors. However, prior studies suggest that it would be, at best, poorly effective.

The second phase of this study demonstrated that there was great individual variation between the dosage of oral isotretinoin required for effective chemoprevention. Some patients had good results on 0.5 mg/kg per day, and the low dosage was associated with less mucocutaneous toxicity and fewer laboratory abnormalities.

Discussion

A primary motivation for the synthesis and study of vitamin A and the synthetic retinoids has been their potential in the treatment and prevention of skin cancer. The studies discussed here demonstrate that, for some XP patients, isotretinoin is effective in the prevention of skin cancers. The benefit is not long lasting, as the frequency of new skin cancer formation returns quickly after the isotretinoin is discontinued. The rapid onset and loss of effect, coincident with therapy, suggests that isotretinoin is acting at a late stage in carcinogenesis. It is probably not acting by correcting the defect in DNA repair. Consequently, patients who did not have XP but are developing many new skin cancers per year may also benefit from this approach.

Many derivatives of vitamin A have been synthesized. These compounds vary in their range of activity and spectrum of toxicity. The synthetic retinoid 4-hydroxyphenyl retinamide (Fenretinide) is effective in the prevention of mammary tumors in rodents and is being studied in the prevention of human cancer (9, 10). Other retinoids may be tailored by manipulation of their chemical structure to be active in the treatment or prevention of specific tumors. There is great promise that in the future retinoid derivatives may be found that will have greater therapeutic efficacy and less toxicity and may be useful in the chemoprevention of not only skin cancer but other malignancies as well.

REFERENCES

1. Scotto J, Fears TR, Fraumeni JF Jr. Incidence of nonmelanoma skin cancer in the United States. Bethesda, Md: Department of Health and Human Services; 1981. DHHS publication no. (NIH) 82-2433.
2. Peck GL, DiGiovanna JJ. Retinoids. In: Fitzpatrick TB, Eisen AZ, Wolff K, Freedberg IM, Austen KF, eds. *Dermatology in General Medicine.* 3rd ed. New York: McGraw-Hill; 1987:2582–2906.
3. Peck GL, Yoder FW, Olsen TG, Pandya MD, Butkus D. Treatment of Darier's disease, lamellar ichthyosis, pityriasis rubra pilaris, cystic acne, and basal cell carcinoma with oral 13-*cis*-retinoic acid. *Dermatologica* 1978;157(suppl 1):11–12.
4. Peck GL, Olsen TG, Butkus D, *et al.* Treatment of basal cell carcinomas with 13-*cis*-retinoic acid. *Proc Am Assoc Cancer Res.* 1979;20:56. abstract.
5. Peck GL, Gross EG, Butkus D, DiGiovanna JJ. Chemoprevention of basal cell carcinoma with isotretinoin. *J Am Acad Dermatol.* 1982;6:815–823.
6. Kraemer KH, Lee MM, Scotto J. Xeroderma pigmentosum: cutaneous, ocular, and neurologic abnormalities in 830 published cases. *Arch Dermatol.* 1987;123:241–250.
7. Kraemer KH, Lee MM, Scotto J. DNA repair protects against cutaneous and internal neoplasia: evidence from xeroderma pigmentosum. *Carcinogenesis.* 1984;5:511–514.

8. Kraemer KH, DiGiovanna JJ, Moshell AN, Tarone RE, Peck GL. Prevention of skin cancer in xeroderma pigmentosum with the use of oral isotretinoin. *N Engl J Med.* 1988;318:1633–1637.
9. Moon RC, Itri LM. Retinoids and cancer. In: Sporn MB, Roberts AB, Goodman DS, eds. *The Retinoids.* Orlando, Fla: Academic Press; 1984;2:327–371.
10. Modiano MR, Dalton WS, Lippman SM, *et al.* Phase II study of fenretinide (N-[4-hydroxyphenyl]retinamide) in advanced breast cancer and melanoma. *Invest New Drugs.* 1990;8:317–319.

C. E. BUTTERWORTH, JR.

Folic Acid Deficiency and Cervical Dysplasia

ABSTRACT

Cervical dysplasia is generally regarded as the earliest detectable stage of cervical cancer. It is readily curable, but early detection and treatment place a heavy burden on the health care delivery system; primary prevention would be a desirable alternative. The probable causative agent, human papilloma virus, can be found in some normal biopsies as well as in dysplastic tissue, suggesting differences in viral gene expression. In a recent case-control study of women with the human papilloma virus, the risk of dysplasia was fivefold greater among women in the lower two tertiles of red blood cell folate content than in the highest. Folate deficiency may facilitate incorporation of human papilloma virus genomes into host chromosomes at a folate-sensitive fragile site. Oral folate supplements do not alter the course of established disease. However, evidence suggests that a significant reduction in early cervical cancer could be achieved in up to two-thirds of high-risk populations through improved nutritional intake of folate before exposure to an oncogenic strain of papilloma virus.

Introduction

Cervical dysplasia, or cervical intraepithelial neoplasia (CIN), is generally regarded as the earliest detectable stage of cervical cancer. Preinvasive lesions, including carcinoma in situ, can be successfully eradicated by relatively simple local measures such as excisional biopsy, cryosurgery, and laser-beam microsurgery in the ambulatory setting. Some early cases appear to be self-limited and disappear spontaneously but require careful monitoring. From 1947 to 1984 there was a decline of approximately 70% in cervical cancer mortality in the United

States, attributable largely to the increasing availability of Papanicolaou (Pap) smear screening programs (1). Early detection is undoubtedly the key to successful patient management, but it imposes heavy demands on the health care delivery system. Early detection requires ready access to clinical facilities for examination and management, either through low-cost community-based or private resources. It is also necessary to maintain quality assurance in laboratory programs for accurate interpretation of Pap smears and biopsy specimens. In addition, health professionals as well as the general public must be educated about the importance of regular screening, appropriate treatment, and follow-up. Programs that are presently operating are not without considerable cost and may be reaching the point of diminishing returns.

Even with continued improvement in health care systems the cancer mortality rate for white women in the United States changed very little from 1980 to 1987, declining from 3.6 to 2.9 per 100,000, a drop of only 11% (Fig. 1). For black women mortality declined somewhat more steeply from 10.1 to 7.6 per 100,000 during the same period (2),

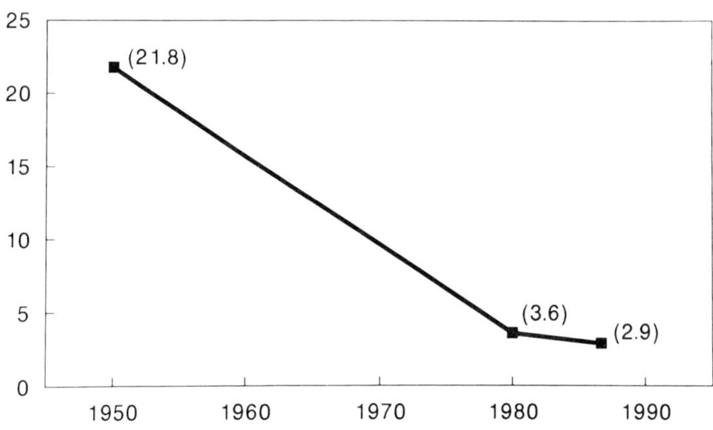

Figure 1. The mortality rate for cervical cancer in the United States declined by approximately 70% from 1947 to 1984. Much of the improvement has been attributed to increased use of the Papanicolaou smear test and better access to facilities for diagnosis and treatment. From 1980 to 1987 the death rate declined by 11%, from 3.6 to 2.9 per 100 000 (1, 2). During this interval the death rate for black women fell from 10.1 to 7.6 per 100 000. However, even in 1987 the mortality rate for black women was 2.6 times that of whites.

a rate of 25%. The relative slowing in the rate of improvement in mortality during the 1980s could be due to saturation of existing resources for early detection and outpatient management. This could be due in part to an actual increase in the number of cases of dysplasia, a relative increase in the rate of detection of earlier lesions, limited access to clinical facilities, and failure to follow suspicious lesions. Promising new techniques for detecting specific viral gene products in peripheral blood samples may facilitate screening procedures and ultimately obviate the need for direct examination of the cervix in some cases.

Until recently the possibility of primary prevention has received little attention. Current evidence suggests that it may be possible to reduce the incidence of cervical dysplasia in certain populations through improving nutritional reserves of folate. Although other approaches, such as greater use of barrier contraceptives, antiviral drugs, and vaccines, may be worthy of consideration, the following discussion will be directed primarily at the possibility of lowering cervical cancer risk by maintaining normal nutritional reserves of folate.

Incidence

In 1987 in the United States cancer of the uterus was the third most common cause of cancer death among women 15 to 34 years of age, and the fourth most common cause in the 35- to 54-year-old age group (3). Approximately half these cases are listed as cancer of the cervix, whereas the remainder are listed as originating in the corpus uteri and unspecified sites, which include the cervix. It is estimated that in 1991 uterine cancer will rank fourth among the six major causes of cancer death among all women (after lung, breast, and colon/rectum) (3). Approximately 50 000 new cases of cervical carcinoma in situ were projected to occur in 1991 (3). However, only 7% would be likely to result in death. This is a reflection of the curability of CIN when detected. It is also a reminder of the large number of women who must undergo pelvic examinations and multiple Pap smear screening to achieve this result.

In parts of the developing world, cervical cancer is the leading cause of cancer deaths among women. In Suriname the age-adjusted death rate for cervical cancer was 22.5 per 100 000 population during 1984–1986 (3). This is the highest recorded rate among 48 countries for which recent mortality statistics are available. Suriname is followed by Costa Rica, Chile, Panama, and Romania in that order. The United States ranked thirty-seventh among the same 48 reporting countries during 1984–1986, with an annual mortality of 3.2 per 100 000. By contrast, the lowest rate reported in recent years was 0.9 per 100 000, in Italy (3). A goal has been proposed for lowering the United States mortality rate to 1.5 per 100 000 by the year 2000 (2). It seems unlikely that this goal can be reached at the present rate of decline.

Epidemiology and Risk Factors

Epidemiologic studies have led to the identification of a variety of risk factors for cervical cancer (4), many of which are related directly or indirectly to sexual activity. These include early age of first sexual intercourse and first pregnancy; total number of live births; number of male sexual partners; and use of oral contraceptive steroid hormones. There is controversy about the last factor, however, since oral contraceptive users may be subject to closer scrutiny than nonusers (5). On the other hand, tissue culture studies have shown that the oncogenic potential for cells exposed to human papilloma virus (HPV) is enhanced in the presence of either progesterone or glucocorticoids (6). Thus the steroid hormones present in oral contraceptives or occurring naturally with pregnancy could influence the course of HPV infection. Other risk factors identified by epidemiologic investigations are cigarette smoking, low socioeconomic status, and immunosuppression (7). The basis for an association between cervical cancer and cigarette smoking is not clear, but it could involve the increased requirements for vitamin C (8) and folate (9) among smokers. Similarly, low socioeconomic status could simply be an indicator of inadequate nutrition as well as limited access to health care.

One of the most significant advances in the epidemiology of cervical cancer in recent years is recognition of HPVs as important etiologic agents (10–15). More than fifty different strains have been identified, of which types 16, 18, 31, 33, and 35 have been found most commonly in association with cancers of the female genital tract. Although infection of cervical epithelial cells with HPV is now regarded as the probable cause of cervical cancer, HPV genomes do appear in normal tissue as well (16). Therefore, it has become necessary to consider various systems that may be involved in the regulation of oncogene expression, including nutritional status and immunity.

Folate Deficiency

Several separate lines of investigation have converged to focus attention on folate deficiency as a potential risk factor for cervical cancer. In 1968, Shojania and colleagues (17) reported the occurrence of low serum folate values among oral contraceptive users. Two years later Streiff described seven women with folate deficiency and megaloblastic anemia associated with use of oral contraceptives (18). In 1973 Whitehead and associates (19) presented evidence that megaloblastic changes can occur in cervical smears of oral contraceptive users even in the absence of anemia and without diminished serum folate levels. They introduced the important concept of localized folate deficiency occurring in target tissue as a result of steroid hormone stimulation and demonstrated that megaloblastic cervical cytology became normal after a few weeks of oral folate supplementation. The concept of selective sex hormone–related changes in cervical epithelium has been confirmed in a group of young women in Shanxi, China, a district in which the frequency of both folate deficiency and cervical cancer is high (20). Dysplastic change, average nuclear diameter, and hyperploidy improved with one to three months of oral folate supplementation in 13 oral contraceptive users from this district (20).

Since 1977 several reports have indicated an increased incidence of cervical cancer among oral contraceptive users (21–24). In 1982 it was noted that there are morphologic similarities between the cytologic features of megaloblastosis and those associated with cervical dysplasia (25). It was also reported at that time that 10 mg daily of oral folate supplements led to improvement in cervical biopsies, and it was suggested that megaloblastic features are sometimes mistaken for dysplasia or are part of the dysplastic process (25). A more extensive trial of supplementation (26) in a group of dysplastic subjects failed to demonstrate improvement in biopsy status at the end of six months (see below). It now seems likely that the beneficial effects of folic acid supplementation observed earlier were due to misclassification of megaloblastic features as dysplasia, or inclusion of subjects with atypia-LTD (less than dysplasia). In an evaluation of 50 subjects with atypia-LTD, Borst *et al.* (27) found a higher-than-normal incidence of positive tests for HPV-16 (46% versus 11.6% among normals). Seven subjects (14%) were found to have CIN by colposcopically directed biopsy. Although approximately 60% of women with mild dysplasia show spontaneous regression to normal (26, 28), current evidence suggests that they, as well as women with atypia-LTD, should be closely monitored to determine if progression occurs. The relationship of HPV-infection and folate deficiency to atypia-LTD needs further clarification.

The general subject of folate deficiency and cancer has been reviewed elsewhere (29, 30). The prevailing view is that folate deficiency is not carcinogenic alone, but acts as a cocarcinogenic factor in the presence of chemical carcinogens or other oncogenic events. The folic acid antagonist methotrexate is capable of acting as a cocarcinogen during the initial stages of carcinogenesis and as an anticancer agent in established cases (31). There is evidence that folate deficiency is associated with increased incidence of malignant or premalignant lesions of the esophagus (32, 33), lung (34), colon (35), and hematopoietic system (36).

Possible Relationship of Folate Deficiency to Oncogene Expression

Most human chromosomes carry at least one protooncogene, many of which are at specific sites and are associated with certain types of malignancy. Sublethal folate deficiency appears to interfere with DNA repair mechanisms in such a way as to permit chromosomal deletions, translocations, and viral gene insertions. As a result, normal regulatory mechanisms based on the function of adjacent genes become disrupted (37). In addition, it has been suggested that undermethylation of DNA, a consequence of folate deficiency, leads to enhanced transcription of genetic information through interference with histone binding sites.

The discovery of the folate-sensitive fragile site on X chromosomes in cases of hereditary mental retardation by Sutherland in 1979 (38) led to renewed interest in folate and DNA repair. In 1984 Yunis and Soreng (39) reported the existence of 51 fragile sites on human chromosomes, 20 of which correlated with breakpoints known to occur in human malignancy. It has been demonstrated in an established line of cultured cells derived from a patient with cervical carcinoma that the DNA genome of HPV-18 is integrated at a single site on chromosome 12 (40). By means of direct in situ DNA hybridization it was shown that the viral genome was present at the same location as a heritable fragile site, which may have facilitated incorporation of genetic material from the virus (40).

Clinical Investigations

My colleagues and I recently completed two closely related interdisciplinary trials covering the period 1985–1990 (26, 41). The first was a case-control study involving 294 cases of dysplasia and 170 controls, derived from screening 726 ambulatory subjects at community family-planning clinics. The population sample was 67% black and 33% white, and had a median annual income of less than $9000, a median age of 25 years, and an average of 12 years of formal education. The second study was a double-blind therapeutic intervention trial in which women identified as cases in the case-control study took part in a six-month follow-up program without biopsy or locally aggressive treatment. They were randomly assigned to receive a daily oral supplement consisting of either 10 mg of folic acid or 10 mg of ascorbate (the latter being regarded as a placebo). After six months, a biopsy was obtained under colopscopic guidance and appropriate therapy was provided if needed.

In the case-control study, logistic regression models were used to compute odds ratios for various risk factors (exposures). As expected, cervical dysplasia was significantly associated with the number of sexual partners, parity, the use of oral contraceptives, and the presence of HPV-16 infection. Infection with HPV-16 proved to be the strongest single risk factor for cervical dysplasia in this series. There was in general no risk associated with multiple laboratory indexes of nutritional status (hematocrit, plasma levels of vitamin C, retinol, carotenoids, folate, B_{12}, iron, copper, zinc, red cell folate, red cell B_6 transaminase activity; lymphocyte dU suppression tests). The absence of an association between plasma nutrient levels and dysplasia can be attributed to the use of nonfasting blood specimens obtained at the time of the clinic visit.

An unexpected finding emerged when upper, middle, and lower tertiles of red cell folate concentration were statistically analyzed for interaction with certain other variables. Unlike plasma folate, the folate content of red blood cells (RBC) is not subject to variation because of recent ingestion of food and is believed to be a more accurate index of body stores. It was observed that women with RBC folate values greater than 660 nmol/L were not at increased risk for dysplasia in association with cigarette smoking, parity, or HPV-16 infection. However, among women in the lower two tertiles (<660 nmol/L) the odds ratios for each of these variables were consistently elevated. In the case of HPV-16 infection the odds ratio (OR) was 5.1 (95% confidence interval [CI] 2.3 to 11.1) for women in the lower tertiles of RBC folate compared with 1.1 (95% CI 0.4 to 3.1) for the upper tertile. The joint effect of low RBC folate and HPV-16 positive status was statistically significantly larger than the sum or product of the independent effects ($P < 0.05$), thus fulfilling the definition of interaction. Although the risk of dysplasia was somewhat greater among oral contraceptive users with low levels of RBC folate (OR 3.5), the risk was present (OR 2.3) among oral contraceptive users with RBC folate levels greater than 660 nmol/L. This can be explained by either an independent effect of oral contraceptives or overrepresentation of current oral contraceptive users in the population sample.

The minimal rates of dysplasia observed among subjects in the upper tertile of RBC folate suggest that normal folate nutriture is protective. Although the mechanism of protection is unknown, it is conceivable that folate and/or dietary factors associated with it could minimize chromosome breakage at fragile sites and the opportunistic insertion of viral oncogenes. Other possible mechanisms include maintenance of normal metabolic pathways for single-carbon transport, repair of epithelial surfaces, and maintenance of normal immune functions.

The clinical intervention trial did not confirm the hypothesis that oral folic acid supplements would exert a beneficial effect on the course of dysplasia during the six-month period of observation (26). At the end of the study the cytologic and histologic findings were not statistically significantly different in folate-supplemented subjects versus those who received the placebo. Biopsies were normal in 66% of those receiving a placebo and 64% of those receiving the folic acid supplement. In keeping with the case-control study, there was a higher incidence of positive HPV-16 tests among cases with low RBC folate values at the initial visit ($P = 0.035$). The incidence of positive HPV-16 tests among all subjects was essentially the same at the end of the trial (33%) as at the beginning (31%). We concluded that folate deficiency may have a cocarcinogenic effect in the presence of exposure to HPV-16. However, folate supplements apparently have little or no effect after infection has occurred (26). This is consistent with the concept of a separate initiation phase that may be followed by a period of latency, regression, or progression of the induced change.

Conclusion

Two aspects of these investigations deserve special comment. First is the large number of subjects apparently at increased risk (41). As much as two-thirds of the population represented by the sample appears to have suboptimal folate nutritional status and might benefit from improved eating habits or supplements or both. This is not surprising in view of reports that 70% of low-income women participating in the second National Health and Nutrition Examination Survey consumed less than 50% of the 1980 recommended dietary allowance for folate (42). The observations concerning dysplasia incidence (41) provide evidence that poor nutritional intake of folate is associated with serious consequences and is not merely an abstract statistical finding.

The second important feature of these investigations is that overt manifestations of folate deficiency were lacking in the cases of dysplasia (41). Subjects were ambulatory and nonanemic, and did not have glossitis or diarrhea. The determination of risk was based on the association of a clinical finding (dysplasia) with red cell folate values in the lower two tertiles of the population under study, not with an arbitrary definition of desirable intake (such as recommended dietary allowance or United States recommended dietary allowance), and not by comparison with blood levels in a selected normal population. Whatever the underlying mechanism, the results suggest that two-thirds of this particular population of low-income women are not consuming adequate amounts of folate.

In an extensive review of the literature on the importance of nutritional status to pregnancy outcome, Bendich (43) stressed both the prevalence of low folate intake among low-income women and the need for adequate micronutrient reserves at the time of conception. The recent report from the Medical Research Council (UK) provides conclusive evidence that folate supplementation prior to pregnancy affords significant protection against the occurrence of a neural tube defect in children born of high-risk mothers (44). Supplementation is not effective if initiated during the middle of the first trimester, which is the time most women become aware of their pregnancy. The central issue seems to be that a transient period of deficiency may be of crucial importance in connection with both neural tube defects and HPV infection. In both cases the key consideration seems to be long-range prevention and maintenance of reserves above some critical level below which increased risks occur.

Bendich (43) concluded that the recent decrease in the recommended dietary allowance for folate (Food and Nutrition Board, 1989) from the previous level of 400 μg to 180 μg should be reversed for women of childbearing age. The findings in connection with cervical dysplasia (26, 41) support this conclusion. The accumulated evidence suggests that improved folate intake could significantly lower the incidence not only of birth defects but also of cervical dysplasia and cervical cancer in certain high-risk populations.

REFERENCES

1. Devesa SS, Silverman DT, Young JL, *et al.* Cancer incidence and mortality trends among whites in the US, 1947–84. *J Natl Cancer Inst.* 1987;79:701.
2. Centers for Disease Control. Black-white differences in cervical cancer mortality—United States, 1980–1987. *JAMA.* 1990;263: 3001–3002.
3. Boring CC, Squires TS, Tong T. Cancer statistics, 1991. *CA.* a cancer journal for clinicians. 1991;41:19–36.
4. Brinton LA, Fraumeni JF Jr. Epidemiology of uterine cervical cancer. *J Chron Dis.* 1986;39:1051–1065.
5. Irwin KL, Rosero-Bixby L, Oberle MW, *et al.* Oral contraceptives and cervical cancer risk in Costa Rica: detection bias or causal association? *JAMA.* 1988;259:59–64.
6. Pater MM, Hughes GA, Hyslop DE, Nakshatri H, Pater A. Glucocorticoid-dependent oncogenic transformation by type 16 but not type 11 human papillomavirus DNA. *Nature.* 1988;335: 832–835.
7. Brinton LA, Schairer C, Haenszel W, *et al.* Cigarette smoking and invasive cervical cancer. *JAMA.* 1986;255:3265–3269.
8. Pelletier O. Vitamin C and cigarette smokers. *Ann N Y Acad Sci.* 1975;258:156–168.
9. Witter FR, Blake DA, Baumgardner R, *et al.* Folate, carotene and smoking. *Am J Obstet Gynecol.* 1982;144:857.
10. Jenson AB, Lancaster WD. Association of human papillomavirus

with benign, premalignant, and malignant anogenital lesions. Chapter 2, pp. 11–45. In: Pfister H, ed. Papillomaviruses and Human Cancer. Boca Raton, Fla: CRC Press; 1990:11–45.
11. Meisels A, Morin C. Human papillomavirus and cancer of the uterine cervix. *Gynecol Oncol.* 1981;12:S111–S123.
12. Durst M, Kleinheinz A, Hotz M, Gissmann L. The physical state of human papillomavirus type 16 DNA in benign and malignant genital tumors. *J Gen Virol.* 1985;66:1515–1522.
13. Crum CP, Ikenberg H, Richart RM, Gissman L. Human papillomavirus DNA from a cervical carcinoma and its prevalence in cancer biopsy samples from different geographic regions. *Proc Natl Acad Sci U S A.* 1983;80:3812–3815.
14. Reeves WC, Brinton LA, Garcia M, *et al.* Human papillomavirus infection and cervical cancer in Latin America. *N Engl J Med.* 1989;320:1437–1441.
15. Lorincz AT, Schiffman MH, Jaffurs WJ, Marlow J, Quinn AP, Temple GF. Temporal associations of human papillomavirus infection with cervical cytologic abnormalities. *Am J Obstet Gynecol.* 1990;162:645–651.
16. Macnab JCM, Walkinshaw A, Cordiner JW, Clements JB. Human papillomavirus in clinically and histologically normal tissue of patients with genital cancer. *N Engl J Med.* 1986;315:1052–1058.
17. Shojania AM, Hornady G, Barnes PH. Oral contraceptives and serum-folate level. *Lancet.* 1968; 1376–1377.
18. Streiff RR. Folate deficiency and oral contraceptives. *JAMA.* 1970; 214:105–108.
19. Whitehead N, Reyner F, Lindenbaum J. Megaloblastic changes in the cervical epithelium: association with oral contraceptive therapy and reversal with folic acid. *JAMA.* 1973;226:1421–1424.
20. Ran JY, Li XF, Rau HL, Wang LY, Herbert V. Selective folate deficiency in one but not another cell line: despite "normal" red cell folate, folate therapy reduced cervical dysplasia and hyperploidy in women using oral contraceptives. *Blood.* 1990;76(10, suppl 1):114a.
21. Peritz E, Ramcharan S, Frank J, Brown WL, Huang S, Ray R. The incidence of cervical cancer and duration of oral contraceptive use. *Am J Epidemiol.* 1977;106:462–469.
22. Stern E. Steroid contraceptive use and cervical dysplasia: increased risk of progression. *Science.* 1977;196:1460–1462.
23. Swan SH, Brown WL. Oral contraceptive use, sexual activity and cervical carcinoma. *Am J Obstet Gynecol.* 1981;139:52–57.

24. Vessey MP, Lawless M, McPherson Y, Yeates D. Neoplasia of the cervix uteri and contraception: a possible adverse effect of the pill. *Lancet.* 1983;ii:930–934.
25. Butterworth CE Jr, Hatch KD, Gore H, Mueller H, Krumdieck CL. Improvement in cervical dysplasia associated with folic acid therapy in users of oral contraceptives. *Am J Clin Nutr.* 1982;35:73–82.
26. Butterworth CE Jr, Hatch KD, Soong SJ, *et al.* Oral folic acid supplementation for cervical dysplasia: a clinical intervention trial. *Am J Obstet Gynecol.* 1992;166:803–809.
27. Borst M, Butterworth CE Jr, Baker V, *et al.* Human papillomavirus screening for women with atypical papanicolaou smears. *J Reprod Med.* 1991;36:95–99.
28. Nasiell K, Roger V, Nasiell M. Behavior of mild cervical dysplasia during long-term follow-up. *Obstet Gynecol.* 1986;67:665–669.
29. Butterworth CE Jr. Folate deficiency and cancer. In: Bendich A, Butterworth CE Jr, eds. *Micronutrients in Health and Disease Prevention.* New York, Marcel Dekker Inc; 1991:165–183.
30. Eto I, Krumdieck CL. Role of vitamin B_{12} and folate deficiencies in carcinogenesis. *Adv Exp Med Biol.* 1986;206:313–330.
31. Barich LL, Schwarz J, Barich D. Oral methotrexate in mice: a co-carcinogenic as well as an anti-tumor agent to methylcholanthrene-induced cutaneous tumors. *J Invest Dermatol.* 1986;39:615–619.
32. Jaskiewicz K, Marasas WFO, Lazarus C, Beyers Ad, van Helden PD. Association of esophageal cytological abnormalities with vitamin and lipotrope deficiencies in populations at risk of esophageal cancer. *Anticancer Res.* 1988;8:711–715.
33. van Helden PD, Beyers Ad, Bester AJ, Jaskiewicz K. Esophageal cancer: vitamin and lipotrope deficiencies in an at-risk South African population. *Nutr Cancer.* 1987;10:247–255.
34. Heimburger DC, Alexander CB, Birch R, Butterworth CE Jr, Bailey WC, Krumdieck CL. Improvement in bronchial squamous metaplasia in smokers treated with folate and vitamin B_{12}: report of a preliminary randomized double-blind intervention trial. *JAMA.* 1988;259:1525–1530.
35. Lashner BA, Heidenreich PA, Su GL, Kane SV, Hanauer SB. Effect of folate supplementation on the incidence of dysplasia and cancer in chronic ulcerative colitis: a case-control study. *Gastroenterology.* 1989;97:255–259.
36. Arthur DC, Danzl TJ, Branda RF. Cytogenetic studies of a family

with a hereditary defect of cellular folate uptake and high incidence of hematologic disease. In: Butterworth CE Jr, Hutchinson ML, eds. *Nutritional Factors in the Induction and Maintenance of Malignancy.* New York: Academic Press; 1983:101–111.

37. Rowley JD. The Philadelphia chromosome translocation: a paradigm for understanding leukemia. In: Fortner JG, Rhoads JE, eds. *Accomplishments in Cancer Research.* Philadelphia: J.B. Lippincott; 1989:105–116.
38. Sutherland GR. Heritable fragile sites on human chromosomes, I: factors affecting expression in lymphocyte culture. *Am J Hum Genet.* 1979;31:125–135.
39. Yunis JJ, Soreng AL. Constitutive fragile sites and cancer. *Science.* 1984;226:1199–1204.
40. Popescu NC, Amsbaugh SC, DiPaolo JA. Human papillomavirus type 18 DNA is integrated at a single chromosome site in cervical carcinoma cell line SW756. *J Virol.* 1987;61:1682–1685.
41. Butterworth CE Jr, Hatch KD, Macaluso MM, *et al.* Folate deficiency and cervical dysplasia. *JAMA.* 1992;267:528–533.
42. Subar AF, Block G, James LD. Folate intake and food sources in the US population. *Am J Clin Nutr.* 1989;50:508–516.
43. Bendich A. Importance of vitamin status to pregnancy outcomes. In: Bendich A, Butterworth CE Jr, eds. *Micronutrients in Health and Disease Prevention.* New York: Marcel Dekker, Inc; 1991:235–262.
44. MRC Vitamin Study Research Group. Prevention of neural tube defects: results of the Medical Research Council Vitamin Study. *Lancet.* 1991;338:131–137.

BRET A. LASHNER

Mucosal Dysplasia of the Colon in Patients with Chronic Ulcerative Colitis

ABSTRACT

Colorectal cancer is the second most common cancer in the United States. The rising incidence makes efforts at risk-factor detection and intervention of prime importance. Well-studied environmental associations include vitamins A, D, and E, as well as dietary calcium, carotene, selenium, fiber, and fat. Patients with ulcerative colitis have a high cancer risk and at times will develop dysplasia, a premalignant lesion that has been used as the criterion for a positive screening test in surveillance programs. The etiology of dysplasia or cancer in ulcerative colitis is unknown but is presumed to be similar to the etiology of sporadic cancer, offering a possible human model to study environmental risk factors on a relatively small group.

This case-control study of ulcerative colitis patients compared cases with dysplasia or cancer with controls without cancer. Red blood cell folic acid was a mean of 66.2 ng/mL lower in cases. The risk of developing dysplasia or cancer was decreased by 18% for each 10 ng/mL increase in red blood cell folic acid (odds ratio 0.82, 95% confidence interval 0.68 to 0.99). Other factors associated with dysplasia and cancer were deficiencies in vitamins A, D, and E and carotene.

Therefore, depressed red blood cell folic acid is associated with an increased risk of dysplasia and cancer in patients with ulcerative colitis. Also, ulcerative colitis patients can serve as useful human models to study risk factors for colorectal cancer.

Colorectal Cancer

Colorectal cancer is the second most common malignancy in the United States, diagnosed in over 150 000 patients per year. The annual incidence of colorectal cancer has risen over the last 40 years, with the most dramatic rises occurring in colon cancer and in men (1). Despite major advances in diagnostic techniques and treatment options, the expected five-year survival has hovered at approximately 50% for 40 years. Earlier diagnosis at a more favorable pathologic stage and better surgical, chemo-, and radiation therapy have failed to favorably affect overall survival rates.

Efforts at primary prevention through risk-factor identification and intervention have received particular attention in recent years. Since colorectal cancer incidence rates vary throughout the world and migrants develop colorectal cancer at the rate of the host country within one generation, colorectal cancer is believed to be caused by one or more environmental factors (2). Another piece of evidence that must be coherent with etiologic hypotheses is that higher colorectal cancer rates in the United States are seen in the northern tier of states, with a concentration in the northeast and the Great Lakes area (1).

Nutritional Risk Factors

Many nutritional risk factors are experimentally and epidemiologically associated with colorectal cancer. Vitamin A and the dimer beta-carotene can suppress neoplastic transformation in cell culture (3). Also, deficiency states have been associated with metaplasia of columnar epithelium in bronchial mucosa (4). Beta-carotene administration has been shown to protect the gastrointestinal tract from dimethylhydrazine-induced malignancies in rats (4, 5). Numerous epidemiologic studies have associated low levels of vitamin A or beta-carotene intake with cancers throughout the body, including the esophagus, stomach, and colon (6–10).

Vitamin E is an intracellular antioxidant and a potential inhibitor of carcinogenesis (4, 5, 11, 12). In the mouse dimethylhydrazine model, vitamin E supplementation has been shown to decrease the number of colonic tumors per animal (4). In a study of patients followed in a hypertension detection program, serum vitamin E levels were reduced by 0.10 mg% (95% confidence interval (CI), 0.22 mg% reduction to 0.02 mg% increase) in patients with cancer of all sites, but especially gastrointestinal malignancies, in which vitamin E was reduced by 0.15 mg% (11).

Selenium is a trace element that regulates the activity of glutathione peroxidase, an intracellular antioxidant. Dietary supplementation has decreased the incidence of spontaneously occurring tumors in mice and dimethylhydrazine-induced colon tumors in rats (4). Geographic areas with decreased soil selenium content are associated with increased incidence of breast and colon cancer in humans (4, 5). This effect is independent of the decreased oral intake often seen in cancer patients, since selenium determinations have been made from banked sera of patients who developed cancer years after collection (13).

Western populations with diets relatively low in fiber have a colon cancer risk that is up to eight times as high as that of populations of developing countries with high fiber intake (4). Most, but not all, correlation analyses have shown that high total fiber consumption of a population is associated with low colon cancer incidence (14–17). The protective effect of fiber is thought to be due to carcinogen binding, alteration of intraluminal intestinal flora, and increased intestinal transit. Rats fed bran had a lower rate of dimethylhydrazine-induced tumors of the colon than rats fed a standard low-fiber chow (4).

The association between consumption of increased dietary total fat, saturated fat, and cholesterol in a population and increased national incidence rates for colon cancer is strong (16–19). A high-fat, low-fiber diet may act synergistically to increase the risk of colon cancer (17). Fat from red meat, as opposed to fat from chicken or fish, confers a high colon cancer risk (20). Dietary total fat and saturated fat have been demonstrated to enhance the colon cancer–producing effect of dimethylhydrazine in rats (4).

In the United States, colon cancer rates are highest in areas of low exposure to natural sunlight (21). The Western Electric Health Study confirmed the epidemiologic protective effect of vitamin D and dietary calcium for colon cancer (22). The relative risk of colon cancer for the highest quartile of vitamin D and dietary calcium compared with the lowest quartile was 2.7 ($P < 0.05$), and there was a dose-response effect. Dietary calcium supplementation can decrease the proliferation rate of colonic crypt cells toward a normal quiescent equilibrium (23). Alternatively, dietary calcium may act as a protective agent by forming inactive calcium soaps from toxic intraluminal fatty acids and free bile acids (24).

Polyps and Dysplasia

Patients with familial polyposis coli or Gardener's syndrome develop a large number of adenomatous polyps. The key pathologic feature of these polyps is mucosal dysplasia, which classifies the polyp as adenomatous. Predictably, patients with polyposis coli will develop colorectal cancer in a short period of time, usually by age 30, unless the polypoid lesions are removed through total colectomy. Similarly, sporadic adenomatous polyps that develop with age are thought to grow and develop into malignancy unless they are removed endoscopically or surgically (25, 26). Also, polyps tend to recur in patients who have had previous colonoscopic removal, and repeated colonoscopic surveillance of such patients often is recommended by physicians and national agencies. However, despite the advent of routine colonoscopy with polypectomy over the last 20 years, cancer incidence rates have steadily increased and mortality rates have remained stable. The effectiveness of reducing colorectal cancer mortality through endoscopic screening and polypectomy has been seriously questioned (26).

Cancer in Ulcerative Colitis

Patients with chronic ulcerative colitis have an increased risk for colon cancer over the general population. The known risk factors for cancer increase with the extent and duration of the disease and with older age at symptom onset (27–31). If the environmental risk factors for colorectal cancer are the same for colitic and noncolitic patients, the ulcerative colitis model in humans represents a unique opportunity to evaluate the effect of important exposures on the development of malignant or premalignant disease in a relatively small sample. Fortunately, the pathologic premalignant lesion for colorectal cancer in ulcerative colitis is mucosal dysplasia, the identical lesion in adenomatous polyps.

Dysplasia in Ulcerative Colitis

Mucosal dysplasia in ulcerative colitis patients has been classified as low-grade and high-grade (32). The lead time between low-grade dys-

20. Willett WC, Stampfer MJ, Colditz GA, Rosner BA, Speizer FE. Relation of meat, fat, and fiber intake to the risk of colon cancer in a prospective study among women. *N Engl J Med.* 1990;323: 1664–1672.
21. Garland CE, Garland FC. Do sunlight and vitamin D reduce the likelihood of colon cancer? *Int J Epidemiol.* 1980;9:227–231.
22. Garland C, Shekelle RB, Barrett-Connor E, *et al.* Dietary vitamin D and calcium and the risk of colorectal cancer: a 19-year prospective study in men. *Lancet.* 1985;1:307–309.
23. Lipkin M, Newmark H. Effect of added dietary calcium on colonic epithelial-cell proliferation in subjects at high risk for familial colonic cancer. *N Engl J Med.* 1985;313:1381–1384.
24. Newmark HL, Wargovich MJ, Bruce WR. Colon cancer and dietary fat, phosphate, and calcium: a hypothesis. *J Natl Cancer Inst.* 1984;72:1323–1325.
25. Fleischer DE, Goldberg SB, Browning TH, *et al.* Detection and surveillance of colorectal cancer. *JAMA.* 1989;261:580–585.
26. Ransohoff DF, Lang CA. Screening for colorectal cancer. *N Engl J Med.* 1991;325:37–41.
27. Lashner BA, Silverstein MD, Hanauer SB. Hazard rates for dysplasia and cancer in ulcerative colitis: results from a surveillance program. *Dig Dis Sci.* 1989;34:1536–1541.
28. Greenstein AJ, Sachar DB, Smith H, *et al.* Cancer in universal and left sided ulcerative colitis: factors determining risk. *Gastroenterology.* 1979;77:290–294.
29. Katzka I, Brody RS, Morris E, Katz S. Assessment of colorectal cancer risk in patients with ulcerative colitis: experience from a private practice. *Gastroenterology.* 1983;85:22–29.
30. Nugent FW, Haggitt RC, Colcher H, Kutteruf GC. Malignant potential of chronic ulcerative colitis. *Gastroenterology.* 1979;76:1–5.
31. Prior P, Gyde SN, Macartney JC, Thompson H, *et al.* Cancer morbidity in ulcerative colitis. *Gut.* 1982:23:490–497.
32. Riddell RH, Goldman H, Ransohoff DF, *et al.* Dysplasia in inflammatory bowel disease: standardized classification with provisional clinical applications. *Human Pathol.* 1983;14:931–968.
33. Lashner BA, Hanauer SB, Silverstein MD. Optimal timing of colonoscopy to screen for cancer in ulcerative colitis. *Ann Intern Med.* 1988;108:274–278.
34. Lashner BA. Colon cancer surveillance in ulcerative colitis. *Semin Gastrointest Dis.* 1991;2:126–131.

35. Collins RH, Feldman M, Fordtran JS. Colon cancer, dysplasia, and surveillance in patients with ulcerative colitis. *N Engl J Med.* 1987;316:1654–1658.
36. Lennard-Jones JE, Ritchie JK, Morson BC, *et al.* Cancer surveillance in ulcerative colitis. *Lancet.* 1983;ii:149–152.
37. Lashner BA, Kane SV, Hanauer SB. Colon cancer surveillance in chronic ulcerative colitis: an historical cohort study. *Am J Gastroenterol.* 1990;85:1083–1087.
38. Alpers DH. Absorption of water-soluble vitamins, folate, minerals, and vitamin D. In: Sleisenger MH, Fordtran JS, eds. *Gastrointestinal Disease.* Philadelphia: WB Saunders Company;1983.
39. Sutherland GR, Jacky PB, Baker E, Manuel A. Heritable fragile sites on human chromosomes: new folate-sensitive fragile sites. *Am J Hum Genet.* 1983;35:432–437.
40. Maltby EL, Higgins S. Folate sensitive site as 10q23 and its expression as a deletion. *J Med Genet.* 1987;25:299.
41. Tommerup N, Neilsen J, Mikkelsen M. A folate sensitive heritable fragile site at 19p13. *Clin Genet.* 1985;27:510–514.
42. Cravo M, Mason JB, Dyal Y, *et al.* Folate deficiency enhances the development of colonic neoplasia in DMH-treated rats. *Gastroenterology.* 1991;100:A356.
43. Cravo M, Mason JB, Salomon RN, *et al.* Folate deficiency in rats causes hypomethylation of liver DNA. *Gastroenterology.* 1991;100:A356.
44. Wainfan E, Dizik M, Stender M, Christman JK. Rapid appearance of hypomethylated DNA in livers of rats and cancer promoting methyl-deficient diets. *Cancer Res.* 1989;49:4094–4097.
45. Heimburger DC, Alexander B, Birch R, Butterworth CE, Baily WC, Krumdiek CL. Improvement in bronchial squamous metaplasia in smokers treated with folate and vitamin B_{12}. *JAMA.* 1988;259:1525–1530.
46. Butterworth CE, Hatch KD, Gore H, Meuller H, Krundiek CL. Improvement in cervical dysplasia with folic acid therapy in users of oral contraceptives. *Am J Clin Nutr.* 1982;35:73–82.
47. Lashner BA, Heidenreich PA, Su GL, Kane SV, Hanauer SB. Effect of folate supplementation on the incidence of dysplasia and cancer in chronic ulcerative colitis. *Gastroenterology.* 1989;97:255–259.
48. Lashner BA. Red blood cell folate is associated with dysplasia or cancer in ulcerative colitis. *Gastroenterology.* 1990;98:A184.

49. Franklin JL, Rosenberg IH. Impaired folic acid absorption in inflammatory bowel disease: effects of salicylazosulfapyridine. *Gastroenterology.* 1973;64:517–525.
50. Selhub J, Dhar GJ, Rosenberg IH. Inhibition of folate enzymes by sulfasalazine. *J Clin Invest.* 1978;61:221–214.
51. Physicians Health Study Research Group. Preliminary report: findings from the aspirin component of the ongoing Physicians' Health Study. *N Engl J Med.* 1988;318:262–264.

PART IV

Vitamins C, E, and B_6

LAWRENCE J. MACHLIN

A Nutritional Perspective on Vitamins E, C, and A and Beta-Carotene

ABSTRACT

Although beta-carotene and vitamins E, C, and A can all function as antioxidants, their transport, tissue and intracellular distribution, metabolism, and mechanisms of action in preventing cancer are distinct. In view of these differences, additive or synergistic effects of these vitamins are certainly possible.

Dietary surveys indicate that a large proportion of the United States population is not consuming the recommended dietary allowances of vitamins C and E. Also, most people are not consuming the amounts of carotene and fruits and vegetables suggested by the dietary guidelines of the National Cancer Institute and the United States Department of Agriculture.

Introduction

Clinical studies concerning vitamins and cancer must address a number of important questions. Specifically, what levels of the vitamins under examination are people consuming in their normal diet? What are the important food sources of these vitamins? What is the dose-response relationship between intake and blood and tissue levels? What are the safety concerns? What interactions occur between these nutrients, and how do they affect cancer trials? This paper addresses these topics briefly, in order to point out some of the issues involved.

Vitamin E

Vitamin E is the major lipid soluble antioxidant (1). The chromanol ring is responsible for its antioxidant function, and the isophytol side chain is thought to help anchor the molecule in cell membranes. Almost all of the vitamin is located in the membrane component of the cell with very little in the cytosol.

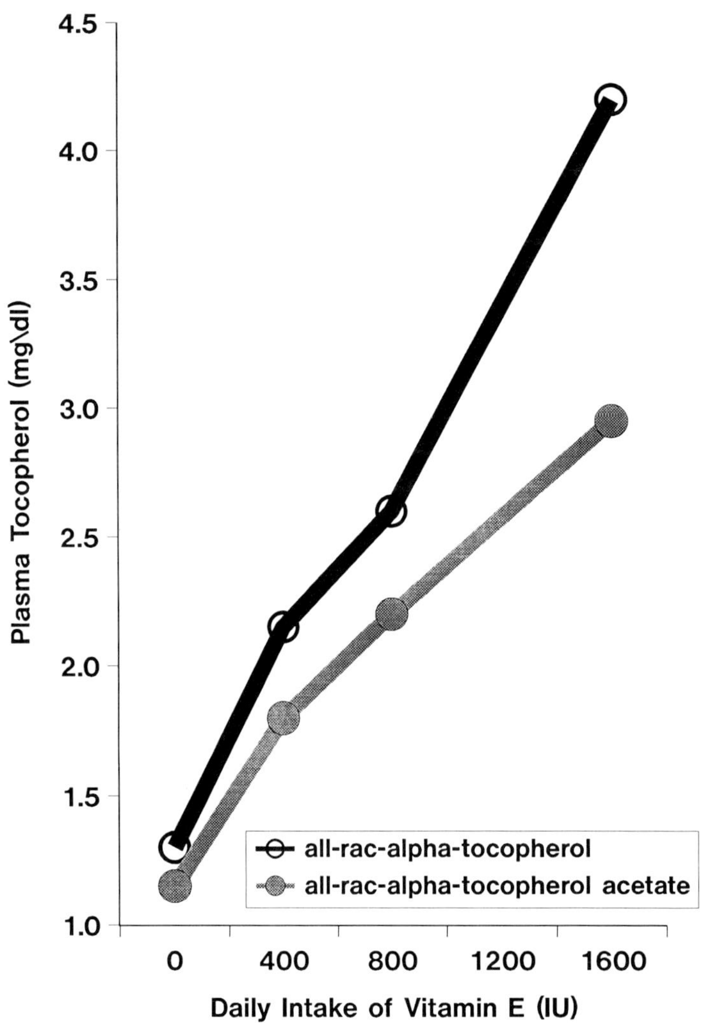

Figure 1. Relationship of intake of vitamin E to plasma levels of tocopherol in adult humans after 21 days of supplementation. "Zero" intake was prior to supplementation.

From Baker *et al.* (2), with permission of Butterworth-Heinemann.

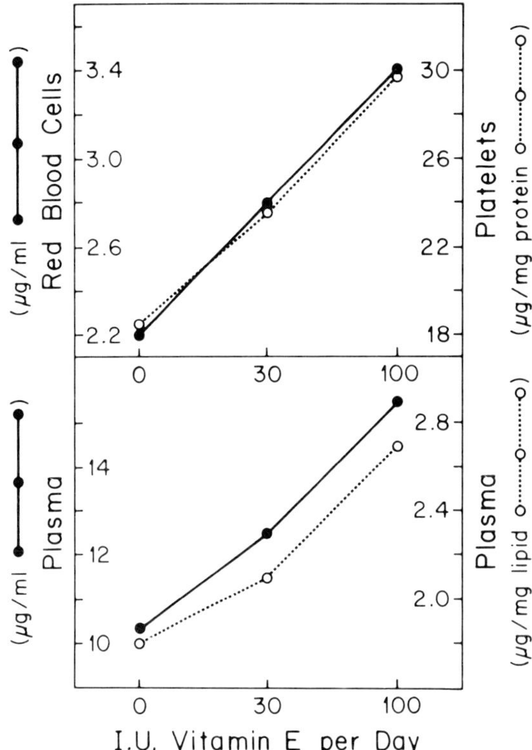

Figure 2. Effect of vitamin E supplements on alpha-tocopherol concentration in human blood.
From Lehman *et al.* (3). © Am. J. Clin. Nutr. American Society for Clinical Nutrition.

Plasma levels increase with increased dosage over a wide range of intakes (2) (Fig. 1). The tocopherol content of the red blood cells and platelets parallels the increase in plasma (3) (Fig. 2). Other studies have shown that there is a high correlation of blood levels of tocopherol to their content in the buccal cells (4) and that the tocopherol content of all tissues can be increased by high intakes of vitamin E, although the rate of increase in individual tissues can vary substantially (5).

Vitamin C

In addition to its classic role as a cofactor in hydroxylation reactions and as a reducing agent, ascorbic acid has an important role as an antioxidant (6). In one summary of many reports, plasma ascorbate

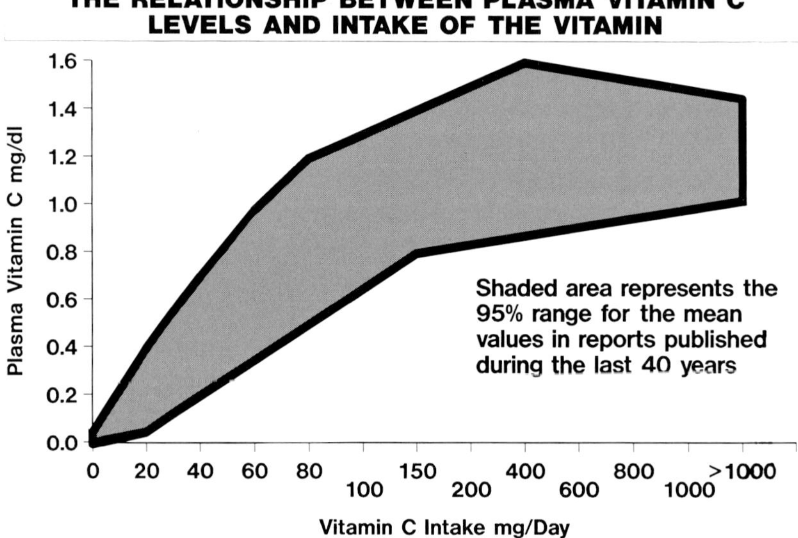

Figure 3. Blood levels of vitamin C.
From Basu *et al.* (7).

evels increase up to 1.6 mg/dL on intake of about 600 mg per day (7) (Fig. 3). However, many other reports show that plasma levels of 2–2.5 mg % are attainable with doses of 2 g or more, particularly if given in divided doses.

Interaction of Vitamins E and C

There is substantial evidence that ascorbate can spare vitamin E by reducing the tocopheryl radical to tocopherol (6, 8). Some studies have shown a sparing effect of vitamin C on vitamin E in vivo, although this may not be demonstrable in all tissues.

Beta-Carotene

Beta-carotene (Fig. 4) is converted to retinal by a beta-carotene dioxygenase, and the retinal is reduced to retinol (Fig. 5). There is also evidence of eccentric cleavage of beta-carotene with production of a number of metabolic products in addition to retinal. Conversion of beta-carotene to retinal is quite inefficient in vivo, and together with

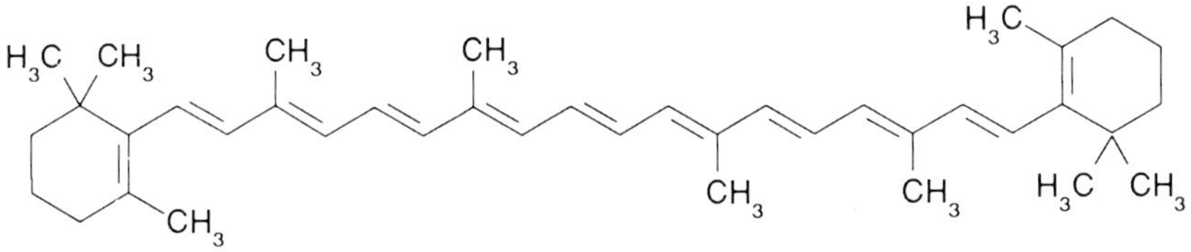

A natural pigment in yellow and green vegetables and fruits

Provitamin A

Partly converted into vitamin A in the body and rest stored as beta carotene

Antioxidant

Singlet oxygen quencher

1 mg of beta carotene = 1667 IU vitamin A activity

Figure 4. Beta-carotene.

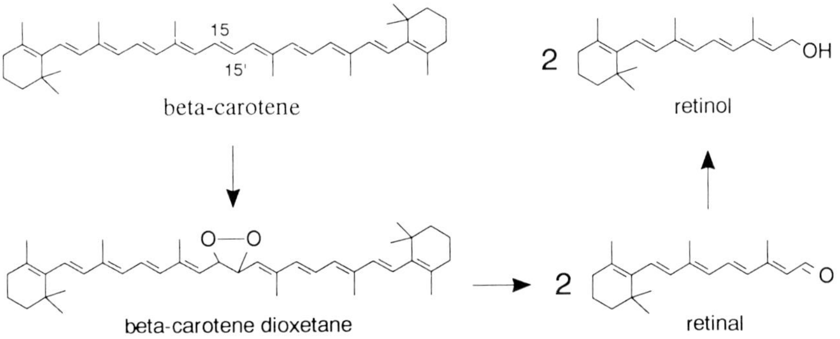

Figure 5. Conversion of beta-carotene to retinol.

the losses in absorption it is presently assumed (1980 recommended dietary allowance [RDA]) that 6 μg of beta-carotene is equivalent to 1 μg of retinol nutritionally.

Because conversion of beta-carotene to retinol is tightly regulated, administration of beta-carotene rarely increases plasma retinol (Fig. 6) unless the subjects are deficient in vitamin A. Furthermore, high levels of beta-carotene cannot result in hypervitaminosis A. The kinetics of uptake and disappearance of beta-carotene from plasma and tissues is quite slow, with as much as two months of treatment necessary to reach maximum plasma values (9). When 15–60 mg per

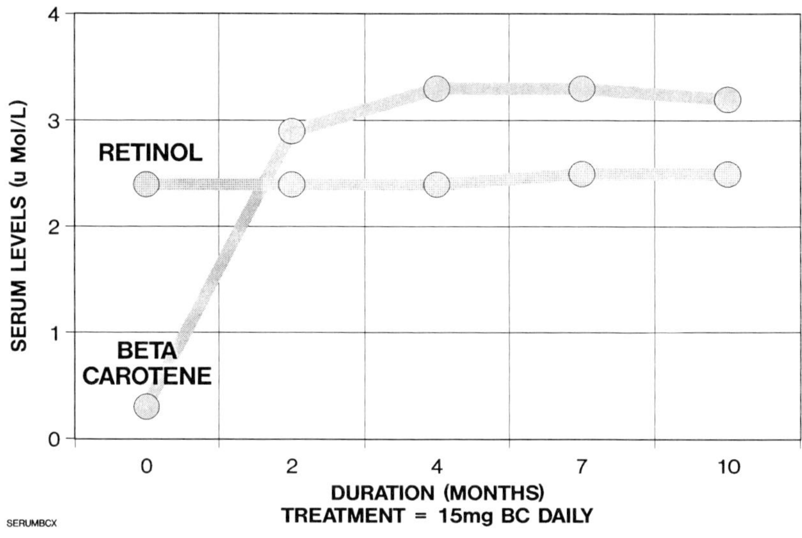

Figure 6. Effect of duration of beta-carotene supplementation on serum levels of beta-carotene and retinol.

From Costantino *et al.* (10). © Am. J. Clin. Nutr. American Society for Clinical Nutrition.

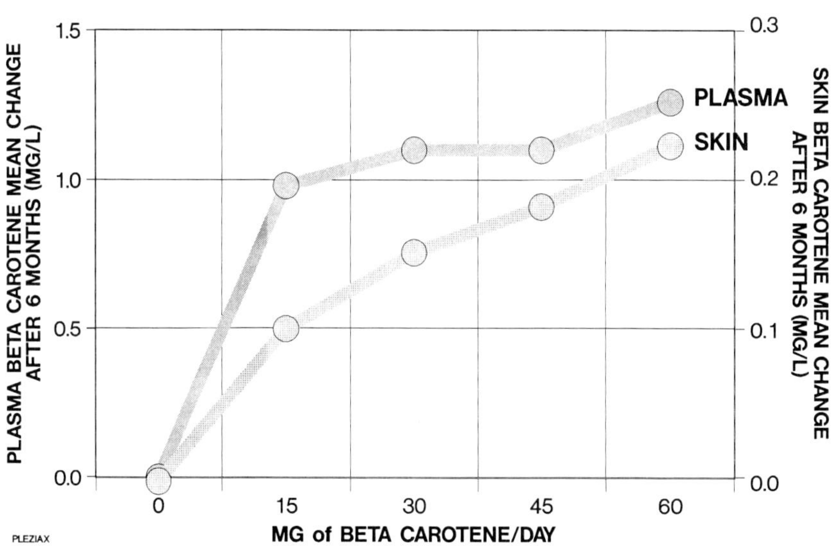

Figure 7. Effect of dose on plasma and skin levels of beta-carotene.

From Plezia *et al.* (9).

day of beta-carotene were administered for six months, plasma levels appeared to level off between 15 mg and 60 mg per day, whereas skin levels continued to increase over the entire range of intakes (10) (Fig. 7).

Beta-carotene is an effective antioxidant, particularly at low oxygen tensions. However, its role as an in vivo antioxidant has not been clearly established. It is an extremely effective quencher of singlet oxygen, a function that may help explain its effectiveness in the treatment of certain light-sensitivity disorders. Vitamin A has only weak antioxidant preparations, and there is no clear evidence that it is an in vivo antioxidant.

Food Sources

Food sources of vitamin A and beta-carotene are quite distinct (Tables 1 and 2). Vitamin A is found in foods of animal origin, such as liver, dairy products, and eggs, whereas beta-carotene is found almost exclusively in vegetables and fruits. Thus, it is relatively easy to

Table 1. Richest Sources of Vitamins

Vitamin A	Beta-Carotene	Vitamin C	Vitamin E
Liver	Carrots	Citrus fruits	Vegetable oils
Butter	Spinach	Melons	Nuts and seeds
Milk	Kale	Strawberries	Fortified cereals
Cheese	Sweet potatoes	Pineapples	Leafy green vegetables
Egg yolks	Butternut squash	Peppers	Wheat germ

Table 2. Most Common Major Sources of Vitamins[a]

Vitamin A	Beta-Carotene	Vitamin C	Vitamin E
Liver	Carrots	Orange juice	Fats, oils
Eggs	Tomatoes, juices	Grapefruit juice	Vegetables
Whole milk	Soups	Tomatoes, juices	Meat, poultry, fish
Margarine	Greens	Fortified fruit drinks	Desserts
Cold cereals	Cantaloupe	Oranges, tangerines	Breakfast cereals
Cheese		Potatoes	

[a]According to the National Health and Nutrition Examination Survey, 1976–1980.

distinguish the two nutrients based on dietary intakes. Epidemiologists should take care to distinguish whether vitamin A or beta-carotene or the total vitamin A activity of a diet is having an impact on the risk of cancer. Several food sources have a sufficiently high content of vitamin C or beta-carotene that even one portion can supply more than one RDA of the nutrient. This is not true of vitamin E, of which few common foods can provide one RDA. This means that it is relatively difficult to substantially increase the intake of vitamin E by dietary manipulations alone and that if a need for higher than RDA levels were established, supplementation or additional fortification of foods may be desirable.

Vitamin Intake

Studies by Block (private communication) (Fig. 8) indicate that a majority of women do not consume even one RDA (8 tocopherol equiva-

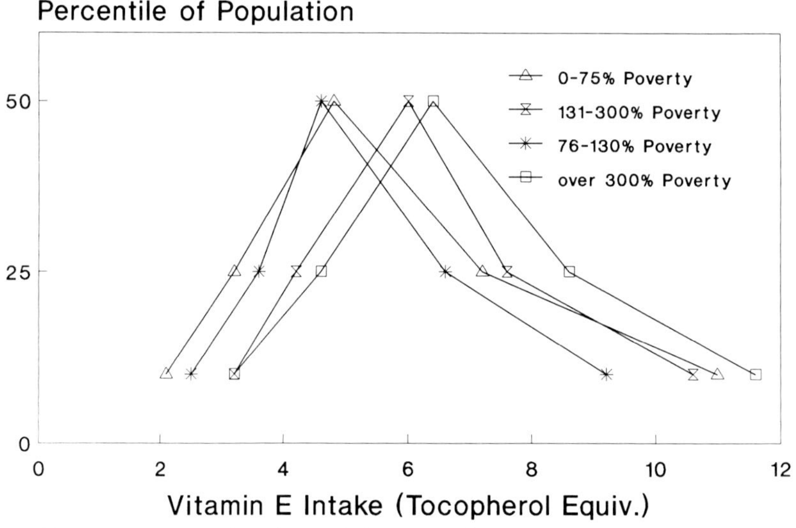

Figure 8. Vitamin E intake distribution, CSFII (1986), in women aged 19 to 50. G. Block, private communication.

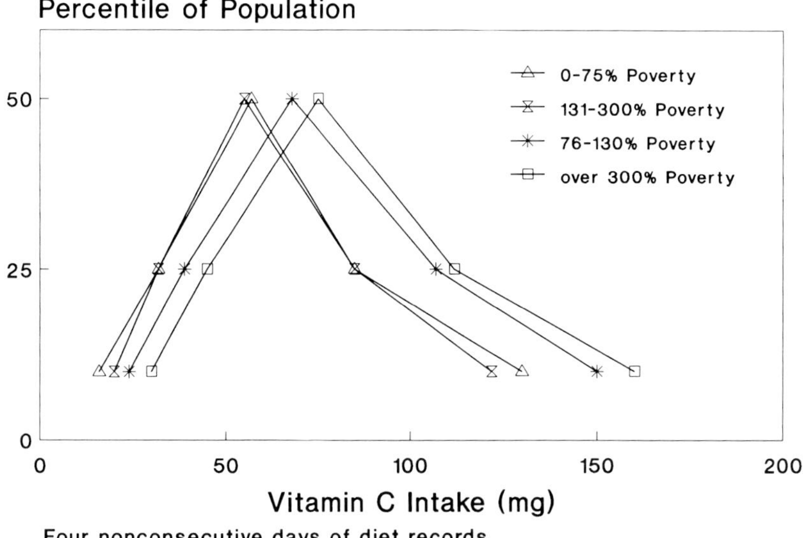

Figure 9. Vitamin C intake distribution, CSFII (1986), in women aged 19 to 50. G. Block, private communication.

lents [TE]) of vitamin E. About one-half the women consumed less than one RDA of vitamin C (60 mg) (Fig. 9). The median intake of carotene was 200 retinol equivalents (RE), which are equivalent to 1.2 mg of carotene (Fig. 10). The diets recommended by the National Cancer Institute and the United States Department of Agriculture generally contain about 6 mg of carotene, suggesting a considerable gap between what people are ingesting and what it may be desirable to ingest for cancer prevention.

Safety

The literature suggests that high-dose supplements of vitamins E and C and beta-carotene are well tolerated, with no significant adverse effects observed in normal adults with levels up to 3000 IU (2000 TE) of vitamin E (11), 10 g of vitamin C (12), and 180 mg of beta-carotene (13). Some individuals experience some gastric distress at

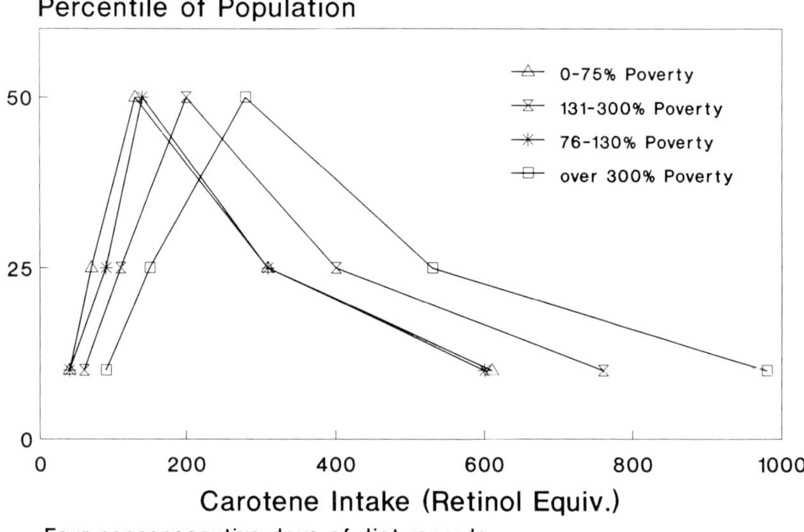

Figure 10. Carotene intake distribution, CSFII (1986), in women aged 19 to 50. G. Block, private communication.

very high intakes of vitamin C. At 25 mg per day of beta-carotene, carotenodermia (yellowing of the skin) starts to occur. This presents no health hazard but jeopardizes the blinding of studies. Vitamin A is known to have toxic effects when consumed for long periods at levels over 50 000 IU per day (14). However, in some cases (15) investigators have administered as much as 300 000 IU per day for two years as a chemopreventive agent with only minimal side effects. Clearly, safety considerations are different in subjects with pathology such as abnormal liver or kidney function.

Interactions

The possible sparing effect of vitamin C on vitamin E has been discussed. Vitamin E is also known to spare vitamin A (16) and to help prevent toxicity from vitamin A (16) and retinoids (17). The mode of action of vitamins E, C, and A and beta-carotene in cancer prevention is not likely to be the same. Although they share the attribute of anti-

Table 3. Relative Risk of Gastric Cancer Associated with Dietary Vitamin C and Vitamin E

		Vitamin C		
		Low	Medium Relative Risk	High
Vitamin E	Low	1.0	0.7	0.8
	Medium	0.9	0.6	0.5
	High	1.0	0.5	0.4

From Biuatti *et al.* (18).

oxidant activity, their antioxidant potency varies considerably, and the tissue and intracellular distribution are unique for each nutrient. They also vary considerably in regard to other mechanisms for prevention of carcinogenesis. For example, vitamins C and E can block nitrosamine formation, whereas vitamin A and beta-carotene do not have any such effect. Vitamin A maintains normal cell differentiation, but the other vitamins do not influence this process. Given the sparing effects between vitamins, different cell and tissue distribution, and different carcinogenesis-inhibiting mechanisms, it would seem logical that combinations of vitamins may be more effective than a single vitamin. Indeed, Buiatti *et al.* have observed that a maximum reduction in relative risk of gastric cancer occurs when there is a high intake of both vitamins E and C (18) (Table 3). Although comparable investigations are difficult to undertake, vitamin interactions such as these would be well worth exploring.

Conclusion

Most people are not adhering to diets presently recommended by the National Cancer Institute or the United States Department of Agriculture. Although vitamins E, C, and A and beta-carotene can all function as antioxidants, their transport, tissue and intracellular distribution and metabolism, and mechanisms of action in preventing cancer are distinct. Thus additive or synergistic effects of these vitamins are certainly possible.

Many intervention studies using both individual vitamins and combinations of vitamins are under way. It is hoped that these will provide some of the information we need to make more useful and realistic recommendations to both high-risk populations and the general public in regard to the role of antioxidant vitamins in the prevention of cancer.

REFERENCES

1. Machlin LJ. Vitamin E. In: Machlin LJ, ed. *Handbook of Vitamins.* New York: Marcel Dekker;1991:99–144.
2. Baker H, Frank O, DeAngelis B, Ferngold S. Plasma tocopherol in man at various times after ingestion of free or acetylated tocopherol. *Nutr Rep Int.* 1980;21:531–536.
3. Lehman J, Rao DD, Canary JJ, Judd JT. Vitamin E and relationships among tocopherols in plasma, platelets, lymphocytes, and red blood cells. *Am J Clin Nutr.* 1988;47:470–474.
4. Yokota K, Tamai H, Mino M. Clinical evaluation of alpha-tocopherol in buccal mucosal cells of children. *J Nutr Sci Vitaminol (Tokyo).* 1990;36:365–375.
5. Machlin LJ, Gabriel E. Kinetics of tissue α-tocopherol uptake and depletion following administration of high levels of vitamin E. *Ann N Y Acad Sci.* 1982;393:48–60.
6. Bendich A, Machlin LJ, Scandurra O, Burton GW, Wayner DM. The antioxidant role of vitamin C. *Adv Free Rad Biol Med.* 1986;2: 419–444.
7. Basu TK, Schorah CJ. *Vitamin C in Health and Disease.* Westport, Conn: The AUI Publishing Co; 1982:83–84.
8. Niki E. Antioxidants in relation to lipid peroxidation. *Chem and Physics Lipids.* 1987;44:227–253.
9. Plezia PM, Alberts DS, Sayers SM, Xu MJ, Peng YM, Ritenbaugh C. Evaluation of plasma and skin concentrations of β-carotene (BC), retinol (ROH), and retinyl palmitate in normal subjects receiving daily doses of BC for 9 months. In: *Proceedings Intl. Assoc. Vitamins and Nutritional Oncology;* July 25–29, 1989; Charleston, SC.
10. Costantino JP, Kuller LH, Begg L, Redmond CK, Bates MW. Serum level changes after administration of a pharmacologic dose and β-carotene. *Am J Clin Nutr.* 1988;48:1277–1283.
11. Bendich A, Machlin LJ. Safety of oral intake of vitamin E. *Am J Clin Nutr.* 1988;48:612–619.

12. Rivers JM. Safety of high level vitamin C ingestion. *Ann N Y Acad Sci.* 1987;498:445–454.
13. Bendich A. The safety of beta carotene. *Nutr Cancer.* 1988;11:207–214.
14. Bendich A, Langseth L. Safety of vitamin A. *Am J Clin Nutr.* 1989;49:358–371.
15. Infante M, Pastorino V, Chesa G, *et al.* Laboratory evaluation during high-dose vitamin A administration: a randomized study on lung cancer patients after surgical resection. *J Cancer Res Clin Oncol.* 1991;117:156–162.
16. Draper HH. Nutrient interrelationships. In: Machlin LJ, ed. *Vitamin E: A Comprehensive Treatise.* New York: Marcel Dekker; 1980: 272–288.
17. Besa EC, Abraham JL, Bartholomew MJ, Hyzinski M, Nowell DC. Treatment with 13-*cis*-retinoic acid in transfusion-dependent patients with myelodysplastic syndrome and decreased toxicity with addition of alpha-tocopherol. *Am J Med.* 1990;89:739–747.
18. Buiatti E, Palli D, DeCarli A, *et al.* A case-control study of gastric cancer and diet in Italy. *Int J Cancer.* 1989;44:611–616.

GEORGE M. SOBALA

Ascorbic Acid in Gastric Juice

ABSTRACT

The concentration of ascorbic acid in gastric juice was selectively determined by high-pressure liquid chromatography in the studies reported on. The relationships between ascorbic acid levels in gastric juice and *Helicobacter pylori* infection, chronic gastritis, intestinal metaplasia, and nitrite and nitrosamine concentrations were examined. There is evidence for secretion of ascorbic acid in high concentrations into the normal stomach. *Helicobacter pylori* infection, which causes chronic gastritis, appears to damage this secretory process. Ascorbic acid concentrations in gastric juice are low in patients with chronic gastritis and especially those with intestinal metaplasia and hypochlorhydria and also in patients living in an area at risk for gastric cancer. Oral vitamin supplementation does not improve fasting gastric juice concentrations in such patients. Preliminary evidence suggests that eradication of *H pylori* may restore ascorbic acid secretion.

Introduction

Vitamin C and ascorbic acid are not synonymous. Both ascorbic acid and dehydroascorbic acid can prevent scurvy and are thus considered to be vitamin C, but only ascorbic acid has antioxidant properties. Dehydroascorbic acid can be recycled back to ascorbic acid intracellularly, but this reaction does not occur in the gastric juice.

Ascorbic acid is potentially important in the prevention of gastric cancer. It may prevent the formation in the stomach of carcinogens such as N-nitroso compounds. A simple view of the chemical reactions involved is that ascorbic acid reacts with nitrite and converts it to nitric oxide, while it is oxidized itself to dehydroascorbic acid. It thus makes nitrite unavailable to participate in N-nitrosation reactions. Ascorbic acid is better suited for this than other antioxidants as the optimum pH for this reaction is said to be around 4.0 (1), approximately that of the postprandial stomach. Experimental evidence supports this hypothesis. Ascorbic acid can reduce nitrite and prevent N-nitroso compound formation in vitro and also in humans in the experimental model of N-nitrosation, the nitroso-proline test. In rats and mice, administration of ascorbic acid reduces tumor formation in response to dietary nitrite and amines.

This simple model serves as a suitable starting point for experimental work, but the chemistry of ascorbic acid and nitrite-derived radicals is probably more complex. The nitric oxide formed by the reduction of nitrite-derived species is not a nitrosating agent, but under aerobic conditions it can be reoxidized to nitrosating agents by dissolved oxygen. Thus the stochiometry of the nitrite/ascorbate reaction varies according to the physical conditions (*e.g.*, dissolved oxygen concentration, mass transfer effects) of the reaction mixture. This topic has been dealt with fully by Licht *et al.* (2, 3).

Until recently, most of the work on ascorbic acid and gastric cancer has focused on the role of diet, and little attention has been paid to concentrations of this vitamin in the gastric juice, although this is clearly where it will exert any chemical effect.

Total vitamin C concentrations in gastric juice have been measured on a few occasions over the last 50 years using techniques that estimate both ascorbic and dehydroascorbic acids together. Misleadingly, some of these studies have reported their measurements of total vitamin C as being those of ascorbic acid itself. The findings of these studies are summarized in Table 1. These data suggest that vitamin C may be present in gastric juice in quite high concentrations in some individuals and that levels may vary according to gastric pathology.

Technical difficulties have up to now prevented the separate measurement of the oxidized and reduced forms of vitamin C in gastric juice. A method of estimation of both these compounds utilizing high-

Table 1. Previous Studies Measuring Total Vitamin C Concentrations in Gastric Juice

Study	Patients	Mean
Peters and Martin (5)	Hospital patients	23 μmol/L
Freeman and Hafkesbring (6)	Normal adults	54 μmol/L
Freeman and Hafkesbring (7)	"Gastritis" patients	17 μmol/L
Singh and Godbole (8)	Peptic ulcer patients	27 μmol/L

pressure liquid chromatography has been developed recently at Leeds University (4). Using this method of analysis, we set out to measure the concentrations of both ascorbic acid and total vitamin C in gastric juice and to assess their significance to gastric pathology and gastric carcinogenesis.

Ascorbic Acid Versus Gastric Histopathology

In our first study we set out to explore the range of ascorbic acid concentrations to be found in gastric juice and hypothesized that levels would vary according to gastric pathology (9).

Method

Gastric juice was obtained from 77 patients at endoscopy and assayed for ascorbic acid and total vitamin C, and these results were analyzed according to the macroscopic findings, antral and body histology, gastric juice pH and culture results, plasma vitamin C levels, and an assessment of dietary intake.

Results

The most important findings were that high concentrations of both ascorbic acid and total vitamin C existed in patients with normal gastric histology (Fig. 1), in whom there was a concentration gradient between gastric juice and plasma. This suggests the presence of a secretory process. Assuming a gastric juice output of 2.5 L per 24 hours and extrapolating from these concentrations, some individuals may secrete as much as 100 mg of ascorbic acid into the stomach each day. Presumably this would be reabsorbed in the small intestine and recycled.

Vitamin C and ascorbic acid levels were significantly lower in the presence of *Helicobacter pylori*–associated chronic gastritis (Fig. 1): in such patients there was no overall plasma-to-juice concentration gradient. In gastric juice of neutral pH little or no ascorbic acid was detectable, although dehydroascorbic acid was present. This may reflect consumption of ascorbic acid by high concentrations of nitrite at neutral pH. Thus we found that patients with chronic gastritis and hypochlorhydria, who by the Correa hypothesis of gastric carcinogene-

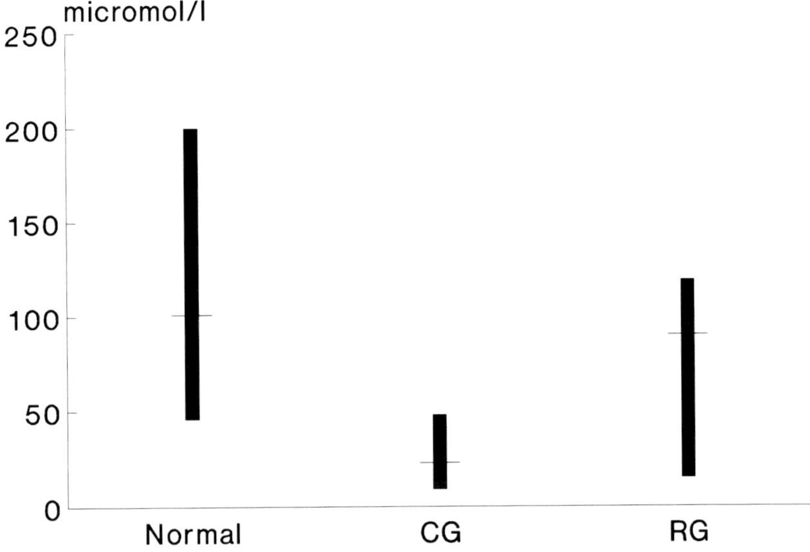

Figure 1. Ascorbic acid concentrations in gastric juice of patients with normal gastric histology, chronic gastritis (CG), and reactive gastritis (RG). Box plots show medians and interquartile ranges.
From Sobala *et al.* (9).

sis are at greatest risk for gastric cancer, did have very low ascorbic acid levels in gastric juice.

Ascorbic Acid, Nitrite, Nitroso Compounds, and Intestinal Metaplasia

We next hypothesized that if they were of relevance to the Correa hypothesis of gastric carcinogenesis, ascorbic acid levels in gastric juice should be lowest in premalignant conditions such as intestinal metaplasia and that they should vary inversely with nitrite and total nitroso compound concentrations [10].

Method

Fifty-six patients underwent endoscopy, and gastric juice was obtained for assay of ascorbic acid, total vitamin C, pH, and bile acids. Nitrite, nitrate, and total N-nitroso compounds were assayed for us by Pignatelli and colleagues at the International Agency for Research on Cancer (IARC), Lyon, France. Antral and body biopsies were taken for histology.

Results

Concentrations of ascorbic acid in gastric juice were lower in patients with both chronic superficial and chronic atrophic gastritis as compared with patients with normal histology. Among patients with gastritis, ascorbic acid levels were lower in the presence of intestinal metaplasia (Fig. 2), a phenomenon that could probably be explained by the higher gastric juice pH in these subjects.

We found no correlations between ascorbic acid concentrations in gastric juice and nitrite and nitroso compound levels. However, the few patients that had substantial concentrations of nitrite did have little or no measurable ascorbic acid, and it is possible that if larger numbers had been studied a relationship would have emerged.

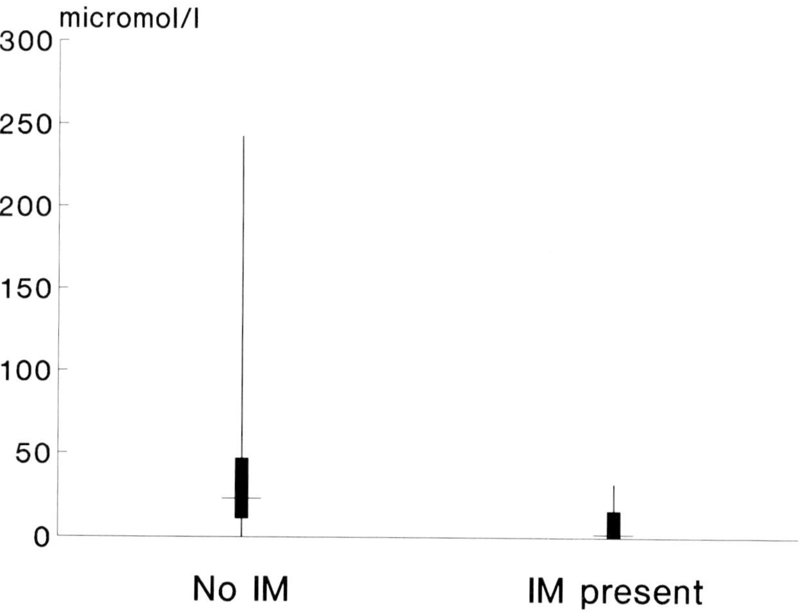

Figure 2. Ascorbic acid concentrations of gastric juice in patients with chronic gastritis and no or coexisting intestinal metaplasia in antral biopsies. Box and whisker plots show medians, quartiles, and ranges.
From Sobala *et al.* (10) by permission of Oxford University Press.

Thus ascorbic acid levels were indeed low in patients with intestinal metaplasia, atrophy, and chronic gastritis. In this study these features were also associated with *H pylori* infection. A negative association with nitrite concentrations was not confirmed but cannot be ruled out by these data.

Ascorbic Acid in a "Cancer Family"

The next hypothesis to be tested was that ascorbic acid levels in gastric juice should be low in other groups of patients at high risk for gastric cancer. Our first opportunity to examine this was in a "cancer family" (11).

Method

In the family studied, two of four siblings had developed intestinal-type gastric cancer before the age of 40, and a third had undergone partial gastrectomy for dysplasia in the gastric antrum. Five of the eight children had *H pylori*–associated chronic gastritis. Three of these had intestinal metaplasia before the age of 35, a most unusual finding in the United Kingdom. Gastric juice was obtained at endoscopy from four of these children with gastritis for assay of ascorbic acid. Nitrite and total N-nitroso compounds were again assayed by IARC.

Results

On rebiopsy, all four children (aged 20 to 34) had *H pylori*–associated chronic atrophic gastritis. Three had intestinal metaplasia on this occasion, and the fourth had intestinal metaplasia on previous biopsy. In all four the gastric juice was of acid pH, and nitrite and total N-nitroso compound concentrations were unremarkable. Unexpectedly, ascorbic acid concentrations in gastric juice were found to correspond to those found in historical controls with normal gastric histology and were significantly higher than those in historical control patients with chronic gastritis, of similar age, and with acid gastric juice. These results were not in accord with the Correa or ascorbic acid hypothesis and possibly suggest that there are significant differences in the cell biology of gastritis in patients genetically at high risk for gastric cancer.

Ascorbic Acid in a High-Risk Geographical Area

We next tested the same hypothesis in patients living in a geographical area with a high incidence of gastric cancer (12).

Methods

With the assistance of Dr. Munoz, IARC, 41 subjects with and without atrophic gastritis from San Cristobal, Venezuela, underwent endoscopy, and gastric juice was obtained for assay of ascorbic acid and total vitamin C.

Results

Irrespective of the presence of glandular atrophy, most subjects had *H pylori* infection. Ascorbic acid levels in gastric juice were found to be significantly lower than those in historical controls in the United Kingdom with normal gastric histology. However, the levels were higher than those found in United Kingdom patients with *H pylori*–associated chronic gastritis. Thus, the high cancer risk in this area cannot be entirely due to low ascorbic acid levels in gastric juice.

Ascorbic Acid and Acute *H pylori* Infection

Our results had indicated that ascorbic acid levels in gastric juice were lower in the presence of *H pylori*–associated gastritis. This suggested that the onset of *H pylori* infection in an individual should be accompanied by a fall in ascorbic acid concentrations in gastric juice. This seemed an untestable hypothesis until I unexpectedly developed symptoms of a similar nature to those reported by Arthur Morris after his voluntary ingestion of *H pylori* (13). Infection with *H pylori* was confirmed by a change in isotope carbon-labeled urea breath testing from negative to positive, seroconversion on enzyme-linked immunosorbent assay to *H pylori*, positive culture of the organism, and the development of initially acute neutrophilic and then chronic *H pylori*–associated gastritis on histology. By chance I had acted as my own subject and undergone aspiration of gastric juice via nasogastric tube before and after intravenous injection of ascorbic acid, 170 days before the onset of symptoms. The same protocol was thus repeated 37 days and 161 days after infection (14).

Pre-infection fasting gastric juice levels were in the low range for a subject with presumed normal histology but not exceptionally so. Levels rose sharply after intravenous injection. Thirty-seven days after infection, gastric juice was of neutral pH and ascorbic acid was nearly undetectable both before and after injection. By 161 days, gastric acid output had returned, but basal ascorbic acid levels remained very low and incremented poorly after intravenous injection (Fig. 3). Although not amenable to rigorous statistical analysis, these serendipitous findings are in keeping with the hypothesis that *H pylori* infection damages the mechanism for gastric secretion of ascorbic acid.

Effects of Oral Supplementation

Method

In collaboration with IARC and to investigate whether oral supplementation with vitamin C can raise low ascorbic acid levels in gastric

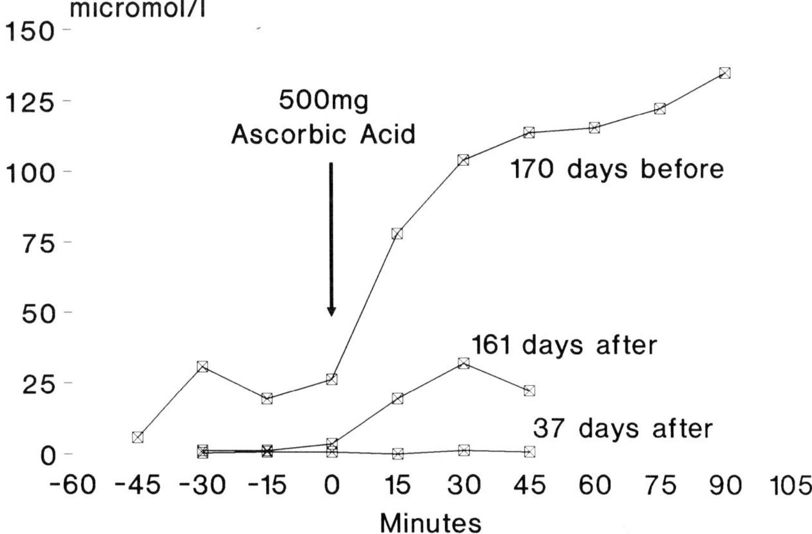

Figure 3. Ascorbic acid concentrations in gastric juice of the author at 15-minute intervals before and after a 500 mg intravenous injection of ascorbic acid approximately 170 days before, 161 days after, and 37 days after spontaneous acute *H pylori* infection.
From Sobala *et al.* (14).

juice, the 41 subjects in Venezuela received one week's treatment with oral vitamin supplements including 500–750 mg of vitamin C (12). Once again they underwent endoscopy, and gastric juice was obtained for ascorbic acid assay.

Results

Although oral supplementation led to a sharp rise in plasma vitamin C levels, there was no change in ascorbic acid levels in gastric juice. Thus enhancement of whole-body vitamin C stores does not increase intragastric secretion of ascorbic acid in subjects with *H pylori*–associated gastritis. Oral supplementation will presumably increase gastric concentrations only transiently following ingestion. These data are in keeping with the results of a study performed years ago (15) in which it was found that a few days of oral high-dose vitamin C supplementation did not increase total vitamin C concentrations in gastric juice in volunteers of unknown gastric histological status.

Effect of Eradication of *H pylori*

If infection with *H pylori* damages the putative secretory mechanism, then eradication of such infection (which is accompanied by resolution of gastritis) may allow recovery of secretion. We are in the process of testing this hypothesis. Gastric juice samples are being obtained for ascorbic acid assay in an ongoing trial from patients with duodenal ulcer disease and *H pylori*–associated gastritis before and after attempted eradication of the bacterium. Results to date suggest that there probably is a gradual recovery of ascorbic acid levels in gastric juice after successful eradication. This hypothesis bears careful further examination.

Conclusion

Ascorbic acid is present in high concentrations in the gastric juice of individuals with normal gastric histology, suggesting a secretory process. *H pylori*–associated gastritis appears to damage the secretion mechanism: acute infection is associated with a fall in levels, and eradication of infection may gradually restore levels. In patients with gastritis, those with neutral gastric juice pH and intestinal metaplasia have the lowest ascorbic acid levels. This probably represents consumption by nitrite-derived species. However, low concentrations of ascorbic acid in gastric juice would seem to be only one factor in explaining high risk for gastric cancer in susceptible populations, as similar levels are found in populations at low risk for the disease. Oral vitamin supplementation in the presence of *H pylori*–associated gastritis is not effective in raising fasting ascorbic acid concentrations in gastric juice.

These findings suggest one mechanism by which *H pylori* infection may predispose certain individuals to developing gastric cancer, although multiple other factors must be involved to account for the wide variation in gastric cancer incidence among different populations with similar prevalences of *H pylori* infection. A reduced ascorbic acid concentration in gastric juice could make individuals more susceptible to certain dietary carcinogens, but the risk would only be realized if such exposure subsequently occurred.

ACKNOWLEDGMENTS

This work has been a collaborative effort with C. J. Schorah, M. Sanderson, and M. F. Dixon in Leeds and B. Pignatelli and N. Munoz from the IARC, Lyon, France, and the Cancer Control Centre, San Cristobal, Venezuela.

REFERENCES

1. Mirvish SS, Wallcave L, Eagan M, Shubik P. Ascorbate-nitrite reaction: possible means of blocking the formation of carcinogenic N-nitroso compounds. *Science.* 1972;177:65–68.
2. Licht WR, Deen WM. Theoretical model for predicting rates of nitrosamine and nitrosamide formation in the human stomach. *Carcinogenesis.* 1988;9:2227–2237.
3. Licht WR, Tannenbaum SR, Deen WM. Use of ascorbic acid to inhibit nitrosation: kinetic and mass transfer considerations for an in vitro system. *Carcinogenesis.* 1988;3:365–372.
4. Sanderson MJ, Schorah CJ. Measurement of ascorbic acid and dehydroascorbic acid in gastric juice by HPLC. *Biomed Chromatogr.* 1987;2:197–202.

5. Peters GA, Martin HE. Ascorbic acid in gastric juice. *Proc Soc Exp Biol Med.* 1937;36:76–78.
6. Freeman JT, Hafkesbring R. Comparative study of ascorbic acid levels in gastric secretion, blood, urine and saliva. *Gastroenterology.* 1951;18:224–229.
7. Freeman JT, Hafkesbring R. Comparative studies of ascorbic acid levels in gastric secretion and blood, III: gastrointestinal disease. *Gastroenterology.* 1957;32:878–886.
8. Singh D, Godbole AG. A study of plasma and gastric juice ascorbic acid in peptic ulcer disease. *J Assoc Physicians India.* 1968; 16:833–837.
9. Sobala GM, Schorah CJ, Sanderson M, *et al.* Ascorbic acid in the human stomach. *Gastroenterology.* 1989;97:357–363.
10. Sobala GM, Pignatelli B, Schorah CJ, *et al.* Simultaneous determination of ascorbic acid, nitrite, total nitrosocompounds and bile acids in fasting gastric juice, and gastric mucosal histology: implications for gastric carcinogenesis. *Carcinogenesis.* 1991;12: 193–198.
11. Sobala GM, Pignatelli B, Schorah CJ, *et al.* Study of gastric juice factors implicated in gastric carcinogenesis in members of a gastric cancer family. *Gut.* 1990;31(10):A1174.
12. Munoz N, Oliver W, Sobala G, *et al.* Prevalence of *Helicobacter pylori* infection and effect of anti-oxidants in a high-risk population for gastric cancer in Venezuela. *Ital J Gastro.* 1991;23(9) (suppl 2):15.
13. Morris A, Nicholson G. Ingestion of *Campylobacter pyloridis* causes gastritis and raised fasting gastric pH. *Am J Gastroenterol.* 1987; 82:192–199.
14. Sobala GM, Crabtree J, Dixon MF, *et al.* Acute *Helicobacter pylori* infection: clinical features, local and systemic immune response, gastric mucosal histology and gastric juice ascorbic acid concentrations. *Gut.* 1991;32:1415–1418.
15. Hafkesbring R, Freeman JT. Comparative studies of ascorbic acid levels in gastric secretion, blood, urine and saliva, II: saturation studies. *Am J Med Sci.* 1952;224:324.

GLADYS BLOCK

Human Data on Vitamin C in Cancer Prevention

ABSTRACT

Over ninety epidemiologic studies of the role of intake of vitamin C (or fruits that supply vitamin C) and cancer have been reviewed. Almost all show a protective relationship, with a median relative risk of about 2 for low compared with high intake, and three-fourths were statistically significant. Evidence is consistent for cancers of the stomach, esophagus, oral cavity, and pancreas, and it is substantial for cancers of the cervix and rectum as well. Increasing evidence supports a role in reducing the risk of lung cancer, and a meta-analysis found a strong role in reduction of breast cancer. National survey data indicate that substantial segments of the United States population are regularly consuming quite low levels of vitamin C. In women under age 45 the median intake is below the recommended dietary allowance, and among persons near the poverty level the median is below the recommended dietary allowance in both men and women. Substantial segments of the population near the poverty level consume far below the recommended dietary allowance. The epidemiologic data suggest that levels well above the recommended dietary allowance may be needed to reduce cancer risk.

Introduction

Extensive epidemiologic evidence indicates an inverse association between intake of vitamin C, or fruits that supply vitamin C, and risk of cancer. Consistently, persons with a high intake of vitamin C or citrus fruit have a lower risk of developing cancer. This paper summarizes that literature and provides some data on the intake of this vitamin in the United States population.

Vitamin C has a number of important biologic functions, including synthesis of neurotransmitters, hormones, collagen, and other biologically important substances. In the area of cancer prevention, however, probably its most important role is as an antioxidant and free radical scavenger. Oxidative damage to DNA and cell membranes is thought to be an important factor in cancer initiation and progression, and there is considerable evidence that ascorbic acid can prevent such damage and participate in its repair. Epidemiologic data can provide the means of examining whether the laboratory data, which provide the biologic mechanisms and rationale, are relevant to the human population.

Methods

Epidemiologic studies that examined the relationship between cancer and intake of vitamin C, or of fruits rich in vitamin C, have been reported in detail elsewhere (1) and are summarized here. Only case-control and cohort studies are included in this summary. In addition, several large, nationally representative surveys of dietary intake have provided data on levels of nutrient intake in the United States and on blood levels of ascorbic acid. These studies were the second National Health and Nutrition Examination Survey (NHANES II) (2) and the Continuing Survey of Food Intakes by Individuals (CSFII) (3), conducted by the United States Department of Agriculture. The nutrient data in NHANES II were collected using a 24-hour recall, which provides good information on the mean and median intake in the population. The CSFII nutrient data reported here consist of four 24-hour recalls obtained for the same individuals in four different seasons of the year. They thus provide not only good information about the mean and median intake but also improved data on the distribution of usual intakes. The NHANES II also obtained serum ascorbate measurements (4), and those data provide information on the distribution of blood levels.

Results

Epidemiologic Data

esophageal and oral cancer

The evidence of a protective role for vitamin C in esophageal and oral cancer is strong. Seven of eight oral cancer studies, all large and well controlled for smoking and alcohol, found low vitamin C intake to be a strong independent risk factor. Frequently, those in the lowest fourth of the distribution of intake had approximately a twofold increased risk of oral cancer compared with those in the highest one-fourth (5, 6). Similar results were seen for esophageal cancer. All four studies that examined an index of intake of vitamin C found increased risk with low intake (7–10), as did most studies that studied intake of fruit. The only studies that did not find a protective effect of high intake were in high-risk populations, in which essentially no one had high intake of fruit. For example, no high-intake protective effect was found in an area of China with an extremely high esophageal cancer rate (11); but the high intake category there consisted of those who ate fruit 35 times per year.

In summary, all nine studies of these cancer sites that examined a vitamin C index found significant protective effects, with a relative risk magnitude of about 2.0. The studies with foods rich in vitamin C were similarly consistent. Carotene was a weaker factor in five of these studies and was not significant.

STOMACH CANCER

In a large cohort study by Stahelin *et al.* (12), plasma samples were obtained before the development of disease and analyzed for ascorbic acid. Persons who developed stomach cancer over the subsequent 12 years had a significantly lower level of ascorbic acid in their plasma at baseline. Seven other investigators have reported on the relationship between dietary vitamin C intake and stomach cancer risk, and all found significant and substantial protection with higher intake. Seven of eight additional studies that examined fruit intake also found significantly reduced risk with higher intakes.

LUNG CANCER

Nine of eleven investigators who studied the role of vitamin C in lung cancer found reduced risk with high intake, even after control for smoking (13, 14), and five of these were statistically significant. Of those five, four found a weaker effect of beta-carotene. The evidence for an important role for carotenoids in reducing the risk of lung cancer is consistent, but recent studies suggest that vitamin C is also a protective factor.

PANCREATIC CANCER

Six of seven studies of risk factors for pancreatic cancer found vitamin C, or fruits rich in vitamin C, to be associated with a significant and substantial reduction in risk. Falk *et al.* (15), for example, found that those who consumed less than 70 mg per day had a relative risk of 2.6 compared with those who consumed 159 mg per day or more. Like esophageal cancer and lung cancer, pancreatic cancer has poor prognosis, and agents that can help reduce the risk are extremely important.

CERVICAL CANCER

Several studies of the precancerous condition cervical dysplasia found greatly increased risk with low intake of vitamin C (16, 17). For example, plasma levels were 0.36 mg/dL in women with the precursor lesion and 0.75 mg/dL in controls, even after control for number of pregnancies, number of sexual partners, and other risk factors. When diet records rather than questionnaires were used to assess intake, it was found that women with intake below 88 mg of vitamin C per day had four times the risk of dysplasia or carcinoma in situ as those with higher intake. (For reference, the recommended dietary allowance is 60 mg per day.) Three of five studies of invasive cervical cancer found significant increased risk with low intake of dietary vitamin C, and at least one of the studies that did not find an effect failed to consider the role of vitamin supplements.

COLORECTAL CANCER

Six of seven studies of rectal cancer found reduced risk with higher intake of vitamin C or foods rich in vitamin C; four were statistically significant. For colon cancer, six of eight studies found reduced risk with higher intake; four of these studies were statistically significant. Macquart-Moulin *et al.* (18), for example, found a relative risk of 1.8 for low- compared with high-intake quartile, in a study with 399 cases and matched controls, after adjustment for age, sex, caloric intake, and body weight. Others have found fruit intake to be protective (19, 20).

BREAST CANCER

Howe *et al.* (21), in a meta-analysis of the role of dietary factors in this cancer, found that "vitamin C intake had the most consistent and statistically significant inverse association with breast cancer risk." The effect was independent of the effect of saturated fat intake. In this analysis vitamin C, or some agent closely associated with vitamin C in fruits and vegetables, was of a magnitude at least equal to that of saturated fat.

OVARIAN, ENDOMETRIAL, AND PROSTATE CANCER

The one study of endometrial cancer and three of ovarian cancer did not find any association with vitamin C intake, although they did find evidence of a beneficial effect of vegetable intake. Although some studies have suggested an increased risk of prostate cancer with increasing carotenoid intake, the evidence is mixed at best even for vegetables or carotenoids. With one exception (22), neither a harmful nor a protective effect has been found for vitamin C.

SUMMARY

About 50 studies involving non–hormone-dependent cancer sites have examined the role of vitamin C intake; virtually all of them found effects in the protective direction, three-fourths of them were protective to a statistically significant degree, and not one was significantly harmful. An additional 30 studies have examined the effect of fruits rich in vitamin C. Virtually all of them indicated a protective effect with higher intake, and two-thirds of these studies were statistically significant. Magnitudes were of the order of twofold, that is, approximately a twofold increased risk for those in the lower compared with those in the higher one-fourth of the distribution.

Among cancers of the ovary, endometrium, and prostate, the evidence is either meager or does not support a beneficial effect of vitamin C intake. For breast cancer, however, the meta-analysis by Howe *et al.* suggests a strong effect of vitamin C in reducing the risk of this disease.

Intakes and Blood Levels

Although vitamin C intake is often thought to be adequate in the United States, a close look at the distributions of intake in national representative surveys suggests that important segments of the population may be consuming insufficient levels, even by the current recommended dietary allowance standards. In the NHANES II data, the median intake among persons above the poverty line was 69 mg per day for men 35 to 44 years of age and 55 mg per day for women in the same age group. That is, 50% consumed less than that amount on the day of the survey. Below the poverty line, however, the levels are even more disturbing. In the same age group, in the NHANES II data, the median intake was 46 mg per day for men and only 32 mg per day for women. More than half of all persons below the poverty line had less than the recommended dietary allowance.

The CSFII data, based on four nonconsecutive days of dietary data, provide a more reliable estimate of intake levels at other points along the distribution. In those data, the median among women below 130% of the poverty level was only 55 mg per day; but more disturbing, 25% of women below 130% of the poverty line had an average intake, averaged over four nonconsecutive days, of only 32 mg per day. Even among women with incomes at 130% to 300% or over 300% of the poverty line, 25% had four-day average daily intakes of only 38 mg or 44 mg of vitamin C per day, respectively. Of women below 130% of the poverty level, 10% had four-day average intakes of only 19 mg per day.

The intake data in the United States are borne out by serum ascorbic acid levels found in NHANES II. Substantial minorities—10% to 15% of white men and 20% to 30% of black men—had serum ascorbate levels of 0.3 mg/dL or less. These are very low blood levels, and they are levels that have been found to be associated with increased risk of stomach cancer and cervical dysplasia. The risk associated with such low blood levels has not yet been established for other cancer sites, but a risk associated with low blood levels would be reasonable to expect, given the associations with low dietary intakes.

These data suggest that substantial groups in the United States do not consume vitamin C even at the level of the recommended dietary allowance. The studies in the epidemiologic literature suggest that for at least some cancers, even intake of the recommended dietary allowance may place individuals in a high-risk group.

Conclusion

Substantial epidemiologic evidence supports a role for vitamin C in reducing the risk of a variety of cancers (1). Such a role is consistent with ascorbate's antioxidant and free radical properties and with the evidence that oxidative damage is an important factor in cancer incidence. The epidemiologic studies mentioned above cannot distinguish with certainty between a role for vitamin C specifically and a role for other nutrients provided by foods rich in vitamin C. Such nutrients include carotenoids, folate, and vitamin E. It is likely, however, that the answer does not lie with a single nutrient and that efforts and arguments aimed at identifying the "right" one are misguided. It is increasingly clear that all of these nutrients are important, perhaps at different physiologic sites or under different carcinogenic challenges. Ascorbic acid may be the first line of defense in some situations (23, 24), but adequate intakes of all nutrients are necessary. In the United States, it would appear that substantial segments of the population do not regularly consume levels of vitamin C that appear to confer a reduced risk of cancer.

REFERENCES

1. Block G. Vitamin C and cancer prevention: the epidemiologic evidence. *Am J Clin Nutr.* 1991;53:270S–282S.
2. Carroll MD, Abraham S, Dresser CM. *Dietary Intake Source Data: United States, 1976–80.* Hyattsville, Md: National Center for Health Statistics; 1983. Dept of Health and Human Services publication PHS 83-1681. Vital and Health Statistics series 11, no. 231.
3. United States Department of Agriculture Human Nutrition Information Service. *Nationwide Food Consumption Survey, Continuing Survey of Food Intakes by Individuals. Women 19-50 and Their Children 1-5 Years, 4 Days.* Washington, DC: US Dept of Agriculture, 1988. NFCS, CSFII 86–3.
4. Fulwood R, Johnson CL, Bryner JD. *Hematological and Nutritional Biochemistry Reference Data for Persons 6 Months–74 Years of Age: United States, 1976–80.* Washington, DC: National Center for Health Statistics; 1982. Dept of Health and Human Services publication PHS 83-1682. Vital and Health Statistics series 11, no. 232.
5. McLaughlin JK, Gridley G, Block G, *et al.* Dietary factors in oral and pharyngeal cancer. *J Natl Cancer Inst.* 1988;80:1237–1243.
6. Winn DM, Ziegler RG, Pickle LW, Gridley G, Blot WJ, Hoover RN. Diet in the etiology of oral and pharyngeal cancer among women from the southern United States. *Cancer Res.* 1984;44:1216–1222.
7. Brown LM, Blot WJ, Schuman SH, *et al.* Environmental factors and high risk of esophageal cancer among men in coastal South Carolina. *J Natl Cancer Inst.* 1988;80:1620–1625.
8. Tuyns AJ. Protective effect of citrus fruit on esophageal cancer. *Nutr Cancer.* 1983;5:195–200.
9. Ziegler RG, Morris LE, Blot WJ, Pottern LM, Hoover R, Frau-

meni JF. Esophageal cancer among black men in Washington, D.C., II: role of nutrition. *J Natl Cancer Inst.* 1981;67:1199–1206.

10. Mettlin C, Graham S, Priore R, Marshall J, Swanson M. Diet and cancer of the esophagus. *Nutr Cancer.* 1980;2:143–147.
11. Li J-Y, Ershow AG, Chen Z-J, *et al.* A case-control study of cancer of the esophagus and gastric cardia in Linxian. *Int J Cancer.* 1989;43:755–761.
12. Stahelin HB, Gey KF, Eichholzer M, *et al.* Plasma antioxidant vitamins and subsequent cancer mortality in the 12-year follow-up of the Prospective Basel Study. *Am J Epidemiol.* 1991;133:766–775.
13. Kromhout D. Essential micronutrients in relation to carcinogenesis. *Am J Clin Nutr.* 1987;45:1361–1367.
14. Fontham ETH, Pickle LW, Haenszel W, Correa P, Lin Y, Falk RT. Dietary vitamins A and C and lung cancer risk in Louisiana. *Cancer.* 1988;62:2267–2273.
15. Falk RT, Pickle LW, Fontham ET, Correa P, Fraumeni JF. Life-style risk factors for pancreatic cancer in Louisiana: a case-control study. *Am J Epidemiol.* 1988;128:324–336.
16. Wassertheil-Smoller S, Romney SL, Wylie-Rosett J, *et al.* Dietary vitamin C and uterine cervical dysplasia. *Am J Epidemiol.* 1981; 114:714–724.
17. Romney SL, Duttagupta C, Basu J, *et al.* Plasma vitamin C and uterine cervical dysplasia. *Am J Obstet Gynecol.* 1985;151:976–980.
18. Macquart-Moulin G, Riboli E, Cornee J, Charnay B, Berthezene P, Day N. Case-control study on colorectal cancer and diet in Marseilles. *Int J Cancer.* 1986;38:183–191.
19. Modan B, Barell V, Lubin F, Modan M, Greenberg RA, Graham S. Low-fiber intake as an etiologic factor in cancer of the colon. *J Natl Cancer Inst.* 1975;55:15–18.
20. Slattery ML, Sorenson AW, Mahoney AW, French TK, Kritchevsky D, Street JC. Diet and colon cancer: assessment of risk by fiber type and food source. *J Natl Cancer Inst.* 1988;80:1474–1480.
21. Howe GR, Hirohata T, Hislop TG, *et al.* Dietary factors and risk of breast cancer: combined analysis of 12 case-control studies. *J Natl Cancer Inst.* 1990;82:561–569.
22. Graham S, Haughey B, Marshall J, *et al.* Diet in the epidemiology of carcinoma of the prostate gland. *J Natl Cancer Inst.* 1983;70: 687–692.
23. Frei B, England L, Ames BN. Ascorbate is an outstanding antioxi-

dant in human blood plasma. *Proc Natl Acad Sci U S A.* 1989; 86:6377–6381.

24. Frei B, Stocker R, Ames BN. Antioxidant defenses and lipid peroxidation in human blood plasma. *Proc Natl Acad Sci U S A.* 1988;85:9748–9752.

CLEMENT IP

Vitamin E and Cancer Prevention in the Experimental Model

ABSTRACT

The interest in the antioxidant activity of vitamin E in cancer prevention can be traced in part to the free radical theory of carcinogenesis. However, little information is available on the effect of low vitamin E intake on tumor development in experimental animals. Most of the studies have involved the effect of an excess of vitamin E administration, which is achieved by addition to the diet, topical application, or repeated oral dosing. This paper reviews the results of vitamin E supplementation on four tumor models induced by carcinogens: oral cancer, skin cancer, breast cancer, and intestinal cancer. In general, vitamin E is effective in preventing oral and skin cancers when applied topically or given by repeat oral dosing. Results of vitamin E administration via the dietary route in the prevention of breast and intestinal tract cancer are much less encouraging. Vitamin E is a powerful antioxidant and can be tolerated in relatively large amounts. In the event that vitamin E by itself proves to have limited utility, the possibility remains that it may potentiate the activity of other anticancer agents as evidenced by the efficacy of the combination treatment of vitamin E and selenite.

Introduction

Vitamin E is a family of fat-soluble compounds that share a common 6-hydroxychroman ring structure and that can be divided into two groups on the basis of the degree of saturation of the side chain. The more important group, the tocopherols, is characterized by a long saturated side chain. There are four members of this group: the alpha-, beta-, gamma-, and delta-tocopherols; they differ in the number and position of methyl groups on the ring (Fig. 1). Tocotrienols

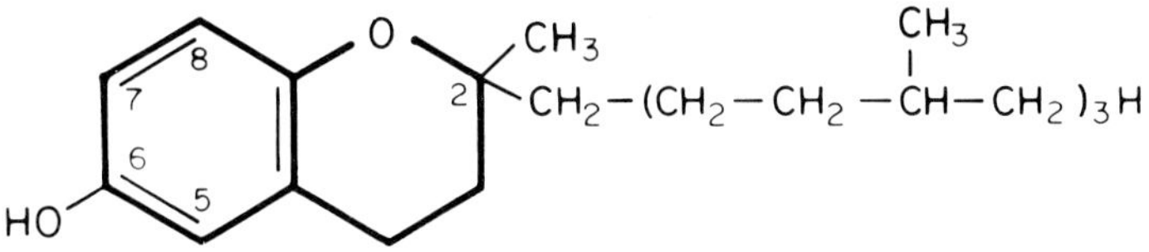

TOCOPHEROL

Tocopherol	Methyl Group
α	5, 7, 8
β	5, 8
γ	7, 8
δ	8

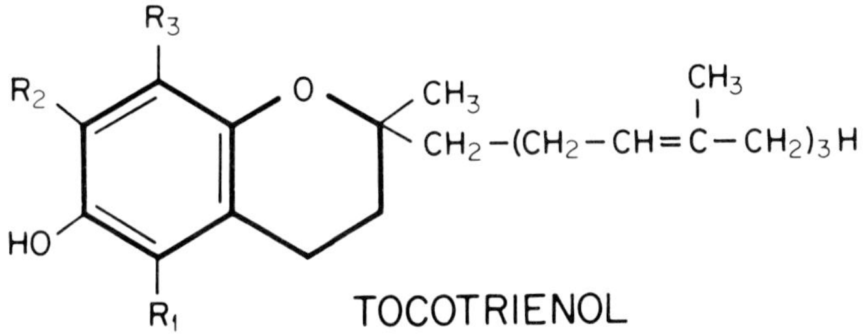

TOCOTRIENOL

Figure 1. Tocopherol and tocotrienol.

represent the second group, which is characterized by an unsaturated side chain. These different forms of vitamin E have different biological activities. Alpha-tocopherol is the most active among them, although it has been estimated that the average American diet contains about 2.5 times more gamma-tocopherol than alpha-tocopherol (1). If the activity of alpha-tocopherol is standardized as 100%, the relative activities of beta-tocopherol, gamma-tocopherol, and delta-tocopherol are in the range of 25% to 50%, 10% to 35%, and less than 5%, respectively (2); the range is due to different types of bioassays. Vitamin E is present in small quantities in a large variety of food. The richest sources are the common vegetable oils and products made from them (such as margarine and shortening), nuts, green leafy vegetables, milk fat, and egg yolk.

Synthetic alpha-tocopherol has several asymmetric centers that can give rise to a mixture of eight stereoisomers, whereas the natural alpha-tocopherol has only one isomer. The current nomenclature has specified that the natural alpha-tocopherol should be designated RRR-alpha-tocopherol (formerly d-alpha-tocopherol), and the synthetic compound should be designated all-rac-alpha-tocopherol (formerly dl-alpha-tocopherol); the activity of the latter is set at 74% of the activity of the former (3). This paper reviews many published studies that examined the effect of different levels of vitamin E on carcinogenesis. The amounts of vitamin E administered to the animals are sometimes expressed in milligrams and sometimes in international units (IU). In order to make it easier for the readers to compare the various studies, let us note here that 1 mg of all-rac-alpha-tocopheryl acetate is equivalent to 1 IU of vitamin E, whereas 1 mg of RRR-alpha-tocopheryl acetate is equivalent to 1.36 IU (4).

A deficiency of vitamin E in rats causes resorption of the fetus in the female and testicular degeneration in the male. The vitamin E–deficient rat also has increased hemolysis, either spontaneous or induced by treatment of the erythrocytes with oxidizing agents. In fact, the criterion of vitamin E requirement in rats is prevention of hemolysis. In a repletion study of vitamin E–deficient rats, Bieri (5) showed that hemolysis was prevented after feeding 20 mg RRR-alpha-tocopheryl acetate per kilogram of diet. This concentration also achieved stable levels of alpha-tocopherol in the tissues within eight weeks of repletion. The AIN-76 diet formulation, which is extensively used in animal nutrition studies, provides 50 IU of vitamin E activity per kilogram of diet in the form of all-rac-alpha-tocopheryl acetate (6). The reason for pointing out the amount of vitamin E in a standardized synthetic diet is to provide a reference base line value comparison with the levels of vitamin E supplementation that will be discussed later.

Antioxidant Function and Protection Against Cancer

The interest in the antioxidant activity of vitamin E in cancer prevention can be traced in part to the free radical theory of carcinogenesis (7, 8). Mounting evidence indicates that the processes of tumor initiation, promotion, and progression can be affected by oxygen radical–mediated events. Vitamin E is known chemically as an antioxidant. Because of its hydrophobic nature, it is better suited to function in the microenvironment of cellular membranes containing a high concentration of lipids. Polyunsaturated fatty acids in the membrane compartment are susceptible to peroxidation induced by free radicals such as peroxyl radical, hydroxyl radical, and superoxide. One of the principal functions of vitamin E is believed to be protection against this type of oxidative damage by acting as a free radical scavenger. Malondialdehyde, an end product of lipid peroxidation, has been shown to cause undesirable bonding of proteins and nucleic acids (9). These cross-linkings of macromolecules may prevent their proper functioning in maintaining cellular homeostasis. In addition, malondialdehyde has also been reported to be a carcinogenic initiator of mouse skin (10) and is found to be mutagenic in the Ames test (11). The free radicals generated during lipid peroxidation could also be involved in the activation of chemical carcinogens. Therefore, lipid peroxidation, although a normal occurrence in animal tissue, can lead to a host of deleterious effects in cells if it remains unchecked. Vitamin E could thus play an important role in lowering the risk of oncogenesis by restricting the extent of peroxidative damage.

Low Vitamin E Intake and Cancer Risk

Surprisingly, little information is available on the effect of low vitamin E intake on tumor development in experimental animals. Our laboratory reported almost ten years ago a study comparing low and normal intakes of dietary vitamin E on the induction of mammary tumors in rats treated with a carcinogen (12). Using the 7,12-dimethylbenz(a)anthracene (DMBA) induced mammary tumor model, we found that a low vitamin E intake (7.5 mg of all-rac-alpha-tocopheryl acetate per kilogram of diet) had minimal effect on carcinoma development in rats fed a 5% stripped corn oil diet, but it resulted in a marked enhancement in tumor incidence and yield in those rats fed a 25% stripped corn oil ration. Control animals in this experiment received an adequate supply of vitamin E (30 mg of all-rac-alpha-tocopheryl acetate per kilogram of diet). Thus the effect of vitamin E deficiency on mammary carcinogenesis apparently is accentuated in rats on a high polyunsaturated-fat diet—an observation similar to that made in studies of selenium deficiency and cancer risk and reported earlier by our laboratory (13). Further studies showed that a low vitamin E intake significantly increased lipid peroxidation in the mammary fat pad, especially in animals fed the high-fat diet (14). Thus in the present model, a high oxidant stress in the target tissue is correlated with an increased susceptibility to mammary carcinogenesis.

Effect of Vitamin E Supplementation on Experimental Tumor Models

This section reviews the results of vitamin E supplementation on four tumor models induced by carcinogens. In the following studies vitamin E was administered in one of three ways: addition of an excess quantity to a diet that already contained an adequate amount of vitamin E to satisfy the nutritional requirement of the animal; topical application to the organ site of interest, for example, oral mucosa or skin; repeated dosing by gavage for a defined period of time. There are also isolated reports about the effect of vitamin E on chemically induced urinary bladder cancer (15), liver cancer (16), and pancreatic cancer (17); however, these will not be included in the following discussion because it is difficult to make any generalized conclusion based on single publications. The inhibitory action of vitamin E on the formation of carcinogenic nitrosamines resulting from the reaction of amines and nitrite has been reviewed recently (18) and will not be covered here. Information on the modulation by vitamin E of cellular proliferation, morphological differentiation, and oncogene expression in the in vitro system is still emerging and is not ready for summary purposes.

Oral Cancer

The chemopreventive activity of vitamin E is most encouraging with the oral cancer model. The studies described below were all carried out in the laboratory of Gerald Shklar. The carcinomas in the buccal pouch of Syrian golden hamsters were induced by topical application of a DMBA solution in mineral oil three times a week for seven weeks. Vitamin E, in the form of all-rac-alpha-tocopherol, has been shown to significantly inhibit the development of epidermoid carcinomas whether given orally (19) or painted directly on the cheek pouch (20). The gavage protocol involved 10 mg of vitamin E given twice per week on alternate days during the period of DMBA administration, whereas the topical application protocol involved painting about

47 mg of vitamin E each time three times a week for four weeks following DMBA administration. Tumors were fewer in number and smaller in size in hamsters receiving vitamin E. Complete prevention of tumor appearance was reported when a low-dose DMBA regimen was used in hamsters given oral doses of vitamin E (21). Shklar *et al.* also showed that direct injection of 250 μg of vitamin E into the tumor-bearing buccal pouch twice a week for four weeks led to significant regression of established tumors (22). Microscopic examination of oral mucosa with regressed tumors revealed a dense infiltration of leukocytes, lymphocytes, and histiocytes. The appearance of these immune cells was associated with an increase in tumor necrosis factor-alpha positive macrophages, suggesting a possible mechanism of tumor destruction (23).

Skin Cancer

The protective effect of vitamin E against skin cancer has also been successfully demonstrated independently by three laboratories. Slaga and Bracken (24) initially showed that in the DMBA and 12-0-tetradecanoylphorbol-13-acetate (TPA) two-stage skin papilloma model in mice, vitamin E (1 mg, form not specified), when applied directly to the skin 5 minutes before DMBA initiation, inhibited tumor development. Several years ago, Perchellet *et al.* (25) found that RRR-alpha-tocopherol also suppressed skin carcinogenesis in the same model system when administered topically 15 minutes before TPA during the tumor-promotion period. In this experiment, TPA treatment was repeated twice a week and continued for 22 weeks. These investigators also showed that RRR-alpha-tocopherol blocked the induction of ornithine decarboxylase activity by TPA. Thus vitamin E appears to be active as a preventive agent in both the initiation and promotion phases of skin carcinogenesis. With the use of ultraviolet (UV) irradiation as the physical carcinogenic agent, Gensler and Magdaleno (26) recently reported that skin cancer incidence in mice was reduced by half if the animals were treated topically with 25 mg of all-rac-alpha-tocopherol three times a week beginning at 3 weeks before UV irradiation and continued for 33 weeks after the first UV exposure. Ultraviolet irradiation is known to induce free radicals and lipid peroxidation in the skin, thus leading to DNA damage, which ultimately results in cancer. The above observation is consistent with that of another study showing that local administration of vitamin E before and after UV exposure reduced malondialdehyde production in the skin (27).

Breast Cancer

In contrast to the results in oral and skin tumorigenesis, the effect of vitamin E on the breast cancer model is rather disappointing. Using DMBA as the carcinogen for tumor induction, Wattenberg failed to detect any protective effect of alpha-tocopherol given in a single 200 mg oral dose at one hour before DMBA (28). Subsequent studies by King and McCay (29) as well as by Horvath and Ip (30) confirmed that all-rac-alpha-tocopheryl acetate, when supplemented at concentrations of 1 g or 2 g per kilogram of diet for the duration of the experiment, did not result in any significant inhibitory response in the development of mammary neoplasia in rats treated with DMBA. Gould and co-workers recently tested alpha-tocopherol and tocotrienol in the methylnitrosourea-induced mammary tumor model (31). This was the first study in which the activity of tocotrienols was evaluated for cancer prevention, although it should be noted that the tocotrienol concentrate was isolated from palm oil and contained only about 60% in the form of alpha-, gamma-, and delta-tocotrienols. Neither tocopherol nor tocotrienol, when supplemented at a level of 3.4 μmol per gram of diet (or about 1.4 g/kg), was found to have any significant inhibitory effect on tumor incidence or number.

Intestinal Cancer

Unlike the results for the breast cancer model, in which vitamin E shows a consistently negative effect, the data on the intestinal cancer model are somewhat confusing. Part of the reason could be certain confounding factors inherent in the design of the experiments. A study by Cook and McNamara (32) is often cited in the literature on the protective effect of vitamin E in colon carcinogenesis. These investigators found fewer numbers of colon adenomas and invasive carcinomas in mice that were treated with dimethylhydrazine (DMH) and given 600 mg of vitamin E per kilogram of diet. Control mice in this experiment were fed only 10 mg of vitamin E per kilogram of diet, a level that could be considered marginally deficient. Thus interpretation of the data could be complicated by comparing mice that were given an excessive amount of vitamin E with those that were given a level of vitamin E that might be below the nutritional requirement. At very high levels of vitamin E supplementation (*i.e.*, 4% of all-rac-alpha-tocopheryl acetate in the diet), Toth and Patil (33) reported increases in tumor development of the duodenum, cecum, colon, rectum, and anus in mice similarly treated with DMH. This level was considerably higher than that used in the breast cancer studies, in which concentrations in the range of 0.1% to 0.2% of vitamin E in the diet were fed to the animals. When lower levels of vitamin E (in the range of 180 to 1750 mg/kg) were used in colon cancer prevention experiments involving either DMH or azoxymethane treatment for tumor induction, three independent reports all came up with negative results (34–36).

Vitamin E Levels in Tissue

As can be seen from the above section, the administration of vitamin E via the diet is not efficacious in preventing cancer that develops in internal organs, such as the mammary gland and the gastrointestinal tract. The reason could be that the effective dose of vitamin E has not been administered, or that the target organ is slow to accumulate this compound. A comprehensive kinetics study on tissue uptake following the feeding of high levels of vitamin E in rats was reported by Machlin and Gabriel almost a decade ago (37). Mature female rats were supplemented with either 1000 or 10 000 mg/kg of all-rac-alpha-tocopheryl acetate in their experiment. Several tissues were analyzed at different time points, including plasma, platelets, the liver, erythrocytes, adipose tissue, the heart, the liver, the lung, skeletal muscle, and the brain. The tocopherol content of all these tissues continued to rise slowly over the duration of the feeding period, which lasted up to 20 weeks. Liver and adipose tissue accumulated tocopherol at a more rapid rate than other tissues, although in all cases a saturation point was not attained even at a dietary level of 10 000 mg/kg after 20 weeks of supplementation. We have observed similar findings in the mammary gland of rats fed 1000 mg of all-rac-alpha-tocopheryl acetate per kilogram of diet for 24 weeks (unpublished data). Thus both the level and the duration of supplementation are important factors in determining the concentration of vitamin E in all tissues. In those previously discussed experiments in which vitamin E failed to exert a cancer-protective effect when added to the diet, the possibility remains that the critical concentration of vitamin E had not been achieved in the target tissue during the course of the studies.

Interaction of Vitamin E and Selenium

There is a considerable body of literature on the anticarcinogenic activity of selenium, particularly that of selenite. Our laboratory has investigated whether the vitamin E status of the animal affects the efficacy of selenite in protection against DMBA-induced mammary tumors. A series of experiments carried out over a period of several years has led to the following observations. First, the chemopreventive action of selenite was attenuated in the presence of a low intake of vitamin E (14). Second, the combination of vitamin E and selenite was more active than the single-agent selenite treatment in suppressing mammary carcinogensis (30). In other words, vitamin E, although supplementation with it alone has no prophylactic effect in the DMBA model, can potentiate the anticarcinogenic action of selenite. Third, subsequent studies indicated that vitamin E would allow the use of lower levels of selenite in chemoprevention (38). For example, a combination of 500 mg/kg of all-rac-alpha-tocopheryl acetate and 1 mg/kg of selenite Se was found to be just as efficacious as 2.5 mg/kg of selenite Se alone. In our experience, a concentration of 1 mg/kg of selenite Se in the diet (in the absence of supplemental vitamin E) normally has minimal effect in tumor suppression. In view of the concern over the toxicity associated with high doses of selenite, the use of vitamin E in enhancing the cancer chemopreventive efficacy of selenite should be further examined.

Since the anticarcinogenic action of selenite is most commonly achieved by administering the test compound at high levels, it is reasonable to suspect that some intermediate (or intermediates) in the normal pathway of selenium detoxification are responsible for the anticarcinogenic effects. Selenite is first reduced to hydrogen selenide, which is then sequentially methylated to methylselenol, dimethylselenide, and trimethylselenonium. At high levels of selenite intake, dimethylselenide is exhaled in the breath, and trimethylselenonium is excreted in the urine (39). There is increasing evidence from our laboratory that the methylated metabolites of selenium, particularly the monomethylated selenide, may be the active species in cancer protection (40, 41). Oxidation of methylselenol and dimethylselenide by microsomal oxygenase in vivo would divert the traffic away from the methylation pathway that would otherwise facilitate the metabolism to dimethylselenide and trimethylselenonium destined for respiratory and urinary excretion, respectively. It is possible that vitamin E stabilizes the microsomal oxygenase system, thereby favoring the oxidation of methylated selenides and decreasing the amount of dimethylselenide available for excretion. Since the oxidized products can be reduced easily back to the starting compounds, the oxidation mechanism may act as a reservoir to retain selenium in the tissues so that a critical concentration of methylselenol will be maintained for a longer period.

Conclusion

Vitamin E is effective in preventing oral and skin cancer in experimental models when applied topically to the mucosal or epidermal surface. Repeated oral dosing with vitamin E has also been found to be successful in protection against oral cancer. At present it is unclear whether these two tissues are particularly sensitive to vitamin E or whether the method of local application allows a greater uptake and concentration of the vitamin in the target cells. Future vitamin E intervention trials may be focused on lesions associated with these two sites, especially in high-risk individuals. Results of vitamin E administration via the diet in the prevention of breast and intestinal tract cancer are much less encouraging. Part of the reason could be a slow accumulation of vitamin E in the tissue when the reagent is given systemically so that an effective concentration may rarely be attained during the course of the experiment. If this is the case, higher levels of vitamin E supplementation need to be evaluated to determine a dose-response relationship or to confirm the possibility that vitamin E is a weak protective agent when given systemically. In the event that vitamin E by itself proves to have limited utility in cancer prevention, the opportunity is still available for investigating the combination of vitamin E and another known inhibitory agent with the objective of increasing the potency of the second agent. The potentiation of the anticarcinogenic activity of selenite by vitamin E appears promising and should be pursued more vigorously in other tumor models. Vitamin E is a powerful antioxidant and can be tolerated in relatively large amounts. The possibility prevails that it may have a permissive effect on other anticancer agents that tend to work more efficiently in a low oxidant stress environment.

REFERENCES

1. Bieri JG, Poukkla-Evarts R. Tocopherols and fatty acids in American diets. *J Am Diet Assoc.* 1973;62:147–151.
2. National Research Council. *Recommended Dietary Allowances: Vitamin E.* 10th ed. Washington, DC: National Academy Press; 1989: 99–107.
3. Diplock AT. Vitamin E. In: *Fat-Soluble Vitamins: Their Biochemistry and Applications.* Lancaster, PA: Technomic Publications Co; 1985: 154–224.
4. Bieri JG, McKenna MC. Expressing dietary values for fat-soluble vitamins: changes in concepts and terminology. *Am J Clin Nutr.* 1981;34:289–295.
5. Bieri JG. Kinetics of tissue alpha-tocopherol depletion and repletion. *Ann N Y Acad Sci.* 1972;203:181–191.
6. American Institute of Nutrition. Report of the American Institute of Nutrition Ad Hoc Committee on Standards for Nutritional Studies. *J. Nutr.* 1977;107:1340–1348.
7. Marnett LJ. Peroxyl free radicals: potential mediators of tumor initiation and promotion. *Carcinogenesis.* 1987;8:1365–1373.
8. Breimer LH. Molecular mechanisms of oxygen radical carcinogenesis and mutagenesis: the role of DNA base damage. *Mol Carcinog.* 1990;3:188–197.
9. Tappel AL. Lipid peroxidation damage to cell components. *Fed Proc.* 1973;32:1870–1874.
10. Shamberger RJ, Andreone TL, Willis CE. Antioxidant and cancer, IV: initiating activity of malonaldehyde as a carcinogen. *J Natl Cancer Inst.* 1974;53:1771–1773.
11. Shamberger RJ, Corlett CL, Beaman KD, Kasten BL. Antioxidants reduce the mutagenic effect of malonaldehyde and propiolactone, part IX: antioxidants and cancer. *Mutat Res.* 1979;66:349–355.
12. Ip C. Dietary vitamin E intake and mammary carcinogenesis in rats. *Carcinogensis.* 1982;3:1453–1456.

13. Ip C, Sinha D. Enhancement of mammary tumorigenesis by dietary selenium deficiency in rats with a high polyunsaturated fat intake. *Cancer Res.* 1981;41:31–34.
14. Ip C. Attentuation of the anticarcinogenic action of selenium by vitamin E deficiency. *Cancer Lett.* 1985;25:325–331.
15. Tamano S, Fukushima S, Shirai T, Hirose M, Ito N. Modification by alpha-tocopherol, propyl gallate, and tertiary butylhydroquinone of urinary bladder carcinogenesis in Fischer 344 rats pretreated with N-butyl-N-(4-hydroxybutyl)nitrosamine. *Cancer Lett.* 1987;35:39–46.
16. Swick RW, Bauman CA. Tocopherol in tumor tissues and effects of tocopherol on the development of liver tumors. *Cancer Res.* 1951;11:948–953.
17. Woutersen RA, Garderen-Hoetmer AV. Inhibition of dietary fat-promoted development of (pre)neoplastic lesions in exocrine pancreas of rats and hamsters by supplemental vitamins A, C and E. *Cancer Lett.* 1988;41:179–189.
18. Mirvish SS. Effects of vitamins C and E on N-nitroso compound formation, carcinogenesis, and cancer. *Cancer.* 1986;58:1842–1850.
19. Shklar G. Oral mucosal carcinogensis in hamsters: inhibition by vitamin E. *J Natl Cancer Inst.* 1982;68:791–797.
20. Odukoya O, Hawach F, Shklar G. Retardation of experimental oral cancer by topical vitamin E. *Nutr Cancer.* 1984;6:98–104.
21. Trickler D, Shklar G. Prevention by vitamin E of experimental oral carcinogenesis. *J Natl Cancer Inst.* 1987;78:165–167.
22. Shklar G, Schwartz J, Trickler DP, Niukian K. Regression by vitamin E of experimental oral cancer. *J Natl Cancer Inst.* 1987;78: 987–992.
23. Shklar G, Schwartz J. Tumor necrosis factor in experimental cancer regression with alpha-tocopherol, beta-carotene, canthaxanthin and algae extract. *Eur J Clin Oncol.* 1988;24:839–850.
24. Slaga T, Bracken WM. The effects of antioxidants on skin tumor initiation and aryl hydrocarbon hydroxylase. *Cancer Res.* 1977;37: 1631–1635.
25. Perchellet JP, Owen MD, Posey TD, Orten DK, Schneider BA. Inhibitory effects of glutathione level-raising agents and D-α-tocopherol on ornithine decarboxylase induction and mouse skin tumor promotion by 12-0-tetradecanoylphorbol-13-acetate. *Carcinogenesis.* 1985;6:567–573.

26. Gensler HL, Magdaleno M. Topical vitamin E inhibition of immunosuppression and tumorigenesis induced by ultraviolet irradiation. *Nutr Cancer.* 1991;15:97–106.
27. Khettab N, Amosy MC, Briand G, *et al.* Photoprotective effect of vitamin A and E on polyamine and oxygenated free radical metabolism in hairless mouse epidermis. *Biochimie.* 1988;70:1709–1713.
28. Wattenberg LW. Inhibition of carcinogenic and toxic effects of polycyclic hydrocarbons by phenolic antioxidants and ethoxyquin. *J. Natl Cancer Inst.* 1972;48:1425–1430.
29. King MM, McCay PB. Modulation of tumor incidence and possible mechanisms of inhibition of mammary carcinogenesis by dietary antioxidants. *Cancer Res.* 1983;43:2485S–2490S.
30. Horvath PM, Ip C. Synergistic effect of vitamin E and selenium in the chemoprevention of mammary carcinogenesis in rats. *Cancer Res.* 1983;43:5335–5341.
31. Gould MN, Haag JD, Kennan WS, Tanner MA, Elson CE. A comparison of tocopherol and tocotrienol for the chemoprevention of chemically induced rat mammary tumors. *Am J Clin Nutr.* 1991; 53:1068S–1070S.
32. Cook MG, McNamara P. Effect of dietary vitamin E on dimethylhydrazine-induced colonic tumors in mice. *Cancer Res.* 1980;40: 1329–1331.
33. Toth B, Patil K. Enhancing effect of vitamin E on murine intestinal tumorigenesis by 1,2-dimethylhydrazine dihydrochloride. *J Natl Cancer Inst.* 1983;70:1107–1111.
34. Chester JF, Gaissert HA, Ross JS, Malt RA, Weitzman SA. Augmentation of 1,2-dimethylhydrazine-induced colon cancer by experimental colitis in mice: role of dietary vitamin E. *J Natl Cancer Inst.* 1986;76:939–942.
35. Temple NJ, El-Khatib SM. Cabbage and vitamin E: their effect on colon tumor formation in mice. *Cancer Lett.* 1987;35:71–77.
36. Reddy BS, Tanaka T. Interactions of selenium deficiency, vitamin E, polyunsaturated fat, and saturated fat on azoxymethane-induced colon carcinogenesis in male F344 rats. *J Natl Cancer Inst.* 1986;76:1157–1162.
37. Machlin LJ, Gabriel E. Kinetics of tissue α-tocopherol uptake and depletion following administration of high levels of vitamin E. *Ann N Y Acad Sci.* 1983;393:48–59.

38. Ip C. Feasibility of using lower doses of chemopreventive agents in combination regimen for cancer protection. *Cancer Lett.* 1988; 39:239–246.
39. Ganther HE. Pathways of selenium metabolism including respiratory excretory products. *J Am Coll Toxicol.* 1986;5:1–5.
40. Ip C, Ganther H. Activity of methylated forms of selenium in cancer prevention. *Cancer Res.* 1990;50:1206–1211.
41. Ip C, Hayes C, Budnick RM, Ganther HE. Chemical form of selenium, critical metabolites, and cancer prevention. *Cancer Res.* 1991;51:595–600.

PAUL KNEKT

Human Data on Vitamin E and Cancer

ABSTRACT

Vitamin E may provide protection against cancer, primarily through its properties as a free radical scavenger and nitrosation blocker. This paper presents current human evidence for this hypothesis from epidemiological studies. The anticancer effect of vitamin E has been examined mainly in observational studies, that is, case-control and nested case-control studies, using dietary recall methods or serum/plasma determinations for the estimation of vitamin E exposure. Several intervention trials have also been initiated, but few results have been reported so far. The most reliable existing evidence comes from nested case-control studies. The focus of these studies has been on all sites of cancer combined and on cancers of the lung, gastrointestinal tract, and breast. Overall, there is a suggestive inverse relationship between the serum vitamin E level and the risk of lung cancer, colorectal cancer, and cancer at all sites. The results from the case-control studies support the lung cancer finding. They also suggest an inverse association with cervical cancer risk; ecological studies suggest a similar association with esophageal cancer risk. Irrespective of study design, none of the studies has provided any evidence for an inverse association between vitamin E exposure and the risk of breast cancer or other hormone-related female cancers. Although there is some evidence of an inverse association between vitamin E levels and some cancers, the findings may have been biased by insufficient control for confounding factors and occult cancer. Thus, the results of ongoing intervention trials are necessary to shed more light on whether a high vitamin E intake protects against cancer in humans.

Introduction

It has been suggested that vitamin E reduces the risk of cancer through its function as a free radical scavenger and as a blocker of nitrosation, and through other mechanisms (1). The most efficient design for testing this hypothesis is an intervention trial. In such a study, individuals who have no history of cancer are randomly assigned to an intervention group receiving vitamin E supplements or to a control group receiving a placebo. The occurrence of cancer within the groups is then monitored for a given time period. The few results published so far have mainly been from small trials concerning breast cancer and colon cancer (2). Several large-scale, randomized, placebo-controlled trials, most of them in groups at high risk of colon, lung, skin, or esophageal cancer, are still ongoing (3). Results from these studies will be available in a few years.

During the last ten years a growing body of observational studies (ecological, case-control, and cohort studies) has reported on the prophylactic effect of vitamin E against cancer in humans (2). The few ecological studies carried out compare mean vitamin E exposure in a number of geographical areas with the incidence of esophageal or gastric cancer in the same areas. The findings from such studies are not very reliable and need to be corroborated by results from studies with other designs. In a case-control study, a group of cancer cases is compared with a group of controls with respect to serum or plasma concentration or dietary intake of vitamin E. Because the presence of cancer may alter a subject's diet and also affect the blood level of vitamin E, it is impossible to know in such studies whether low vitamin E status precedes cancer or vice versa. This shortcoming is minimized in cohort studies, in which a group of cancer-free persons whose vitamin E exposure has been established is followed over time with respect to occurrence of cancer. So far only a few cohort studies on vitamin E exposure and cancer occurrence have been published. One study design almost as effective as a cohort study, but much cheaper to carry out, is a case-control study nested within a cohort study. The aim of this paper is to review the findings of the nested case-control studies and to compare these findings with those from studies with other designs.

Materials and Methods

In a nested case-control study, the cancer cases arising during the follow-up period in an originally cancer-free cohort are compared with controls selected from the entire cohort. This study design is

Table 1. Nested Case-Control Studies of the Relationship Between Serum Vitamin E Level and Cancer Risk

Study	Cohort Size	Cancer Cases (no.)	Sex	Age at Entry (yrs)	Follow-Up (no. of yrs)	Cancer Site(s)	Storage Temp. (°C)	Control Mean Vitamin E (mg/L)
Basel study, Switzerland (4)	4224	115	Male	26–71	7–9	All, 3 sites	Fresh	16.2
Guernsey study, England (5, 6)	10 090	69	Female	26–88	7–14	Breast	−20	6.1
Hypertension Detection and Follow-up Program, U.S. (7)	4480	111	Male and female	30–69	5	All, 5 sites	−70	12.6
Honolulu Heart Program, U.S. (8)	6860	284	Male	52–71	10	5 sites	−75	12.3
Eastern Finland Heart Survey, Finland (9)	12 155	51	Male and female	30–64	4	All, 2 sites	−20	5.0
Washington County study, U.S. (10–15)	25 802	395	Male and female	11–98	8–12	5 sites	−73	12.0
Zoetereer study, the Netherlands (16)	10 532	69	Male and female	5–99	6–9	All, lung	−20	8.5
British United Provident Association, England (17)	22 000	271	Male	35–64	2–9	All, 6 sites	−40	10.3
Malmö study, Sweden (18)	10 000	25	Male	46–48	3–8	All	−20	3.0
Social Insurance Institution study, Finland (19–22)	36 265	766	Male and female	15–99	7–10	All, 19 sites	−20	9.1
Multiple Risk Factor Intervention Trial, U.S. (23)	12 866	156	Male	35–57	10	All, lung	−50	13.0

particularly effective when stored serum or plasma samples are available for the entire cohort at the end of the follow-up; it would be very expensive to analyze samples from all the participants.

The association between serum or plasma levels of vitamin E and the subsequent risk of cancer has been studied using this design in eleven cohorts (Table 1). The sizes of the cohorts ranged from a little over 4000 to more than 36 000, and the number of cancer cases occurring during 2-year- to 14-year-long follow-up periods ranged from 25 to 766. Altogether, over 150 000 persons were monitored, and over 2300 cancer cases occurred. The serum samples of the persons participating in the studies were taken at the base line and, in most cases, were stored frozen at −20°C to −75°C. The mean serum vitamin E levels varied from 3 to 16.2 mg/L. At the end of follow-up, vitamin E determinations were made from the serum samples of cancer patients and selected controls. In most studies, controls were selected by pair matching, using sex, age, and date of blood collection as the matching variables. Other central confounding factors, such as serum cholesterol and smoking, were generally adjusted for by modeling. One drawback in several of the studies was the small number of cancer cases, allowing evaluation only of all sites of cancer combined and of the most incident sites of cancer.

One trial involving a study population large enough to allow extension of the study to more uncommon sites of cancer was the cancer follow-up of the Finnish Mobile Clinic Health Examination Survey (19–22). During the period 1968–1972, multiphasic screening examinations were carried out in various parts of Finland. As part of that survey, serum samples were taken from 36 265 persons and stored at −20°C. Ten years after the base-line examination, a longitudinal study was undertaken to investigate the association between serum vitamin E level and the incidence of cancer. Cancer incidence data from the nationwide Finnish Cancer Registry were linked to the health examination data set. During a mean follow-up of eight years, cancer was diagnosed in 766 perons. In total, 1419 controls were selected by pair matching using sex, age, and place of residence (including date of blood collection) as matching factors. The serum vitamin E levels were determined by high-pressure liquid chromatography. The association between serum vitamin E and cancer incidence was estimated for 19 different cancer sites.

Results

There was a significant inverse association between serum vitamin E level and all sites of cancer in the Finnish survey (19–22) (Fig. 1). This association was pronounced for cancers of the gastrointestinal tract, with significant inverse associations for stomach and pancreas cancers among men, and suggestive inverse associations for colorectal and cervical cancers among women and for esophageal cancer among men and women combined. Occurrence of melanoma was significantly inversely associated with serum vitamin E level among men and women combined.

Most of the nested case-control studies reporting on all sites of cancer combined found lower serum vitamin E levels in cancer cases than in controls (Table 2). However, the differences were significant in the total cohort only in the Finnish survey (19–20) and one other study (16). Similarly, in addition to the site-specific significant associations observed in the Finnish survey, only one of the studies on lung cancer (10) and one on breast cancer (5) reported a significant

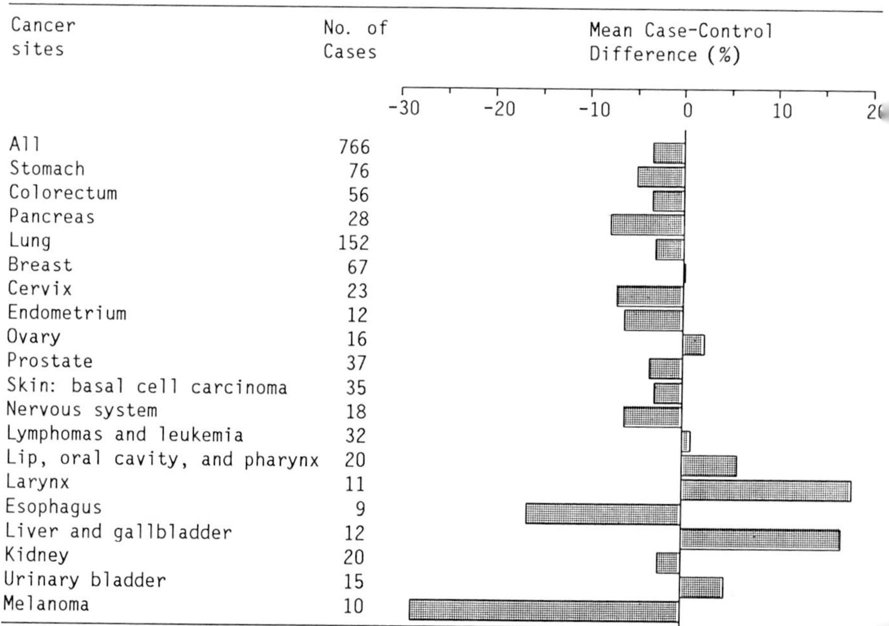

Figure 1. Mean differences in serum vitamin E levels between cancer cases and controls in the cancer follow-up of the Finnish Mobile Clinic Health Survey.

Table 2. Serum Vitamin E Level of Cancer Patients as a Percentage of the Level in Corresponding Controls in Nested Case-Control Studies

		Percentage by Cancer Site(s)							
Country	Study	All	Lung	Colorectum	Stomach	Breast	Bladder	Prostate	Pancreas
Switzerland	(4)	94	88	87	100				
England	(5, 6)					78[a], 105			
U.S.	(7)	92	110		88	87		93	
U.S.	(8)		104	99, 94	99		103		
Finland	(9)	98							
U.S.	(10–15)		88[b]	92, 93		104	90	91	109
Netherlands	(16)	85[a]	91						
England	(17)	98	96	96	105		102		
Sweden	(18)	89							
Finland	(19–22)	97[a]	96	97	95	100	104	97	92
U.S.	(23)	102	96						

Test for difference from 100%:
[a] $P < 0.01$.
[b] $P < 0.001$.

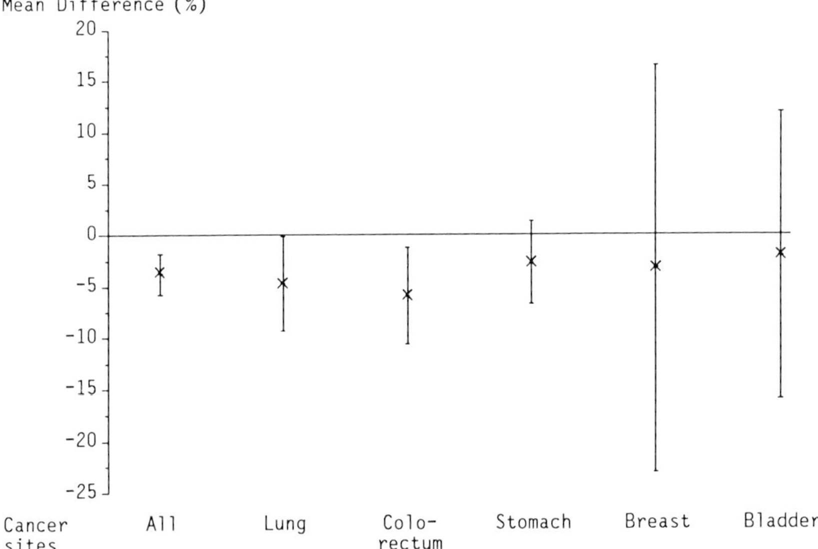

Figure 2. Mean percentage differences in serum vitamin E levels between cancer cases and controls; combination of results from different nested case-control studies. The overall average for studies was calculated as the average of the individual mean differences, each weighted inversely according to its variance.

inverse association. None of the studies on colorectal or bladder cancer found any significant associations between vitamin E and cancer.

One reason for the nonsignificance of the associations might be the small number of cancer cases, which causes a wide confidence interval for the individual studies. Further, the low reliability of serum determinations and changes in the serum vitamin E concentrations during the follow-up may weaken the associations. Another possible cause of the weak association is that the studies may not have included a sufficient range of vitamin E levels for the difference to be noticeable. In accordance with these hypotheses, a combination of the results from the individual studies suggested a significant association in respect to colorectal cancer (24), lung cancer, and all sites of cancer combined (Fig. 2). Combining the results of the other sites included in at least four individual studies—that is, of the stomach, breast, and bladder—however, produced nonsignificant associations between vitamin E level and cancer occurrence.

The relatively weak associations observed in the individual studies may also be due to the presence of the possible preventive effect only in subgroups of the populations. Exposure to different risk factors or intake of some nutrients may modify the vitamin E requirement, and the association may thus vary depending on the level of these factors. So far, associations in different subgroups of populations have rarely been studied. In studies of smokers and nonsmokers conducted separately, an inverse association was pronounced among nonsmokers (9, 17, 20). Similarly, subjects with both low serum selenium and low serum alpha-tocopherol levels were reported to have an elevated risk of cancer of all sites combined (7, 9, 16) and of hormone-related cancers (19).

Discussion

Cancer of All Sites

The overall finding of the nested case-control studies of a suggestive inverse association between serum vitamin E level and the risk of all sites of cancer combined is in agreement with the hypothesis of an anticancer effect of vitamin E. This result was supported by a similar finding from a cohort study (25). Another cohort study, however, gave a similar result during the first seven years of follow-up (26) but not during longer periods (27). It is thus possible that undiagnosed cancer at the base-line examination may have depressed the serum vitamin E level of subsequent cancer cases, causing an association during short follow-ups. This suggestion is supported by the finding of one nested case-control study (17) that patients with cancer at the beginning of the study and that those diagnosed with cancer within the first few years of follow-up had lower serum vitamin E levels than cancer cases diagnosed later. On the other hand, most of the nested case-control studies that have addressed this issue have not reported any strong relationship between the strength of the vitamin E and cancer association and the length of follow-up (5, 10, 11, 16, 20). It is also possible that the low serum vitamin E level is an indicator of some other causal factor. Although the results of the studies have generally been adjusted for age, date of blood collection, smoking, serum cholesterol, and different demographic factors, and in some studies (9, 16, 19, 20) also for serum retinol, beta-carotene, and selenium levels, it is still possible that the results were confounded by a failure to adjust for certain factors, dietary factors associated with vitamin E intake in particular.

Lung Cancer

The finding of significantly lower serum vitamin E levels among lung cancer cases than among corresponding controls in the combined nested case-control material was supported by a cohort study that reported an inverse association between vitamin E intake and lung cancer among nonsmokers (28). The majority of the case-control studies reported similar results, presenting significant, or considerable but nonsignificant, lower mean vitamin E intakes or serum levels among the cancer cases than among the controls (29–35). Only a few studies reported very small differences in vitamin E levels (36–37). Although the inherent potential for bias in the case-control studies may overestimate the association, the possibility of the association cannot be excluded.

Colorectal Cancer

Although single nested case-control studies did not show an association between serum vitamin E level and colorectal cancer risk (4, 8, 11, 15, 17, 20), a meta-analysis of the results presented a weak, significant inverse association (24). In one nested case-control study (38) and in the few case-control studies reported (39, 40), the vitamin E intake of colorectal cancer cases did not differ from that of corresponding controls, however. Although trials on the recurrence rate of colorectal polyps reported a small, nonsignificant inhibitory effect of vitamin E supplementation (41, 42), they did not convincingly confirm the hypothesis of a protective effect of vitamin E against colorectal cancer. The association, if any, between vitamin E exposure and colorectal cancer risk seems to be weak.

Esophageal Cancer

An inverse association was suggested in a nested case-control study that included a small number of esophageal cancer cases (22). This finding was supported by a case-control study in which vitamin E intake among the cancer patients was significantly lower than among controls (43); another case-control study revealed no association (34). A protective effect was also suggested by ecological studies reporting lower vitamin E intake or serum levels in populations with a high risk of esophageal cancer (44–46). Although the associations were generally significant, the findings of such studies are not very reliable and need to be confirmed by results from studies using other designs.

Stomach Cancer

With the exceptions of one study in men (20), stomach cancer cases presented no significant associations in the nested case-control studies (4, 7, 8, 17). Two studies of the same cohort gave a significant association for a shorter follow-up (26) and no association for a longer one (27). Case-control studies reported both significantly lower vitamin E intake among cancer cases (47) and no differences in vitamin E exposure between cases and controls (31, 48). The results are thus inconsistent.

Pancreatic Cancer

One nested case-control study (20) reported a significantly increased risk of cancer of the pancreas among men with low serum vitamin E levels. This may, however, be due to the exceptionally high serum vitamin E levels of the controls in that study. Another nested case-control study reported a nonsignificant decreased risk of pancreatic cancer among individuals with low vitamin E levels (12). One of the case-control studies (49) found an inverse association, whereas two others revealed no differences in vitamin E levels between cases and the corresponding controls (50, 51). The results here too are thus inconsistent.

Breast Cancer

One nested case-control study reported a significant inverse association between serum vitamin E level and breast cancer incidence (5). One potential source of bias in studies based on stored serum samples is the possible degradation of the vitamin E levels during storage, and it was concluded that the observed association was due to different levels of vitamin E loss between case and control samples during storage (6, 52). Accordingly, other nested case-control studies found no association (7, 15, 19). Although one case-control study reported a significant association (34), others found either that breast cancer cases had significantly higher serum vitamin E levels than controls (53–54) or no difference in vitamin E status between cases and controls (55–57). On the basis of several trials using a limited number of patients with mammary dysplasia, it was suggested that the risk of breast cancer may be reduced by vitamin E supplementation (58). Later, however, larger double-blind, randomized, placebo-controlled trials on benign breast disease failed to confirm these results (59, 60, 61). Studies on other hormone-related gynecological cancers, such as those of the endometrium (19) and ovary (19, 62), yielded similar results. Thus, there is no evidence that vitamin E provides protection against breast cancer or other hormone-related gynecological cancers.

Cervical Cancer

The only gynecological cancer inversely associated with vitamin E status was cervical cancer. One nested case-control study presented an elevated risk among persons with a low serum vitamin E level compared with persons with higher levels (19). In accordance with that finding, serological (34, 64) and, with one exception (65), dietary case-control studies (66–67) have reported significantly lower vitamin E intake among cancer patients than among controls. Thus, current information suggests an inverse association between vitamin E exposure and the risk of cervical carcinoma.

Prostate Cancer

The nested case-control studies failed to detect an association between serum vitamin E level and prostate cancer risk (7, 14, 20); a serological case-control study reported similar results (68). Thus there is no evidence of an association between vitamin E level and prostate cancer risk.

Bladder Cancer

One of the nested case-control studies reported a nonsignificant protective effect of vitamin E against bladder cancer (13). Other studies

(8, 17, 20), however, found no association. Two case-control studies (34, 69) reported a suggestive, nonsignificantly lower vitamin E level among cases than among controls. The results are therefore somewhat inconsistent.

Melanoma

A small number of melanoma patients and corresponding controls presented an inverse association between serum vitamin E level and occurrence of the disease in one nested case-control study (22). This finding was not verified in a similar study (15). A single case-control study (70) reported a significant inverse association for dietary intake of vitamin E but not for the serum level. The results of the few studies made are therefore inconsistent.

Cancer of Other Sites

Individual nested case-control studies on cancers of the kidney (22), liver (22), thyroid (71), larynx (22), lip, oral cavity, pharynx (22), and brain (17, 22), or leukemias and lymphomas (7, 22), reported no significant associations between serum vitamin E level and cancer incidence. Similar results were reported from case-control studies on leukemias and lymphomas (34) and cancers of the larynx (34, 72) and vulva (73); inconsistent results were reported for cancers of the pharynx (34, 74) and oral cavity (34, 75).

Conclusion

Some human studies have suggested that vitamin E provides protection against cancer. The most consistent associations have been reported for cancers of the lung, cervix, esophagus, and colorectum. In contrast, hormone-related gynecological cancers generally have not been found to be associated with vitamin E status.

The associations do not convincingly satisfy criteria for causality, generally being weak and inconsistent in different populations. The inconclusiveness of the results may be due partly to the interaction of the preventive effect of vitamin E with other causes of cancer and its subsequent concealment in some populations. Furthermore, the esophageal associations are based mainly on ecological studies and thus should be confirmed in other studies.

To define risk groups in which vitamin E may have a protective effect, results are needed from large-scale observational studies on different sites of cancer carried out under varying circumstances. Furthermore, adjustment for intake of other micronutrients should be made. Meta-analyses should be carried out, pooling data from existing nested case-control studies to obtain results with a higher power. Until the results of such studies and ongoing intervention trials are available, no definite conclusions as to the protective effect of vitamin E against cancer should be drawn.

REFERENCES

1. Packer L. Protective role of vitamin E in biological systems. *Am J Clin Nutr.* 1991;53:1050s–1055s.
2. Knekt P. Role of vitamin E in the prophylaxis of cancer. *Ann Med.* 1991;23:3–12.
3. DeWys WD, Malone WF, Butrum RR, Sestili MA. Clinical trials in cancer prevention. *Cancer.* 1986;58:1954–1962.
4. Stähelin HB, Rösel F, Buess E, Brubacher G. Cancer, vitamins, and plasma lipids: prospective Basel Study. *J Natl Cancer Inst.* 1984;73:1463–1468.
5. Wald NJ, Boreham J, Hayward JL, Bulbrook RD. Plasma retinol, beta-carotene and vitamin E levels in relation to the future risk of breast cancer. *Br J Cancer.* 1984;49:321–324.
6. Russell MJ, Thomas BS, Bulbrook RD. A prospective study of the relationship between serum vitamin A and E and risk of breast cancer. *Br J Cancer.* 1988;57:213–215.
7. Willett WC, Polk BF, Underwood BA, *et al.* Relation of serum vitamins A and E and carotenoids to the risk of cancer. *N Engl J Med.* 1984;310:430–434.
8. Nomura AMY, Stemmermann GN, Heilbrun LK, Salkeld RM, Vuilleumier JP. Serum vitamin levels and the risk of cancer of specific sites in men of Japanese ancestry in Hawaii. *Cancer Res.* 1985;45:2369–2372.
9. Salonen JT, Salonen R, Lappeteläinen R, Mäenpää PH, Alfthan G, Puska P. Risk of cancer in relation to serum concentrations of selenium and vitamins A and E: matched case-control analysis of prospective data. *BMJ* 1985;290:417–420.

10. Menkes MS, Comstock GW, Vuilleumier JP, Helsing KJ, Rider AA, Brookmeyer R. Serum beta-carotene, vitamins A and E, selenium, and the risk of lung cancer. *N Engl J Med.* 1986;315:1250–1254.
11. Schober SE, Comstock GW, Helsing KJ, *et al.* Serologic precursors of cancer, I: prediagnostic serum nutrients and colon cancer risk. *Am J Epidemiol.* 1987;126:1033–1041.
12. Burney PGJ, Comstock GW, Morris JS. Serologic precursors of cancer: serum micronutrients and the subsequent risk of pancreatic cancer. *Am J Clin Nutr.* 1989;49:895–900.
13. Helzlsouer KJ, Comstock GW, Morris JS. Selenium, lycopene, alpha-tocopherol, beta-carotene, retinol, and subsequent bladder cancer. *Cancer Res.* 1989;49:6144–6148.
14. Hsing AW, Comstock GW, Abbey H, Polk BF. Serologic precursors of cancer: retinol, carotenoids, and tocopherol and risk of prostate cancer. *J Natl Cancer Inst.* 1990;82:941–946.
15. Comstock GW, Helzlsouer KJ, Bush TL. Prediagnostic serum levels of carotenoids and vitamin E as related to subsequent cancer in Washington County, Maryland. *Am J Clin Nutr.* 1991;53: 260S–264S.
16. Kok FJ, van Duijn CM, Hofman A, Vermeeren R, de Bruijn AM, Valkenburg HA. Micronutrients and the risk of lung cancer. *N Engl J Med.* 1987;316:1416.
17. Wald NJ, Thompson SG, Densem JW, Boreham J, Bailey A. Serum vitamin E and subsequent risk of cancer. *Br J Cancer.* 1987;56: 69–72.
18. Fex G, Pettersson B, Åkesson B. Low plasma selenium as a risk factor for cancer death in middle-aged men. *Nutr Cancer.* 1987; 10:221–229.
19. Knekt P. Serum vitamin E level and risk of female cancers. *Int J Epidemiol.* 1988; 17:281–286.
20. Knekt P, Aromaa A, Maatela J, *et al.* Serum vitamin E and risk of cancer among Finnish men during a 10-year follow-up. *Am J Epidemiol.* 1988;127:28–41.
21. Knekt P, Aromaa A, Maatela J, *et al.* Serum vitamin E, serum selenium and the risk of gastrointestinal cancer. *Int J Cancer.* 1988; 42:846–850.
22. Knekt P, Aromaa A, Maatela J, *et al.* Serum alpha-tocopherol, beta-carotene, retinol, retinol-binding protein and selenium and risk of cancers of low incidence in Finland. *Am J Epidemiol.* 1991; 134:356–361.

23. Connett JE, Kuller LH, Kjelsberg MO, *et al.* Relationship between carotenoids and cancer: the Multiple Risk Factor Intervention Trial (MRFIT) Study. *Cancer.* 1989;64:126–134.
24. Longnecker M, Martin-Moreno J-M, Knekt P, *et al.* Serum alpha-tocopherol in relation to subsequent colorectal cancer in pooled data from five cohorts. *J Natl Cancer Inst.* 1992;84:430–435.
25. Friedman GD, Selby JV. Epidemiological screening for potentially carcinogenic drugs. *Agents Actions Suppl.* 1990;29:83–96.
26. Gey KF, Brubacher GB, Stähelin HB. Plasma levels of antioxidant vitamins in relation to ischemic heart disease and cancer. *Am J Clin Nutr.* 1987;45:1368–1377.
27. Stähelin HB, Gey KF, Eichholzer M, *et al.* Plasma antioxidant vitamins and subsequent cancer mortality in the 12-year follow-up of the prospective Basel Study. *Am J Epidemiol* 1991;133:766–775.
28. Knekt P, Järvinen R, Seppänen R, *et al.* Dietary antioxidants and the risk of lung cancer. *Am J Epidemiol.* 1991;134:471–479.
29. Lopez-S A, LeGardeur BY. Vitamins A, C, and E in relation to lung cancer incidence. *Am J Clin Nutr.* 1982;35:851. Abstract.
30. Miyamoto H, Araya Y, Ito M, *et al.* Serum selenium and vitamin E concentrations in families of lung cancer patients. *Cancer.* 1987; 60:1159–1162.
31. Yeum KJ, Lee-Kim YC, Lee KY, Kim BS, Russell RM. The serum levels of retinol, beta-carotene and alpha-tocopherol of cancer patients in Korea. In: *Proceedings of the 14th International Congress of Nutrition.* Seoul, Korea; 1989;665. Abstract.
32. LeGardeur BY, Lopez-S A, Johnson WD. A case-control study of serum vitamins A, E, and C in lung cancer patients. *Nutr Cancer.* 1990;14:133–140.
33. Rougereau A, Person O, Rougereau G. Fat-soluble vitamins and cancer localization associated to an abnormal ketone derivative of D3 vitamin: carcinomedin. *Int J Vitam Nutr Res.* 1987;57:367–373.
34. Skulchan V, Ong-Ajyooth S. Serum vitamin E in Thai cancer patients. *J Med Assoc Thai.* 1987;70:280–283.
35. Harris RWC, Key TJA, Silcocks PB, Bull D, Wald NJ. A case-control study of dietary carotene in men with lung cancer and in men with other epithelial cancers. *Nutr Cancer.* 1991;15:63–68.
36. Atukorala S, Basu TK, Dickerson JWT, Donaldson D, Sakula A. Vitamin A, zinc and lung cancer. *Br J Cancer.* 1979;40:927–931.
37. Byers TE, Graham S, Haughey BP, Marshall JR, Swanson MK.

Diet and lung cancer risk: findings from the Western New York Diet Study. *Am J Epidemiol.* 1987;125:351–363.

38. Heilbrun LK, Nomura A, Hankin JH, Stemmermann GN. Diet and colorectal cancer with special reference to fiber intake. *Int J Cancer.* 1989;44:1–6.
39. Graham S, Marshall J, Haughey B, *et al.* Dietary epidemiology of cancer of the colon in Western New York. *Am J Epidemiol.* 1988; 128:490–503.
40. Freudenheim JL, Graham S, Marshall JR, Haughey BP, Wilkinson G. A case-control study of diet and rectal cancer in Western New York. *Am J Epidemiol.* 1990;131:612–624.
41. McKeown-Eyssen G, Holloway C, Jazmaji V, Bright-See E, Dion P, Bruce WR. A randomized trial of vitamins C and E in the prevention of recurrence of colorectal polyps. *Cancer Res.* 1988;48: 4701–4705.
42. DeCosse JJ, Miller HH, Lesser ML. Effect of wheat fiber and vitamins C and E on rectal polyps in patients with familial adenomatous polyposis. *J Natl Cancer Inst.* 1989;81:1290–1297.
43. Tuyns AJ, Riboli E, Doornbos G, Péquignot G. Diet and esophageal cancer in Calvados (France). *Nutr Cancer.* 1987;9:81–92.
44. Yang CS, Sun Y, Yang Q, *et al.* Vitamin A and other deficiencies in Linxian, a high esophageal cancer incidence area in Northern China. *J Natl Cancer Inst.* 1984;73:1449–1453.
45. van Helden PD, Beyers AD, Bester AJ, Jaskiewicz K. Esophageal cancer: vitamin and lipotrope deficiencies in an at-risk South African population. *Nutr Cancer.* 1987;10:247–255.
46. Guo W, Li J-Y, Blot WJ, Hsing AW, Chen J, Fraumeni JF, Jr. Correlations of dietary intake and blood nutrient levels with esophageal cancer mortality in China. *Nutr Cancer.* 1990;13:121–127.
47. Buiatti E, Palli D, Decarli A, *et al.* A case-control study of gastric cancer and diet in Italy, II: association with nutrients. *Int J Cancer.* 1990;45:896–901.
48. Risch HA, Jain M, Choi NW, *et al.* Dietary factors and the incidence of cancer of the stomach. *Am J Epidemiol.* 1985;122:947–959.
49. Baghurst PA, McMichael AJ, Slavotinek AH, Baghurst KI, Boyle P, Walker AM. A case-control study of diet and cancer of the pancreas. *Am J Epidemiol.* 1991;134:167–179.
50. Ghadirian P, Simard A, Baillargeon J, Maisonneuve P, Boyle P.

Nutritional factors and pancreatic cancer in the francophone community in Montreal, Canada. *Int J Cancer.* 1991;47:1–6.

51. Zatonski W, Przewozniak K, Howe GR, Maisonneuve P, Walker AM, Boyle P. Nutritional factors and pancreatic cancer: a case-control study from South-West Poland. *Int J Cancer.* 1991;48: 390–394.
52. Wald NJ, Nicolaides-Bouman A, Hudson GA. Plasma retinol, beta-carotene and vitamin E levels in relation to the future risk of breast cancer. *Br J Cancer.* 1988;57:235.
53. Gerber M, Cavallo F, Marubini E, *et al.* Liposoluble vitamins and lipid parameters in breast cancer: a joint study in Northern Italy and Southern France. *Int J Cancer.* 1988;42:489–494.
54. Gerber M, Richardson S, Crastes de Paulet P, Pujol H, Crastes de Paulet A. Relationship between vitamin E and polyunsaturated fatty acids in breast cancer: nutritional and metabolic aspects. *Cancer.* 1989;64:2347–2353.
55. Basu TK, Hill GB, Ng D, Abdi E, Temple N. Serum vitamins A and E, beta-carotene, and selenium in patients with breast cancer. *J Am Coll Nutr.* 1989;8:524–528.
56. Toniolo P, Riboli E, Protta F, Charrel M, Cappa APM. Calorie-providing nutrients and risk of breast cancer. *J Natl Cancer Inst.* 1989;81:278–286.
57. Lee HP, Gourley L, Duffy SW, Esteve J, Lee J, Day NE. Dietary effects on breast-cancer risk in Singapore. *Lancet.* 1991;337:1197–1200.
58. London RS, Murphy L, Kitlowski KE. Hypothesis: breast cancer prevention by supplemental vitamin E. *J Am Coll Nutr.* 1985;4: 559–564.
59. Ernster VL, Goodson WH, Hunt TK, Petrakis NL, Sickles EA, Miike R. Vitamin E and benign breast "disease": a double-blind, randomized clinical trial. *Surgery.* 1985;97:490–494.
60. London RS, Sundaram GS, Murphy L, Manimekalai S, Reynolds M, Goldstein PJ. The effect of vitamin E on mammary dysplasia: a double-blind study. *Obstet Gynecol.* 1985;65:104–106.
61. Meyer EC, Sommers DK, Reitz CJ, Mentis H. Vitamin E and benign breast disease. *Surgery.* 1990;107:549–551.
62. Heinonen PK, Koskinen T, Tuimala R. Serum levels of vitamins A and E in women with ovarian cancer. *Arch Gynecol.* 1985;237: 37–40.

63. Cuzick J, De Stavola BL, Russell MJ, Thomas BS. Vitamin A, vitamin E and the risk of cervical intraepithelial neoplasia. *Br J Cancer.* 1990;62:651–652.
64. Palan PR, Mikhail MS, Basu J, Romney SL. Plasma levels of antioxidant beta-carotene and alpha-tocopherol in uterine cervix dysplasias and cancer. *Nutr Cancer.* 1991;15:13–20.
65. Ziegler RG, Brinton LA, Hamman RF, *et al.* Diet and the risk of invasive cervical cancer among white women in the United States. *Am J Epidemiol.* 1990;132:432–445.
66. Verreault R, Chu J, Mandelson M, Shy K. A case-control study of diet and invasive cervical cancer. *Int J Cancer.* 1989;43:1050–1054.
67. Slattery ML, Abott TM, Overall JC Jr, *et al.* Dietary vitamins A, C, and E and selenium as risk factors for cervical cancer. *Epidemiology.* 1990;1:8–15.
68. Hayes RB, Bogdanovicz JFAT, Schroeder FH, *et al.* Serum retinol and prostate cancer. *Cancer.* 1988;62:2021–2026.
69. Riboli E, Gonzalez CA, Lopez-Abente G, *et al.* Diet and bladder cancer in Spain: a multi-centre case-control study. *Int J Cancer.* 1991;49:214–219.
70. Stryker WS, Stampfer MJ, Stein EA, *et al.* Diet, plasma levels of beta-carotene and alpha-tocopherol, and risk of malignant melanoma. *Am J Epidemiol.* 1990;131:597–611.
71. Glattre E, Thomassen Y, Thoresen SO, *et al.* Prediagnostic serum selenium in a case-control study of thyroid cancer. *Int J Epidemiol.* 1989;18:45–49.
72. Drozdz M, Gierek T, Jendryczko A, Piekarska J, Pilch J, Polanska D. Zinc, vitamins A and E, and retinol-binding protein in sera of patients with cancer of the larynx. *Neoplasma.* 1989;36:357–362.
73. Romppanen U, Tuimala R, Punnonen R, Koskinen T. Serum vitamin A and E levels in patients with lichen sclerosus and carcinoma of the vulva: effect of oral etretinate treatment. *Ann Chir Gynaecol.* 1985;74(suppl 197):27–29.
74. McLaughlin JK, Gridley G, Block G, *et al.* Dietary factors in oral and pharyngeal cancer. *J Natl Cancer Inst.* 1988;80:1237–1243.
75. Krishnamurthy S, Jaya S. Serum alpha-tocopherol, lipoperoxides, and ceruloplasmin and red cell glutatione and antioxidant enzymes in patients of oral cancer. *Indian J Cancer.* 1986;23:36–42.

GERALD LITWACK

Vitamin B_6 and Glucocorticoid Receptor Function

ABSTRACT

The biologically active form of vitamin B_6, pyridoxal phosphate, interacts with the glucocorticoid receptor to inhibit steroid binding and subsequent DNA binding. Inhibition involves the unoccupied, unactivated receptor complex with respect to steroid binding and the activated form with respect to DNA binding, suggesting that a lysine residue at each site becomes pyridoxylated. Mathematical analysis of the inhibition suggests that effective concentrations of pyridoxal phosphate for either site occur within the range of "free" or dissociable levels of pyridoxal phosphate in the cell, predicting that this inhibition should be demonstrable in the intact cell.

Experiments using animals and cells in culture indicate that the status and levels of vitamin B_6 and pyridoxal phosphate in the cell affect the regulation of the glucocorticoid receptor mechanism. Furthermore, studies in intact cells by indirect immunofluorescence of receptor monoclonal antibodies demonstrate that pyridoxal phosphate can prevent receptor translocation into the cellular nucleus. In effect, the biologically active form of vitamin B_6, under certain conditions, can function as an antiglucocorticoid.

Introduction

Vitamin B_6 can be supplied in the diet in various forms, the most common of which is pyridoxine (PN). When PN is taken up in the liver, it is converted to a phosphorylated form and then oxidized to pyridoxal phosphate (PLP), the biologically active form of the vitamin. These interrelations and the handling of other forms of the vitamin are shown dynamically in Figure 1. Here it is obvious that the various forms of the vitamin are metabolized to PLP in a single step in the case of pyridoxal (PL) and in two steps in the case of PN. Pyri-

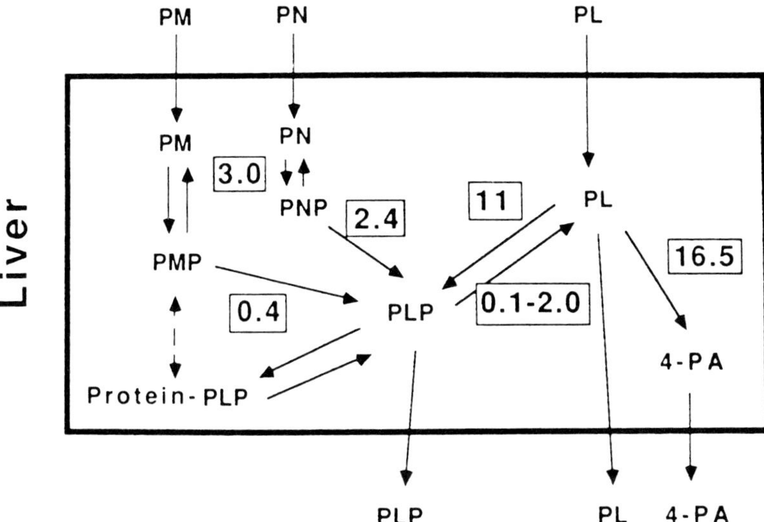

Figure 1. Metabolism of vitamin B_6 by human liver. The estimated rates of the major reactions are given in the boxed numbers and refer to nmol/min/g liver. PM = pyridoxamine; PN = pyridoxine; PL = pyridoxal; PNP = pyridoxine phosphate; PLP = pyridoxal phosphate; PMP = pyridoxamine phosphate; 4-PA = 4-pyridoxic acid.
Reproduced with permission from Merrill and Henderson (1).

doxal phosphate then associates with various enzymes and proteins in such a manner that there may exist a pool of PLP that is available for competitive reactions, although little is understood about how this works in the cell.

Let us briefly describe the physiological context in which the glucocorticoid receptor operates. This is shown in overview in Figure 2. Environmental stress or internal signals influence the limbic system, mainly the hippocampus, which then signals the hypothalamus to release corticotrophic-releasing hormone (CRH) from the CRH-containing neurons. Corticotrophic-releasing hormone enters by fenestrations and then travels down the closed portal system connecting the hypothalamus and the pituitary. It is released through fenestrations in the secondary plexus, searches the environment of a high affinity receptor residing on the surface of the corticotrophic cell of the anterior pituitary, and after binding to it sets off a chain of reactions that leads to the release of corticotropin (ACTH) and other hormones to the general circulation. Then ACTH binds to receptors on the cell

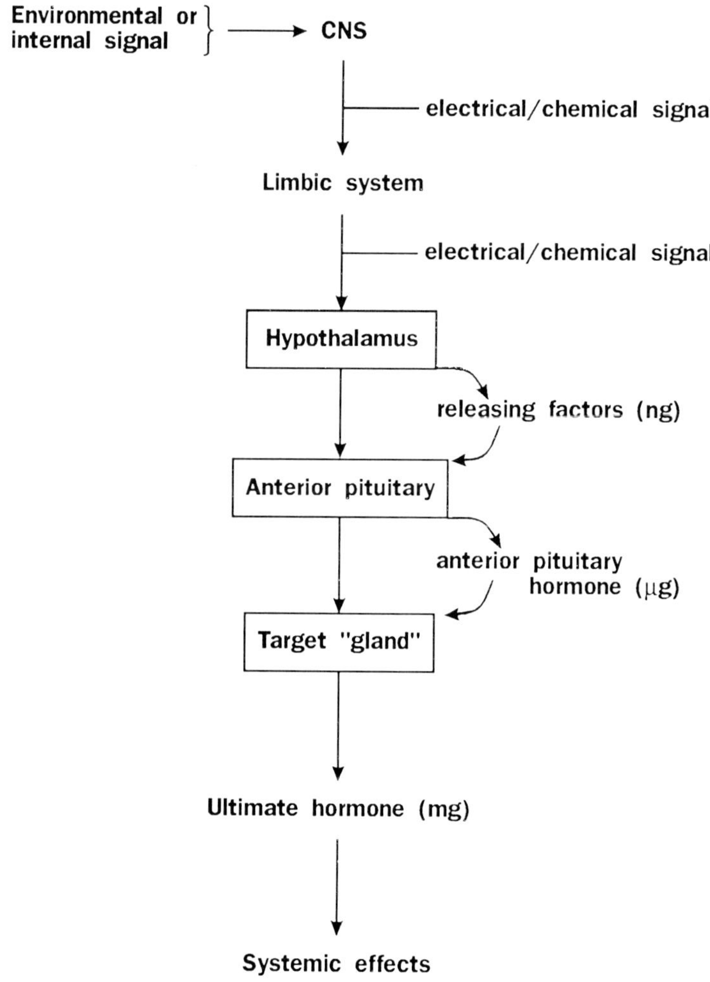

Figure 2. Overview of the humoral route of transmission of signals that initiate many hormonal systems.

Reproduced from Norman and Litwack (2) with permission.

membrane of the inner layer of cells of the adrenal cortex, resulting in the increased synthesis and release of cortisol, the principal glucocorticoid in man. Cortisol is transported in the bloodstream by the protein transcortin. A small amount of the steroid dissociates from transcortin and is taken up by the cells of the body and retained in those that have glucocorticoid receptors (most cells), and can actually be concentrated above the blood concentration in cells that have a relatively high level of the receptor (liver). The increased level of cortisol in the blood has a negative feedback effect on the tissues responsible for the intermediary hormones in the overall process, so that the secretions of CRH and ACTH are shut down until the next signal occurs to initiate the system all over again.

Once inside the cell (Fig. 3), cortisol binds to the unoccupied receptor to form the unactivated complex (or the non-DNA binding form). This becomes activated to the free receptor form that is able to translocate to the nucleus and activate genes that bear glucocorticoid-responsive elements in or near their promoters. The corresponding mRNAs are formed, transported into the cytoplasm, and translated into proteins that alter cellular functions and constitute the cellular response to the hormone.

To understand which forms of the receptor are affected by PLP, we need to go into more detail about the mechanism of activation that accounts for the appearance of the various forms of the glucocorticoid receptor (Fig. 4). On the left in Figure 4 is shown a model of the unactivated, non-DNA binding form of the receptor complex. The DNA binding domain appears to be blocked from any interaction with DNA based on the presence of a dimer of the 90 000 molecular weight heat shock protein (hsp90). A molecule of cortisol, after crossing the cell membrane, binds to the unoccupied receptor complex to form the liganded unactivated receptor. Some as-yet-unidentified molecular event follows that results in the release of a modulator, a small molecule that bridges the receptor to the dimer of hsp90 and also releases the hsp dimer. This may generate an intermediate, if indeed there is also an RNA molecule protecting the DNA binding domain, although the evidence for this is not yet rigorous. Finally, the RNA is released in the second step of the mechanism to generate the DNA binding form of the receptor shown on the right-hand side of the figure. The forms of major importance for the interaction with PLP are the unactivated complex on the far left and the activated form on the far right.

Original Experiments Showing the Activity of PLP

Originally we showed (3, 4) that the ability of the activated receptor complex in cytosol to bind to DNA cellulose could be inhibited by PLP (Fig. 5). This inhibition was specific because PN, pyridoxamine, and

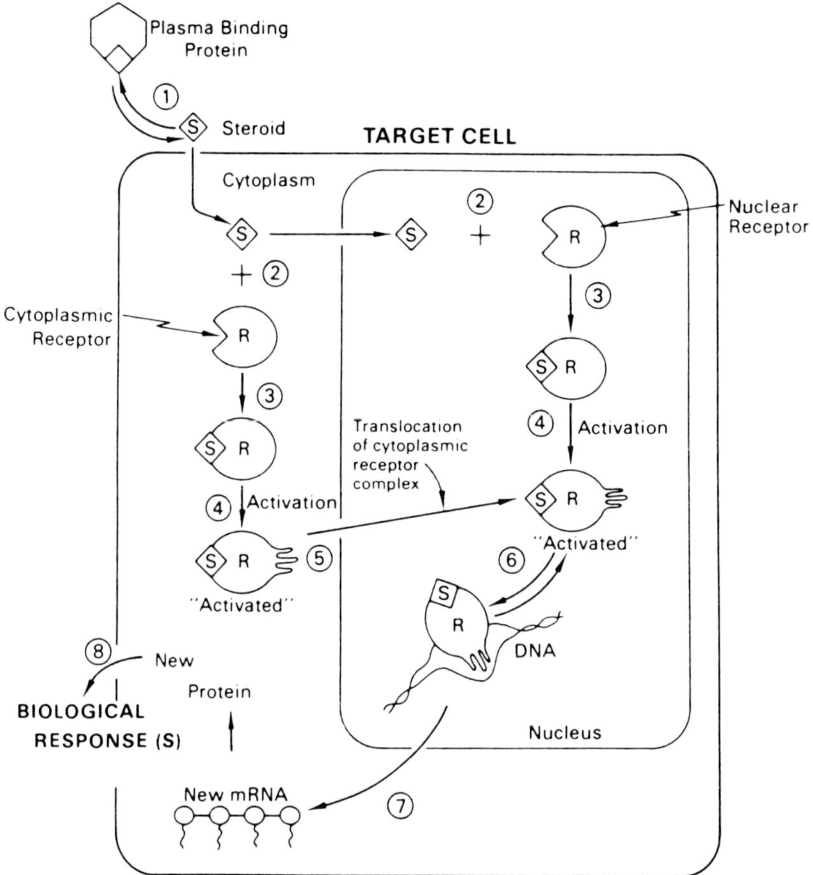

Figure 3. Overview of the cellular actions of steroid receptors. A steroid enters the target cell, probably by free diffusion (1), and binds to its unoccupied receptor (2, 3), either in the cytoplasm or in the nucleus. The glucocorticoid receptor resides in the cytoplasm in the unoccupied form; the mineralocorticoid receptor may also be located in the cytoplasm. However, other members of this gene family are thought to reside in the nucleus. Both pathways are presented in this figure. The steroid-receptor complex then becomes activated (4) and translocates to the nucleus, where it activates transcription of specific genes (5, 6). The mRNAs thus produced are translocated to the cytoplasm (7), where they are translated, and the increases in specific proteins alter the activities of the cell.

Reproduced from Norman and Litwack (2) with permission.

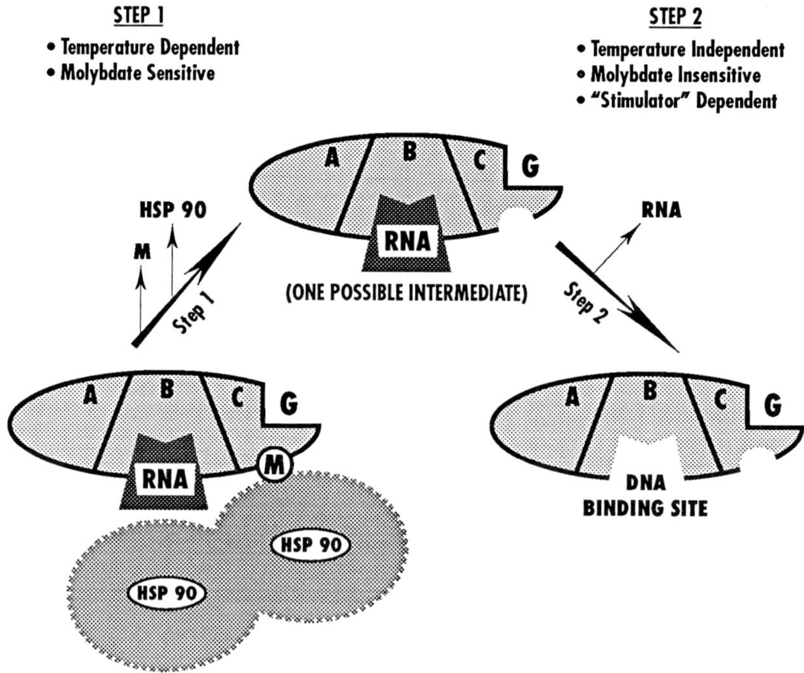

	UNACTIVATED	INTERMEDIATE(S)	ACTIVATED
SEDIMENTATION COEFFICIENT:	8 - 10 S	5 - 7 S	4 - 5 S
STOKES RADIUS:	70 - 80 A	60 - 80 A	50 - 60 A
MOLECULAR WEIGHT:	300,000 - 310,000	130,000 - 180,000	94,000
DNA BINDING:	5%	10 - 20%	30 - 40%
DEAE ELUTION POSITION:	250 mM KP	50 mM KP	50 mM KP

Figure 4. Overview of the speculated steps in the activation of the glucocorticoid receptor. A = N-terminal domain of the receptor; B = DNA binding domain; C = steroid binding domain; G = glucocorticoid hormone; M = modulator; hsp90 = heat shock protein of 90 000 molecular weight. In step one, the small molecule modulator is released causing the release of the nonhomologous proteins of the unactivated complex on the left. This may form an intermediate bound by RNA that occludes the DNA binding domain. In step two, the fully active DNA binding form of the receptor appears and is now able to translocate to the nucleus and interact with hormone-responsive elements.

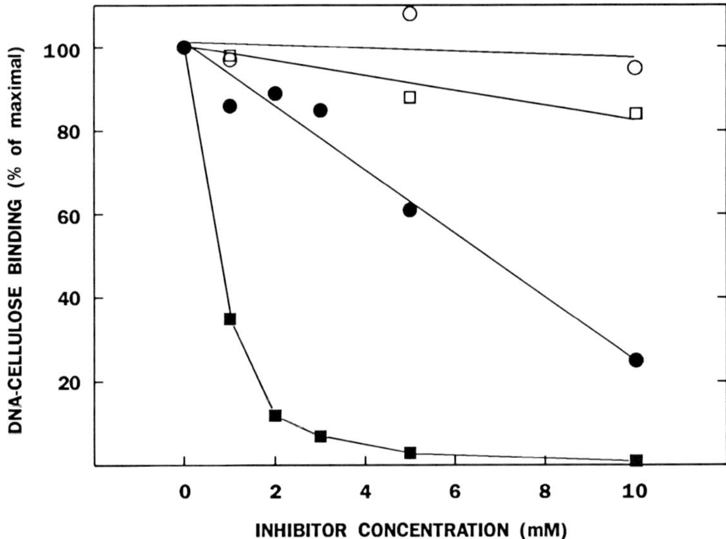

Figure 5. Inhibition of DNA binding of the activated glucocorticoid receptor in cytosol. The uppermost line represents PM and PMP. The middle line represents PL, and the lower curve is for PLP.
Reproduced with permission from Cake *et al.* (3).

pyridoxamine phosphate were without effect and PL had little effect. We also showed later on that nonspecific aldehydes had little effect. We were prompted to carry out this work because we had been probing the amino acid residue side chains that were involved in the activities of the receptor, and we used PLP as a reagent to probe for lysine side chains (5) since the side chain amine is well known to form a Schiff base with PLP. Although the amounts of PLP were in the millimolar range to produce the inhibition, it should be noted that a wide variety of proteins bind PLP, so that in crude and partially purified systems the concentration of PLP added to the reaction will never reflect its "free" concentration but only a small fraction of it.

Inhibition of Steroid Binding by PLP

Using partially purified unactivated receptor preparations obtained from adrenalectomized rats so that the endogenous steroid concentration was very low, we measured ability of the receptor to bind radioactive steroid ([^{3}H]triamcinolone acetonide) as a function of increasing concentrations of PLP. In one case the receptor was pretreated with unlabeled steroid to generate the occupied unactivated form, whereas in the other case the receptor preparation was not exposed to steroid for this purpose. The unoccupied unactivated form was far more sensitive to the inhibition of subsequent radioactive steroid binding than was the occupied unactivated form. Double reciprocal plots were developed for various concentrations of PLP as functions of steroid concentration and specific binding of radioactive steroid. When we replotted the slopes of these curves as a function of the added PLP concentration, we obtained a parabolic inhibition curve. Solution of the equation describing parabolic inhibition for each concentration of PLP led to interesting results that will be discussed in a subsequent section.

PLP Inhibition of DNA Binding by the Activated Receptor

In these experiments we used partially purified (about 200-fold) activated receptor. Although the level of specifically bound steroid was unaffected by PLP in the activated receptor complex, there was marked inhibition of ability of the activated receptor to bind to DNA cellulose. The data were taken at various concentrations of PLP, and then double reciprocal plots were constructed from experiments carried out with respect to steroid concentration and DNA binding at various concentrations of PLP. Replotting the slopes of these curves as a function of PLP concentration produced a parabolic curve of inhibition similar to curves produced when steroid binding was studied using the unoccupied unactivated receptor complex. Experiments were carried out extensively to demonstrate that when PLP was incubated with DNA before the introduction of the receptor there was no effect on subsequent binding of the activated receptor complex to DNA, indicating that PLP does not bind to DNA in a manner to occlude subsequent binding of the receptor and, more important, PLP does not produce this inhibition by binding to DNA and blocking acceptor activity.

Solution of Parabolic Inhibition Curves

The parabolic curves for both inhibition of steroid binding of the unoccupied unactivated receptor complex and inhibition of DNA binding by partially purified activated glucocorticoid receptor are described by the equation

$$K_i \text{ slope} = \frac{K_i^2}{2K_i + [I]}$$

When the equation was solved, first for the series for inhibition of steroid binding and then for the series for inhibition of DNA binding at each concentration of PLP used, the values of K_i were in the range of 1 μM to 4 μM with respect to steroid binding inhibition and about 9 μM with respect to DNA binding inhibition. These concentrations are deemed to be within the concentration range of "free" PLP in the cell (6). Consequently, this information predicts that levels of PLP reached within the cell may be effective for the regulation of the glucocorticoid receptor mechanism.

Effect of the Level of Purification on the Inhibition of DNA Binding by PLP

To confirm that the form of the receptor binding to DNA was the activated form, we quantified the receptor complex by ion exchange chromatography, where its elution position is well known. We first carried experiments out with receptor complexes partially purified by a deoxycorticosterone affinity resin (7). The activated receptor complex, without prior treatment with DNA cellulose, eluted in its characteristic position from DEAE cellulose such that about 430 000 disintegrations per minute (dpm) of specifically bound [^{3}H]dexamethasone mesylate were recovered. This form of the synthetic glucocorticoid was used because it forms a covalent bond with the receptor (8) and losses occurring from steroid dissociation are absent. When we treated the activated receptor complex with DNA cellulose before chromatography, we recovered about 26% of the original amount of specifically bound radioactive steroid in the position of the activated receptor complex, indicating that about 74% of the receptor complex had bound to the DNA. When the same experiment was carried out except that the receptor had been exposed to PLP, 83% of the receptor complex was recovered after DNA treatment, indicating that PLP had inhibited binding to DNA by about 70%. We conducted a similar experiment except that the activated receptor complex was purified to 5000-fold to 10 000-fold over cytosol by affinity chromatography, gel filtration, and ion exchange chromatography (7). Under this condition, about 197 000 dpm were recovered in the characteristic position of the activated receptor complex. After treatment with DNA cellulose, 32% of the control specifically bound radioactivity from [^{3}H]dexamethasone mesylate was recovered. After pretreatment with PLP, the recovery was increased to 76%, indicating an inhibition of DNA binding of the activated receptor complex of 65%, a result fully comparable to that obtained with the lesser purified preparation of the receptor. Thus in crude, partially purified, and highly purified preparations of the activated receptor complex, PLP inhibited DNA binding to the same extent, indicating that PLP must be interacting directly with the receptor and not with some other regulator in the receptor mechanism.

Does PLP Inhibit the Activated Receptor Complex when Binding to a Specific Glucocorticoid-Responsive Element in the DNA Acceptor?

The glucocorticoid-responsive element, a 15-mer (6), was synthesized by J. K. deRiel in our former laboratory in the double-stranded form as shown in Figure 6. Binding of the partially purified activated glucocorticoid receptor complex to this DNA element was determined by gel retardation analysis as shown in Figure 7 (6). These analyses show that PLP also inhibits the activated receptor complex when binding to the glucocorticoid-responsive element, about 40% to 50% inhibition at levels of PLP from the millimole level to as low as 200 μM. This result supports the conclusion that PLP is interacting directly with the glucocorticoid receptor.

```
GRE            G↓  ↓↓↓  ↓nn  n↓↓  ↓↓↓  ↓
 5´    GATC CTG TAC AGG ATG TTC TAG CTA CG        3´
            ||| ||| ||| ||| ||| ||| ||| ||
 3´         GAC ATG TCC TAC AAG ATC GAT GC CTAG   5´
```

Figure 6. Structure of a 27mer double-stranded oligodeoxynucleotide containing the 15mer glucocorticoid-responsive element, indicated by arrows.

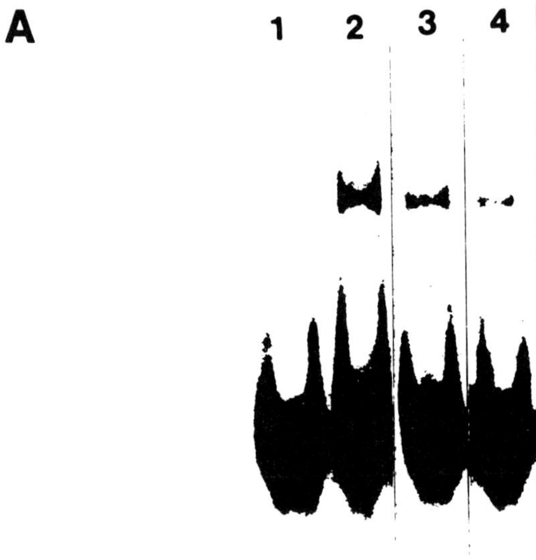

B

	RELATIVE BAND INTENSITY	%	(Δ)	SPECIFIC BINDING TO DNA-CELLULOSE	%	(Δ)
LANE 2	1,932.0	100		74,422.67 [a]	100	
LANE 3	1,236.5	64	(−36)	ND [b]	ND	
LANE 4	933.8	48	(−52)	40,136.67	54	(−46)

[a] dpm

[b] Not determined

Figure 7. *A.* PLP inhibition of activated receptor binding to a specific GRE. Activated receptor complexes were purified about 200-fold from cytosol and concentrated. Receptors were used directly or preincubated at 20°C for 30 minutes with PLP. They were bound to ^{32}P end-labeled GRE for 30 minutes at room temperature and loaded onto nondenaturing gels and electrophoresed. The dried gel was autoradiographed for 20 hours at −80°C. Receptor binding is indicated by the shifted band above in lanes 2–4. Lane 1 = GRE alone; lane 2 = receptor + GRE; lane 3 = receptor + 200 μM PLP; lane 4 = receptor + 2 mM PLP. *B.* Quantitation of the data presented in *A.*

Reproduced from Maksymowych *et al.* (6) with permission.

Ability of PLP to Elute Glucocorticoid Receptor Complexes from DNA and Nuclei

Because of the competitive nature of the inhibition of glucocorticoid receptor binding to DNA by PLP with respect to DNA concentration (3), we were able to predict that PLP should elute the receptor complex from DNA and therefore possibly from cell nuclei (9). Signal experiments are reviewed in Figures 8 and 9. Here it is shown that millimolar levels of PLP specifically elute the glucocorticoid receptor complex from DNA, and the same levels specifically elute the receptor complex from nuclei previously bound with the receptor. The application of this finding proved to be instrumental in the isolation and purification of the androgen receptor (10).

Levels of PLP in Cells in Culture and in Animal Tissues *In Vivo*

To extend our in vitro findings to biological systems, we decided to study the well-known glucocorticoid induction of tyrosine aminotransferase (TAT) in FAZA (liver-derived) cells (11). Minimal Eagle's medium (MEM), containing a full vitamin supplement, was used. Addition of 5 μM of PN caused a slight increase in the constitutive TAT activity. When the medium was treated with 1 μM of triamcinolone acetonide, there was a 5-fold induction of TAT activity as expected. However, when the same experiment was conducted, except that 5 μM of PN were added to the medium, there was only a little more than 2-fold induction of the activity, indicating a 60% decrease in the inductive effect of the steroid. Clearly, the added PN that was metabolized by the cell to PLP had inhibited the function of the glucocorticoid receptor complex that was required for gene activation and production of TAT mRNA. We next repeated this experiment except that the vitamin mixture used to make up the medium was deficient in PN. When the PN-free medium was compared with the complete medium, there was no difference in the level of the constitutive TAT activity. On the other hand, when the steroidal inducer was present, there was a 2.5-fold increase in TAT activity in the complete medium compared with a 3-fold increase in the absence of PN; thus the presence of PN depressed the level of induction by the steroid, even though the difference in concentrations of PN was very small, and

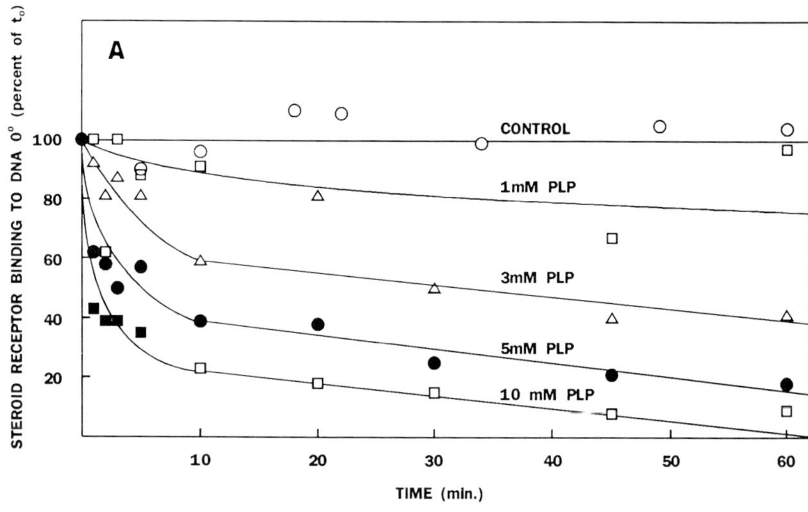

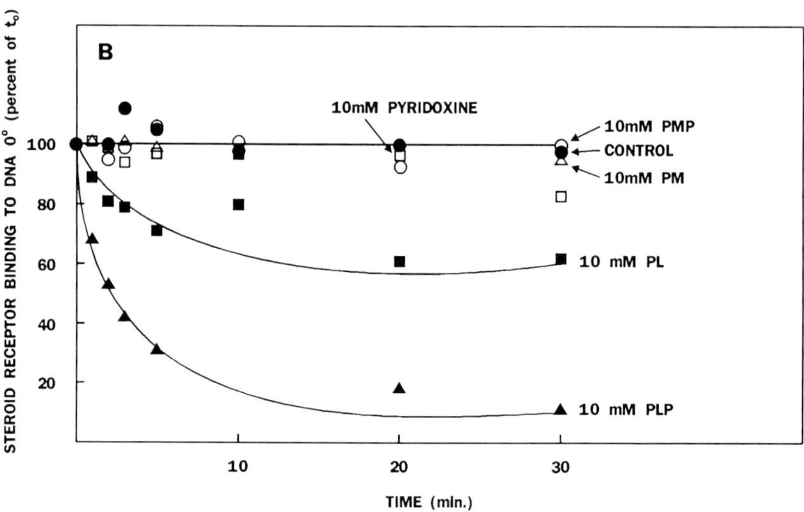

Figure 8. Ability of PLP to dissociate glucocorticoid receptor-DNA complexes. *A* shows the effects of increasing concentration of PLP. Using 10 mM for 1 hour completely releases all of the receptor complex from DNA cellulose. *B* shows the specificity of this activity. No effect is seen with PMP or PM; a partial effect is observed with PL, and a major effect is seen with PLP. Reproduced from Dolan *et al.* (12) with permission.

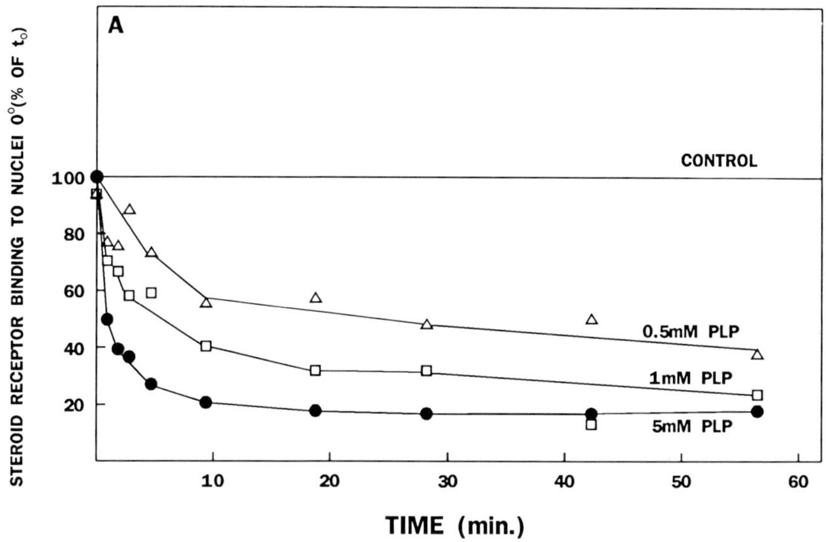

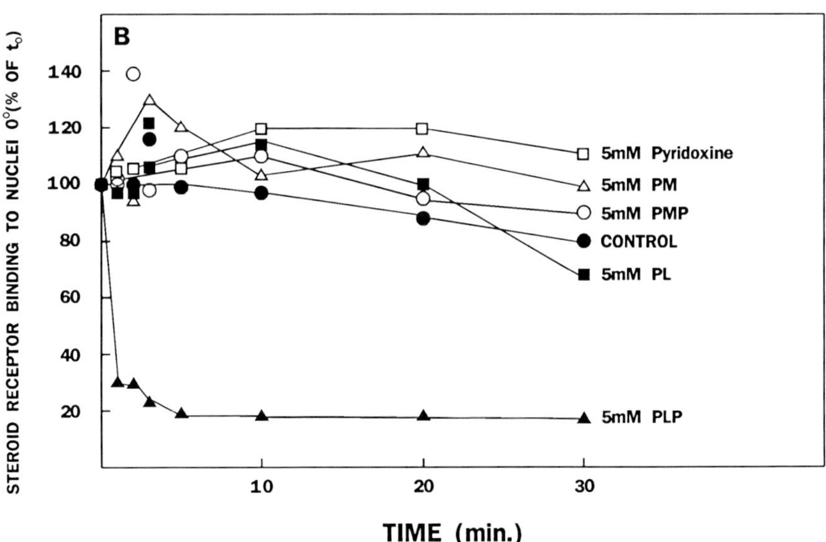

Figure 9. Ability of PLP to remove glucocorticoid-receptor complexes from liver nuclei. *A.* The effects of PLP at various concentrations over a 60-minute period. *B.* The specificity of the effect. PLP is specific with no activity demonstrated by PN, PM, or PMP and very little activity of PL.

Reproduced from Dolan *et al.* (12) with permission.

PLP may play an additional role in the synthesis of TAT, since the enzyme contains PLP as a cofactor.

We carried out a more direct series of experiments for eight weeks in rats made deficient in vitamin B_6 (13). Controls received the deficient diet but received 50 μg of PN per milliliter of drinking water, so that by the end of the eight-week period control animals weighed an average of 290 g and the deficient animals weighed an average of 162 g. Upon supplementation with PN, the test animals grew at the same rate as the controls. Deficiency was also established by the status of liver TAT, where it was demonstrated that the deficient animals had lost 75% of the TAT holoenzyme, restorable by the addition of PLP in vitro. Animals were adrenalectomized three days before use to reduce the endogenous level of steroid-bound receptor. Liver cytosols were prepared from the B_6-deficient rats, and the level of specific steroid binding to receptor, after addition of [^{3}H]triamcinolone acetonide, was equal in samples from both groups. However, there was a marked difference in the rate and extent of binding of the activated receptor complex to DNA such that more than three times as many receptor molecules were activated and bound to DNA in the cytosols from B_6-deficient animals compared with controls. A similar study was done comparing binding to isolated cell nuclei. In this study, 74% of steroid-receptor complexes from deficient cytosol were bound to nuclei after 15 minutes of incubation, whereas 29% of receptor complexes in the control cytosol were bound to nuclei in the same time period. After 30 minutes of incubation the values were 65% and 40% respectively. Thus it is clear that the lack of PLP in cytosols from deficient animals provided a receptor complex that was more activatable and translocatable to the nucleus. Finally, nuclear transfer of the glucocorticoid receptor complex was studied in vivo by injecting the radioactive steroid and isolating cytosols and nuclei (13). These experiments showed that the extent of nuclear translocation was similar in deficient and control samples, whereas the amount of radioactive triamcinolone acetonide taken up by the liver cell was drastically reduced in animals in the vitamin-deficient state. When the concentrations of the receptor complex localized in the nuclei were expressed as the percentage of steroid specifically labeled receptors in the cytosol, the deficient state produced a much more efficient nuclear translocation process than did the controls. In fact, after 40 minutes of incubation of the radioactive steroid in vivo, there were about

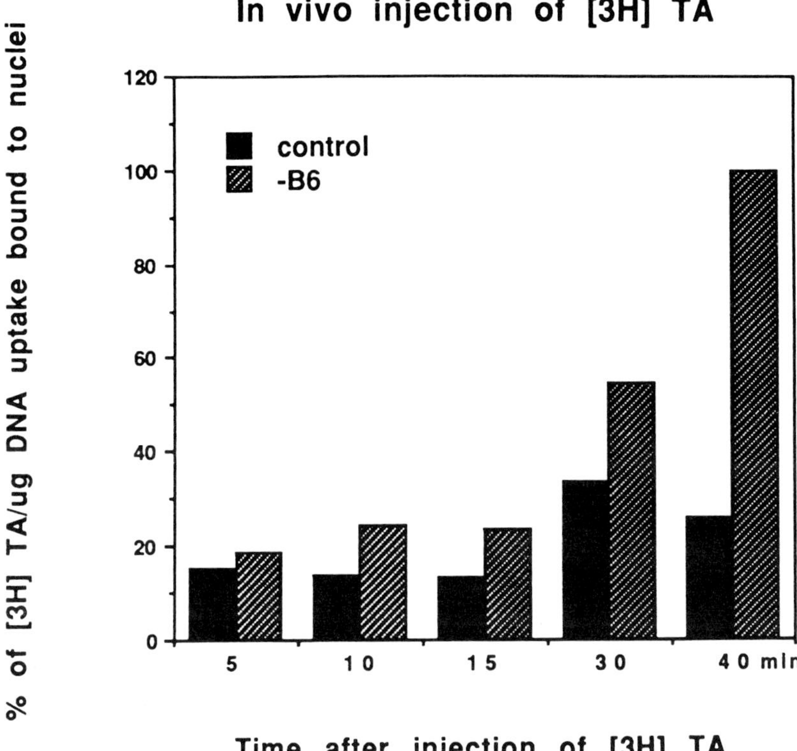

Figure 10. *In vivo* experiment with adrenalectomized–vitamin B_6 deficient rats showing the percent of radioactive triamcinolone (TA) taken up by liver nuclei as a function of time. For purposes of illustration the maximum accumulation of radioactivity in the nucleus was arbitrarily set at a value of 100. After 40 minutes in vivo, the translocation of the glucocorticoid receptor in the deficient animals is much more efficient than in the controls. These data were recalculated from those presented by DiSorbo *et al.* (13).

75% more receptor complexes within nuclei of deficient animals compared with controls (Fig. 10) (13).

Indirect Immunofluorescence with Antireceptor Monoclonal Antibodies

We have studied intact melanoma cells using indirect immunofluorescence to localize the glucocorticoid receptor (14). Using this technique we have shown that the translocation of the glucocorticoid receptor from the cytoplasm to the nucleus is blocked by treatment with PL and all of the fluorescence attributable to the receptor remains in the cytoplasm, whereas in the control (without PL) the receptor is nearly quantitatively translocated to the nucleus. We now are taking advantage of confocal microscopy to continue these experiments. This result represents the first direct demonstration of the inhibition of nuclear transfer by PLP in the intact cell.

ACKNOWLEDGMENTS

Research in this laboratory related to this topic is supported by research grant DK 13531 from the National Institutes of Health and research grant 87B73 from the American Institute for Cancer Research.

REFERENCES

1. Merrill AH, Henderson JM. Vitamin B_6 metabolism by human liver. *Ann N Y Acad Sci.* 1990;585:110–117.
2. Norman AW, Litwack G. *Hormones.* Orlando, Fla: Academic Press, 1987.
3. Cake MH, DiSorbo DM, Litwack G. Effect of pyridoxal phosphate on the DNA binding site of activated hepatic glucocorticoid receptor. *J Biol Chem.* 1978;253:4886–4891.
4. Litwack G, Cake MH. DNA binding site of activated glucocorticoid receptor: interaction with pyridoxal-P. *Fed Proc.* 1977;36:911.
5. DiSorbo DM, Phelps DS, Litwack G. Chemical probes of amino acid residues affect the active sites of the glucocorticoid receptor. *Endocrinology.* 1980;106:922–928.
6. Maksymowych AB, Daniel V, Litwack G. Pyridoxal phosphate as a regulator of the glucocorticoid receptor. *Ann N Y Acad Sci.* 1990;585:438–451.
7. Grandics P, Miller A, Schmidt TJ, Mittman D, Litwack G. Purification of unactivated glucocorticoid receptor to apparent homogeneity. *J Biol Chem.* 1984;259:3173–3180.
8. Simons SS Jr, Miller PA. Comparison of DNA binding properties of activated, covalent and noncovalent glucocorticoid receptor-steroid complexes from HTC cells. *Biochemistry.* 1984;23:6876–6882.
9. Dolan KP, Diaz-Gil JJ, Litwack G. Interaction of pyridoxal 5′-

phosphate with the liver glucocorticoid receptor-DNA complex. *Arch Biochem Biophys*. 1980;201:476–485.
10. Rowley DR, Tindall DJ. Androgen receptor protein: purification and molecular properties. *Biochem Actions Hormones*. 1986;13:305–324.
11. DiSorbo DM, Litwack G. Changes in the intracellular levels of pyridoxal 5′-phosphate affect the induction of tyrosine aminotransferase by glucocorticoids. *Biochem Biophys Res Commun*. 1981; 99:1203–1208.
12. Dolan KP, Diaz-Gil JJ, Litwack G. Interaction of pyridoxal 5′-phosphate with the liver glucocorticoid receptor-DNA complex. *Arch Biochem Biophys*. 1980;201:476–485.
13. DiSorbo DM, Phelps DS, Ohl VS, Litwack G. Pyridoxine deficiency influences the behavior of the glucocorticoid receptor complex. *J Biol Chem*. 1980;255:3866–3870.
14. Lindemeyer S, Robertson N, Litwack G. Glucocorticoid receptor monoclonal antibodies define the biological action of RU38486 in intact B16 melanoma cells. *Cancer Res*. 1990;50:7985–7991.

PART V

Vitamin A and Beta-Carotene

RICHARD C. MOON

Vitamin A, Retinoids, and Animal Tumorigenesis

ABSTRACT

Vitamin A and synthetic analogues of vitamin A (retinoids) are effective inhibitors of chemical carcinogenesis in the mammary gland, lung, and bladder of experimental animals. Modification of the basic retinoid structure has produced retinoids with increased target organ specificity, resulting in increased anticancer activity with reduced systemic toxicity. Combining retinoid treatment with hormonal manipulation results in a synergistic inhibition of mammary carcinogenesis; this combination approach also inhibits development of additional breast cancers following surgical removal of the first breast cancer. Combination chemoprevention has also been effective in inhibiting lung and bladder cancer. Retinoids are most effective when administered shortly after the carcinogenic insult; however, even when retinoid treatment is delayed, the compounds are still effective cancer chemopreventive agents for the mammary gland and bladder. The length of time that retinoid exposure can be delayed and retain an anticancer effect is directly related to tumor latency, with a longer delay permissible against tumors with long latent periods.

Introduction

The rationale for the use of retinoids (vitamin A and its analogues) as chemopreventive agents or inhibitors of carcinogenesis dates back seventy years. In 1922 Mori (1) observed that a deficiency in vitamin A led to metaplastic changes of the epithelium of the respiratory tract; the normal ciliated columnar epithelium became flattened, lost nuclei, and became cornified, and the underlying cells exhibited typical keratohyalin granules. Subsequent studies by Wolbach and Howe (2) extended these observations to epithelia of the gastrointestinal and urinary tracts. These observations on the development of retinoid-deficient squamous metaplasia indicated a process closely akin to that induced by certain chemical carcinogens (3). A more direct link between retinoids and cancer appeared in 1926 when Fujimaki (4) observed the development of carcinomas of the stomach in rats maintained on a diet deficient in vitamin A. More recently, other investigators have shown that animals fed a diet deficient in retinoids and subsequently exposed to chemical carcinogens develop a greater than normal incidence of cancers and putative precursors to these malignancies (5, 6).

In addition to the relationship between retinoid deficiency and neoplasia, other studies have indicated that retinoids can reverse premalignant changes in the epithelium of mouse prostate glands in organ culture (7) and suppress malignant transformation in cells in vitro irrespective of whether the transformation is induced by ionizing radiation (8), chemical carcinogens (9), or transforming polypeptides (10). Retinoids have also been shown to be potent inhibitors of phorbol ester–induced tumor promotion (11). Inasmuch as retinoids inhibit several aspects of the carcinogenic process (transformation, metaplasia, promotion), investigators have extended these studies to show that exogenous retinoids can inhibit tumor formation in vitro in epithelia at several different organ sites.

In this paper we summarize the available information on the chemopreventive effectiveness of retinoids in the several tumor models. Mammary carcinogenesis is emphasized since this is the only process in which the chemopreventive activity of retinoids has been studied in any detail.

Nomenclature, Structure, and Specificity

Retinoid is a general term for any natural or synthetic compound with vitamin A activity. Chemically, the retinoids are defined as diterpenoids derived from a monocyclic parent compound containing five carbon-carbon double bonds and a functional group at the terminus of the acyclic portion. However, this definition does not account for more potent, newer synthetic retinoids such as tri- or tetra-cyclic retinoidal benzoic acid derivatives (Fig. 1), which may not be diterpenoids or may not be derived from a monocyclic parent compound. Recently, Sporn and Roberts (12) have proposed a general definition of *retinoid:* "a substance that can elicit specific biological responses by binding to and activating a specific receptor or set of receptors."

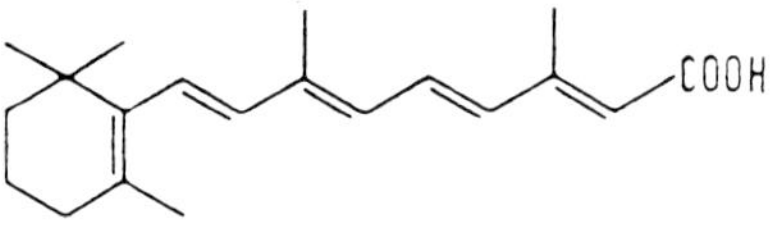

Figure 1. Structures of retinoids: retinoic acid, all-transretinoic acid (monocyclic); TTNPB, (E)-4-[2-5,6,7,8-tetrahydro-5,5,8,8-tetra-methyl-2-naphthalenyl)-1-propenyl]benzoic acid (tricyclic); and TTNN, 5′, 6′, 7′,8′-tetrahydro-5′,5′,8′,8′tetramethyl-[2,2′-binaph-thalene]-6-carboxylic acid (tetracyclic). Reprinted with permission from Moon and Mehta (48).

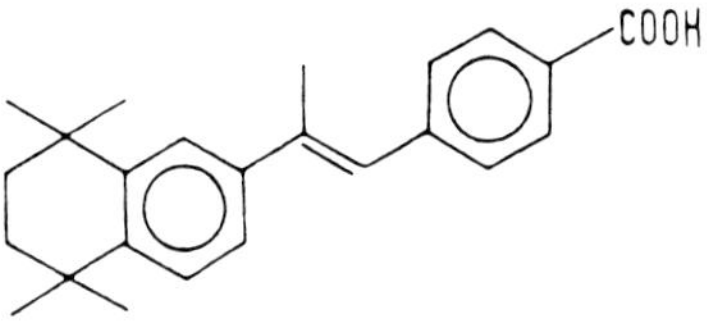

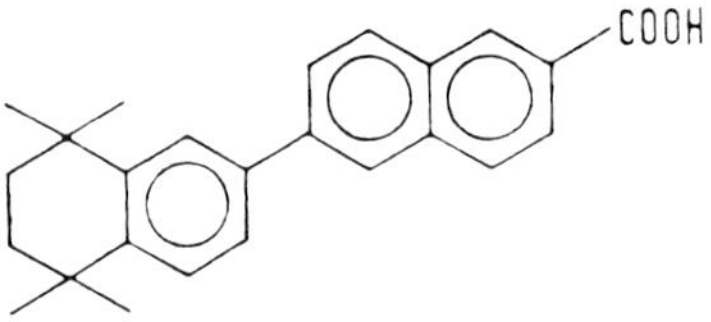

Structures of certain retinoids derived from monocyclic structures, such as retinol or retinoic acid, as well as multicyclic structures such as retinoidal benzoic acid, can be modified to yield almost an unlimited number of retinoids. More than 1000 retinoids have been synthesized, and many have been screened for biological activity by Sporn and his colleagues (13) using the tracheal organ culture assay.

The efficacy of retinoids, active in vitro, has been subsequently tested for anticancer activity in several animal tumor models, and studies in these models have demonstrated that retinoids possess a high degree of target organ specificity and, in some cases, species specificity. Thus, the inhibition expressed at one organ site does not necessarily imply efficacy of the retinoid for inhibiting carcinogenesis of another epithelial tissue. For example, 13-*cis*-retinoic acid is an effective inhibitor of carcinogen-induced urinary bladder cancer in rats (14) and mice (15), but it is without effect against breast cancer in the

Table 1. In Vivo Carcinogenesis Specificity of Retinoids

Target Organ	Carcinogen	Effective	Noneffective
Mammary gland	MNU, DMBA	Retinyl acetate	13-*cis*-retinoic acid
Bladder	OH-BBN	13-*cis*-retinoic acid	TMMP ethyl retinoate
Skin	DMBA + TPA	TMMP ethyl retinoate	Retinyl acetate

Reprinted with permission from Moon and Mehta (48).

rat (Table 1). The trimethylmethoxyphenyl (TMMP) analogue of ethyl retinoate is highly effective against mouse skin carcinogenesis (11) but ineffective against either bladder carcinogenesis in mice or breast cancer in rats. On the other hand, retinyl acetate is extremely active in the rat breast cancer model (16) but exhibits little chemopreventive protection against two-stage skin tumorigenesis (17) or mammary carcinogenesis in mice (18).

Experimental Carcinogenesis and Retinoids

As indicated above, the anticarcinogenic activity of retinoids has been demonstrated in several in vitro experimental tumor models. However, most of the in-depth work has been done using the skin, urinary bladder, and breast cancer models with other model systems being used infrequently.

Bladder Cancer

Sporn *et al.* (19) were the first to demonstrate an effect of retinoids in the inhibition of bladder carcinogenesis in experimental animals, a multistage process involving initiation, promotion, and propagation (20). These workers found that 13-*cis*-retinoic acid not only inhibited the incidence but also reduced the severity of bladder neoplasms induced by the intravesicle administration of methylnitrosourea (MNU) to rats. However, in this study the intravesicle administration of MNU resulted in a high percentage of the malignancies that were classified as squamous-cell carcinomas. In humans, the majority of bladder cancers that develop are of a transitional nature rather than the squamous type. Thus, Moon and Itri (21) conducted several studies to determine the efficacy of retinoids in experimental systems in which the tumors that developed were almost entirely transitional-cell carcinomas. Early work by these investigators showed that 13-*cis*-retinoic acid reduced the incidence and severity of transitional-cell carcinoma as well as that of a number of other bladder proliferative lesions resulting from the intragastric administration of N-butyl-N-(4-hydroxybutyl)nitrosamine (OH-BBN) to either F344 rats or C57BL/6 x DBA/$2F_1$ mice. Subsequent studies indicated that the administration of this retinoid could be delayed for some time following the last carcinogenic exposure without loss of ability to inhibit bladder carcinogenesis.

Subsequent to the studies utilizing the natural retinoid and 13-*cis*-retinoic acid, several other analogues have been shown to have anti-carcinogenic activity in the rodent bladder. Particularly notable among these compounds are the retinamides, a group of retinoids in which the terminal carboxyl group of retinoic acid is replaced by an N-substituted carboxy amide group. In contrast to the natural retinoids, retinamides have the desirable quality of reducing toxicity while retaining much or all of the in vitro biological activity from the natural compounds. Several of the retinamides that have been evaluated for chemopreventive activity against urinary cancer in rats and mice are listed in Table 2.

In contrast to the retinamides, some of which have proved highly effective in inhibiting bladder carcinogenesis when administered after completion of the carcinogen dosing, TMMP ethyl retinoate was apparently more effective in inhibiting OH-BBN–induced bladder neoplasms in rats, if the animals were treated with the retinoid before rather than during or after the administration of the carcinogen (22). In line with these results, Schmahl and Habs (23) indicated that TMMP ethyl retinoate has little effect on OH-BBN–induced bladder carcinogenesis when the retinoid and carcinogen were administered concomitantly.

The above studies demonstrate that several retinoids effectively inhibit development of carcinogen-induced bladder cancer in rats and mice. It is also apparent that several synthetic retinoids, particularly the retinamides, are less toxic and more effective than natural retinoids for this purpose. Although some retinoids may be effective in preventing initiation of bladder carcinogenesis, the majority are apparently more active during the progression phase of the carcino-

Table 2. Retinoids Evaluated for Chemopreventive Activity Against Bladder Cancer in Rats and Mice[a]

Active	Inactive
Retinoic acid	Retinyl palmitate
13-*cis*-retinoic acid	N-(4-carboxyphenyl)retinamide
Retinyl acetate	N-(4-carboxypropyl)retinamide
N-ethylretinamide	N-(3-hydroxypropyl)retinamide
N-ethyl-13-*cis*-retinamide	N-(2,3-dihydroxypropyl)retinamide
N-(2-hydroxyethyl)retinamide	N-(n-butyl)retinamide
N-(2-hydroxyethyl)-13-*cis*-retinamide	N-(4-hydroxybutyl)retinamide
N-(4-hydroxyphenyl)retinamide	N-(4-hydroxybutyl)-13-*cis*-retinamide
N-(4-hydroxyphenyl)-13-*cis*-retinamide	N-(5-tetrazolyl)-13-*cis*-retinamide
N-(2-hydroxypropyl)retinamide	Motretinid
N-(5-tetrazolyl)retinamide	
Etretinate	

Reprinted with permission from Moon and Itri (21).

[a]For details, see (21).

genic response. If such compounds are to be used as chemopreventive agents for bladder cancer in man, then the ability of retinoids to delay tumor growth in urothelium already neoplastically transformed is of critical importance.

Breast Cancer

Experimental evidence obtained over the past 15 years from our laboratory clearly indicates that certain retinoids inhibit development of both MNU and dimethylbenz(a)anthracene (DMBA)-induced mammary cancers in the rat. A host of retinoids have been tested for such activity, and a summary of this work in our laboratory as well as that of other investigators have been reviewed by Moon and Itri (21) and Moon *et al.* (24). We can draw several conclusions from these studies: (a) retinoids increase the latency of the first tumor appearance; (b) retinoids reduce the overall tumor incidence and, more dramatically, reduce tumor multiplicity; (c) some retinoids are apparently species specific; retinyl acetate, which is an effective retinoid against MNU- and DMBA-induced rat breast cancer, is ineffective against mouse mammary carcinogenesis; and (d) N-4-hydroxyphenyl retinamide (4-

HPR) is thus far the most active and least toxic retinoid available for experimental mammary carcinogenesis. Moreover, 4-HPR is active in both mice and rats as well as in inhibition of bladder carcinogenesis.

The efficacy of nontoxic doses of several retinoids in the inhibition of mammary carcinogenesis induced in the rat by MNU is indicated in Table 3. Retinyl acetate and 4-HPR are highly effective in reducing breast cancer incidence and increasing the latency of induced breast cancers (25). In addition, the number of mammary carcinomas is also significantly reduced by the administration of either of these retinoids. However, 13-*cis*-retinoic acid has little effect upon the appearance of MNU-induced mammary carcinomas. Retinyl methyl ether is somewhat effective in inhibiting MNU-induced cancers and extremely effective against DMBA-induced mammary carcinogenesis. Thus, it is readily apparent that minor alterations in the basic retinoid

Table 3. Effect of Retinoids on Mammary Carcinogenesis in Rats

Carcinogen	Retinoid	Effect
DMBA	Retinyl palmitate	None
DMBA	Retinyl acetate Retinyl mether ether 4-HPR Temaroten	Inhibition of carcinogenesis
MNU	Retinyl acetate Retinyl methyl ether 4-HPR Axerophthene All-trans-retinoic acid N-(4-hydroxyphenyl)-13-*cis*-retinamide Temaroten	Inhibition of carcinogenesis
MNU	13-*cis*-retinoic acid Retinyl butyl ether N-ethylretinamide Retinylidene dimedone Retinylidene acetylacetone Etretinate (R010-9359) TMMP analogue of retinyl methyl ether	None
Benzo(a)pyrene	Retinyl acetate	Inhibition of carcinogenesis

structure can alter significantly the activity of the molecule with respect to the inhibition of chemical carcinogenesis of the mammary gland.

The toxicity induced by a retinoid is of extreme importance in long-term chemoprevention studies. As an example, retinyl acetate and 4-HPR are both effective inhibitors of chemical carcinogenesis of the rat mammary gland, but the patterns of metabolism and organ distribution of the two compounds are quite different (25). Chronic dietary administration of high doses of retinyl acetate results in an accumulation of retinyl esters in the liver, a process frequently accompanied by significant hepatic toxicity (26). Dietary administration of 4-HPR results in a much higher level of retinoid in the mammary gland but with relatively little liver accumulation (25). Thus, on the basis of its organ distribution, it would appear that 4-HPR is preferable to retinyl acetate for use in the prevention of breast cancer.

Although retinoids are most effective in inhibiting mammary carcinogenesis when administered shortly after carcinogen treatment, they are still effective cancer-chemopreventive agents if the administration is delayed for some time after the carcinogenic insult (27). The length of time that retinoid treatment can be delayed is largely a function of tumor latency. In animals given a carcinogen dose that induces tumors with a mean induction time of approximately 60 days (27), retinyl acetate administration begun at one week postcarcinogen is highly effective in cancer inhibition. The retinoid treatment is somewhat less effective if initiated 4 weeks after administration of the carcinogen, and beginning the retinoid at 8 weeks after carcinogen treatment has no effect on tumor induction. By contrast, at a carcinogen dose inducing breast cancers with a mean induction time of approximately 240 days (27), retinyl acetate administration can be delayed as long as 16 weeks and still retain its chemopreventive efficacy. Only when the initiation of retinyl acetate treatment is delayed 20 weeks does the retinoid show a loss of cancer-inhibitory activity. The ability of the retinoid to significantly inhibit breast cancer formation when administered at some time after the carcinogenic insult is of the utmost clinical importance, since the initiation of carcinogenesis in humans is largely unknown.

Recent studies by several investigators have demonstrated a significant interaction between retinoids and other modifiers of mammary carcinogenesis. Combined treatment, in most cases, affords greater protection against mammary carcinogenesis than either treatment alone. Carcinogen-induced rat breast cancer models are subject to inhibition both by retinoids and by modification of host hormonal status. As is well known, ovarian hormone–dependent tumors regress following ovariectomy of the tumor-bearing animal. Similarly, if animals are ovariectomized shortly after carcinogen administration, only the ovarian hormone–independent tumors appear and cancer incidence is low. The combination of ovariectomy (two weeks postcarcinogen) and retinyl acetate results in a synergistic inhibition of tumor incidence and multiplicity (28). Similar results were obtained with 4-HPR. In a more recent study, Moon *et al.* (29) clearly demonstrated that tamoxifen and 4-HPR, when used in combination, were much more effective in inhibiting mammary carcinogenesis than was either agent alone. A similar synergistic inhibition has been demonstrated in the MNU-induced mammary carcinogenesis model by concomitant administration of retinyl acetate and 2-bromo-a-ergocryptine, an inhibitor of pituitary prolactin secretion (30). Since the blood prolactin levels of rats treated with retinyl acetate were similar to those of control animals, the enhanced combination effect probably was not due to a further suppression of prolactin secretion but due to an effect at the level of the mammary parenchymal cell. Although hormonal modifications of experimental mammary tumorigenesis are well established, it now appears from the evidence cited above that the retinoids also effectively alter mammary tumorigenesis. These data suggest the existence of populations of preneoplastic and/or neoplastic cells displaying differential sensitivity to the retinoids and hormones. Whether retinoids preferentially suppress the growth of hormone-independent cell population, reverse the neoplastic potential of these cells, or induce terminal differentiation of preneoplastic cells as has been shown for the C3H 10T½ cells (31) is presently unknown.

Combination chemoprevention has also been demonstrated with retinoids and other agents that inhibit development of breast cancer. Thompson *et al.* (32) were the first to show an enhanced inhibition of MNU-induced rat mammary carcinogenesis with retinyl acetate and selenium. The effect was confirmed by Ip and Ip (33) using the DMBA-induced mammary tumor model. Although both groups of workers found that the combined effect of retinyl acetate and selenium was substantially greater than that of either treatment alone, both studies were complicated by the significant reduction in food intake and body weight gain in animals receiving these chemopreventive agents. Attempts to use combined modalities for prevention of breast cancer are not always successful. For example, 4-HPR and the maleic anhydride-divinyl ether copolymer (MVE-2), an immunostimulatory agent, are both effective inhibitors of mammary carcinogenesis induced in rats by MNU. However, combined administration of 4-HPR and MVE-2 was no more effective in cancer inhibition than was the use of either agent alone (34).

Other Epithelial Cancers

A majority of the studies involving retinoids and skin carcinogenesis have been conducted in the laboratories of Bollag and Matter (35) and Boutwell (36). These workers utilized the two-stage carcinogenesis model, in which a carcinogen is applied to the skin of the backs of mice; this initiation leads to the appearance of few, if any, tumors in the animal. However, the application of 12-0-tetradecanoyl-phorbol-13-acetate (TPA) following initiation results in high incidence of papillomas and carcinomas. Such studies have shown conclusively that retinoids inhibit TPA-promoted skin carcinogenesis. Bollag and Matter (35) have established a therapeutic index for retinoids in which the efficacy against skin carcinogenesis related to toxicity is determined; this, in turn, allows the comparison of the effectiveness of one retinoid with that of another. Some analogues such as 13-*cis*-retinoic acid, TMMP ethyl retinoate, and tricyclic retinoidal benzoic acid have a greater therapeutic index than that of all-transretinoic acid and also are more effective against skin carcinogenesis. Although the therapeutic index has proved of value in studies of structure-function relationships, it has provided little insight into the anticancer potential of retinoids in tumor systems other than the skin.

A few reports have appeared relative to retinoids and carcinogen-induced tracheobronchial carcinogenesis. Nettesheim and his colleagues (37) showed an inhibitory effect of retinyl acetate on 3-methylcholanthrene–induced metaplastic lung nodules in rats, whereas 13-*cis*-retinoic acid proved an effective inhibitor of hamster tracheobronchial carcinoma induced by the Saffiotti procedure (38). However, enhancement of MNU-induced tracheobronchial carcinogenesis has been noted in the hamster with 13-*cis*-retinoic acid, ethyl retinamide, and 4-HPR (39). N-4-hydroxyphenyl retinamide was inactive in the MNU hamster model in that it neither enhanced nor inhibited tracheobronchial carcinogenesis (40). Recently, however, we have found 4-HPR to effectively inhibit diethylnitrosamine-induced lung carcinogenesis in hamsters (Table 4). However, the studies with MNU do not utilize an initiation-promotion design.

The effectiveness of retinoids as inhibitors of chemical carcinogenesis of the epithelia of the digestive tract has been somewhat disappointing, although positive results have been obtained in studies of forestomach, esophageal, liver, and pancreatic carcinogenesis. Chu and Malmgren (41) found that the oral administration of retinyl ester prevented the occurrence of stomach papillomas and carcinomas of hamsters receiving polycyclic hydrocarbons. Similar results were obtained by other workers (42, 43).

Nitrosamine-induced esophageal carcinogenesis can also be markedly inhibited by the administration of retinyl ester. Subsequent studies have shown that the synthetic retinoids TMMP ethyl retinoate and 13-*cis*-retinoic acid also exert a protective effect against the induction of esophageal tumors with nitroso compounds (21).

Although several carcinogens and retinoids have been used in

Table 4. Effect of Retinoids on Lung Carcinogenesis In Vivo

Strain	Carcinogen	Retinoid	Effect
Syrian golden hamsters	BP + FEO_2	Retinyl palmitate 13-*cis*-retinoic acid	Reduced incidence of respiratory tract tumors
		Retinyl acetate	None
	MNU	4-HPR 13-*cis*-retinoic acid	None
		Ethyl retinamide Ethylamide of TMMP	Enhancement of carcinogenesis
	DEN	4-HPR	Reduced incidence of adenosquamous carcinomas
Fisher 344 rats	3MC	Retinyl acetate	Decreased incidence of metaplastic nodules
Sprague/Dawley rats	DBN	Retinyl palmitate	None

chemoprevention studies of colon carcinogenesis, the results indicate that for the most part retinoids have been ineffectual in inhibiting chemically induced colon tumorigenesis. Neither the natural nor the synthetic retinoids had an effect upon colon carcinogenesis induced with aflatoxin (43), dimethylhydrazine (42), or MNU (44).

The few studies on liver carcinogenesis have indicated that the retinol esters are ineffectual in modulating aflatoxin-induced liver tumors in rats. However, Daoud and Griffin (45) found 13-*cis*-retinoic acid to be highly effective in reducing the incidence of liver tumors induced by 3-methyl-4-dimethylaminoazobenzene. Similar findings have been reported for hepatomas arising spontaneously in mice given various doses of retinyl ester (18).

Inhibition of pancreatic carcinogenesis with retinoids was first reported by Longnecker *et al.* (46), who found that several synthetic retinoids inhibited the development of azaserine-induced pancreatic tumors when administered during the promotional phase of carcinogenesis. On the other hand, Birt *et al.* (47) found that such synthetic retinoids did not influence significantly the development of N-nitrosobis-(2-oxopropyl)amine–induced pancreatic cancer in hamsters. Whether the differences between the two studies were due to the pathogenesis of the tumors induced by the two different carcinogens or to species differences in metabolizing the retinoids is not known at present.

Conclusion

It is apparent from the studies cited above that a variety of retinoids demonstrate anticancer activity in several experimental models for cancer and that minor modifications of the retinoid molecule can have striking effects on organ distribution and the cancer-chemopreventive activity of a compound. Additive or synergistic interactions between retinoid and other modulators of carcinogenesis have also been demonstrated, particularly in experimental models of the breast and skin. Research should continue to identify retinoids with increased anticancer activity, to assess effects of combined administration of retinoids and other modifiers of carcinogenesis, and to investigate the mechanisms by which retinoids inhibit carcinogenesis. However, several retinoids are presently available for use in well-designed clinical trials, particularly for bladder and breast cancer.

REFERENCES

1. Mori S. The changes in the para-ocular glands which follow the administration of diets low in fat-soluble A; with notes of the effects of the same diets on the salivary glands and the mucosa of the larynx and trachea. *Johns Hopkins Hosp Bull.* 1922;33:357–359.
2. Wolbach SD, Howe PR. Tissue changes following deprivation of fat-soluble A vitamin. *J Exp Med.* 1925;42:753–777.
3. Harris CC, Sporn MB, Kaufman DG, Smith JM, Jackson FE, Saffiotti U. Histogenesis of squamous metaplasias in the hamster tracheal epithelium caused by vitamin A deficiency or benzo(a) pyrene-ferric oxide. *J Natl Cancer Inst.* 1972;48:743–761.
4. Fujimaki Y. Formation of carcinoma in albino rats fed on deficient diets. *J Cancer Res.* 1926;10:469–477.
5. Rogers AE, Herndon BJ, Newberne PM. Inducation by dimethylhydrazine of intestinal carcinoma in normal rats fed high and low levels of vitamin A. *Cancer Res.* 1973:1003–1009.
6. Cohen SM, Wittenberg JF, Bryn GT. Effect of avitaminosis A and hypervitaminosis A on urinary bladder carcinogenesis of N-[4-(5-nitrofuryl)-2-thozolyl)] formamide. *Cancer Res.* 1976;36:2334–2339.
7. Lasnitzki I, Goodman DS. Inhibition of the effects of methylcholanthrene on mouse prostate in organ culture by vitamin A and its analogues. *Cancer Res.* 1974;34:1564–1571.
8. Harisiadis L, Miller RC, Hall EJ, Borek C. A vitamin A analogue inhibits radiation-induced oncogenic transformation. *Nature.* 1978; 274:486–487.
9. Merriman RL, Bertram JS. Reversible inhibition by retinoids of 3-methyl-cholanthrene–induced neoplastic transformation in C3H/10T1/2 C18 cells. *Cancer Res.* 1979;39:1661–1666.
10. Todaro GJ, DeLarco JE, Sporn MB. Retinoids block phenotypic cell transformation produced by sarcoma growth factor. *Nature.* 1978;272–274.
11. Verma AK, Shapas BG, Rice HM, Boutwell RK. Correlation of the inhibition by retinoids of tumor promoter-induced mouse epidermal ornithine decarboxylase activity and of skin tumor promotion. *Cancer Res.* 1979;39:419–425.
12. Sporn MB, Roberts AB. Introduction: what is a retinoid? In: Ciba Foundation Symposium 113. *Retinoids, Differentiation and Disease.* London: Pitman; 1985:1–5.

13. Clamon GH, Sporn MB, Smith JM, Saffiotti U. Alpha and beta retinyl acetate reverse metaplasia of vitamin A deficiency in hamster trachea in organ culture. *Nature.* 1974;250:64–66.
14. Grubbs CJ, Moon RC, Squire RA, *et al.* 13-*cis*-retinoic acid: inhibition of bladder carcinogenesis induced by N-butyl-N-(4-hydroxybutyl) nitrosamine. *Science.* 1977;198:743–744.
15. Becci PJ, Thompson HJ, Strum JM, Brown CC, Sporn MB, Moon RC. N-butyl-N-(4-hydroxybutyl) nitrosamine–induced urinary bladder cancer in C57BL/6 x DBA/$2F_1$ mice as useful model for study of chemoprevention of cancer with retinoids. *Cancer Res.* 1981;41:927–932.
16. Moon RC, Grubbs CJ, Sporn MB, Goodman DG. Retinyl acetate inhibits mammary carcinogenesis induced by N-methyl-N-nitrosourea. *Nature.* 1977;267:620–621.
17. Verma AK, Boutwell RK. Vitamin A acid (retinoic acid), a potent inhibitor of 12-0-tetradecanoyl-phorbol-13-acetate–induced ornithine decarboxylase activity in mouse epidermis. *Cancer Res.* 1977;37:2196–2201.
18. Maiorana A, Gullino P. Effect of retinyl acetate on the incidence of mammary carcinomas and hepatomas in mice. *J Natl Cancer Inst.* 1980;64:655–663.
19. Sporn MB, Squire RA, Brown CC, Smith JM, Wenk ML, Springer S. 13-*cis*-retinoic acid: inhibition of bladder carcinogenesis in the rat. *Science.* 1977;195:487–489.
20. Hicks RM. Multistage carcinogenesis in the urinary bladder. *Br Med Bull.* 1980;36:39–46.
21. Moon RC, Itri L. Retinoids and cancer. In: Sporn MB, Roberts AB, Goodman DS, eds. *The Retinoids.* Orlando, Fla: Academic Press; 1984:327–371.
22. Murasaki G, Miyata YL, Babaya K, Arai M, Fukushima S, Ito N. Inhibitory effect of an aromatic retinoic acid analogue on urinary bladder carcinogenesis in rats treated with N-butyl-N-(4-hydroxybutyl) nitrosamine. *Gann.* 1980;71:333–340.
23. Schmahl D, Habs M. Experiments on the influence of an aromatic retinoid on the chemical carcinogenesis in rats by butyl-butanol-nitrosamine and 1,2-dimethylhydrazine. *Arzneimittelforschung.* 1978;28:49–51.
24. Moon RC, Mehta RG, McCormick DL. Retinoids and mammary

gland differentiation. In: Ciba Foundation Symposium 113. *Retinoids, Differentiation and Disease.* London: Pittman; 1985:156–167.

25. Moon RC, Thompson HJ, Becci PJ, *et al.* N-(4-hydroxyphenyl) retinamide, a new retinoid for prevention of breast cancer in the rat. *Cancer Res.* 1979;39:1339–1346.
26. Smith FR, Goodman DS. Vitamin A transport and human vitamin A toxicity. *N Engl J Med.* 1976;294:805–808.
27. McCormick DL, Moon RC. Influence of delayed administration of retinyl acetate on mammary carcinogenesis. *Cancer Res.* 1982;42: 2639–2643.
28. Moon RC, Mehta RG. Retinoid binding in normal and neoplastic mammary tissue. In: Leavit WW, ed. *Hormones and Cancer.* New York: Plenum Press; 1982:231–249.
29. Moon RC, McCormick DL, Mehta RG. Retinoid and hormone interaction in mammary carcinogenesis. In: Proceedings of the 13th International Congress of Chemotherapy, SE 12.8.2-10, 1983.
30. Welsch CW, Brown CK, Goodrich-Smith M, Chuisano J, Moon RC. Synergistic effect of chronic prolactin suppression and retinoid treatment in the prophylaxis of N-methyl-N-nitrosourea–induced mammary tumorigenesis in female Sprague-Dawley rats. *Cancer Res.* 1980;40:3095–3098.
31. Bertram JS. Inhibition of neoplastic transformation *in vitro* by retinoids. *Cancer Surv.* 1983;3:243–262.
32. Thompson HJ, Meeker LD, Becci PJ. Effect of combined selenium and retinyl acetate treatment on mammary carcinogenesis. *Cancer Res.* 1981;41:1413–1416.
33. Ip C, Ip MM. Chemoprevention of mammary tumorigenesis by a combined regimen of selenium and vitamin A. *Carcinogenesis.* 1981;2:915–918.
34. McCormick DL, Becci PJ, Moon RC. Inhibition of mammary and urinary bladder carcinogenesis by a retinoid and a maleic anhydride-divinyl ether copolymer (MVE02). *Carcinogenesis.* 1982; 3:1473–1477.
35. Bollag W, Matter A. From Vitamin A to retinoids in experimental and clinical oncology: achievements, failures and outlook. *Ann N Y Acad Sci.* 1981;359:9–23.
36. Boutwell RK. Diet and anticarcinogenesis in the mouse skin two stage model. *Cancer Res.* 1983;43:2465s–24658s.

37. Nettesheim P, Care MN, Snyder C. The influence of retinyl acetate on the post-initiation phase of preneoplastic lung nodules in rats. *Cancer Res.* 1976;36:996–1002.
38. Port CD, Sporn MB, Kaufman DG. Prevention of lung cancer in hamsters by 13-*cis*-retinoic acid. *Proc Am Assoc Cancer Res.* 1975; 16:21.
39. Stinson SP, Reznik G, Donahoe R. Effect of three retinoids on tracheal carcinogenesis with N-methyl-N-nitrosourea in hamsters. *J Natl Cancer Inst.* 1981;66:947–951.
40. Grubbs CJ, Becci PJ, Moon RC. Characterization of 1-methyl-1-nitrosourea (MNU)–induced tracheal carcinogenesis and the effect of feeding the retinoid N-(4-hydroxyphenyl) retinamide (4-HPR). *Proc Am Assoc Cancer Res.* 1980;21:102.
41. Chu EW, Malmgren RA. An inhibitory effect of vitamin A on the induction of tumors of forestomach and cervix in the Syrian hamster by carcinogenic hydrocarbons. *Cancer Res.* 1965;25:884–895.
42. Rogers AE, Herndon BJ, Newberne PM. Induction by dimethylhydrazine of intestinal carcinoma in normal rats and rats fed high or low levels of vitamin A. *Cancer Res.* 1973;33:1003–1009.
43. Newberne PM, Suphakarn V. Prevention role of vitamin A in colon carcinogenesis in rats. *Cancer.* 1977;40:2553–2556.
44. Silverman J, Katayama S. Zelenakas K, *et al.* Effect of retinoids on the induction of colon cancer in F344 rats by N-methyl-N-nitrosourea or by 1,2-dimethylhydrazine. *Carcinogenesis.* 1981;2: 1167–1172.
45. Daoud AH, Griffin AC. Effect of retinoic acid, butylated hydroxytoluene, selenium and sorbic acid on azo dye hepatocarcinogenesis. *Cancer Lett.* 1980;9:299–304.
46. Longnecker DS, Curphey TJ, Kuhlmann ET, Roebuck BD. Inhibition of pancreatic carcinogenesis by retinoids in azaserine-treated rats. *Cancer Res.* 1982;42:19–24.
47. Birt DF, Sayet S. Davies MH, Pour P. Sex differences in the effects of retinoids on carcinogenesis by N-nitrosobis (2-oxopropyl) amine in Syrian hamsters. *Cancer Lett.* 1981;14:13–21.
48. Moon RC, Mehta RG. Anticarcinogenic effects of retinoids in animals. In: Poirier LA, Newberne PM, Pariza MW, eds. *Essential Nutrients in Carcinogenesis.* New York: Plenum Publishing Corp; 1986:399–411.

THOMAS E. MOON

Vitamin A and Cancer Prevention in Humans

ABSTRACT

The natural and synthetic vitamin A compounds, retinoids, have been the subject of substantial interest and controversy as micronutrients associated with cancer risk. Human studies provide mixed indications that retinoids may have a cancer-prevention effect. Initial chemopreventive trials generally suggest a role for retinoids and possibly for beta-carotene in the prevention of aerodigestive-tract cancers. The value of retinoids as chemopreventive agents against other cancers and levels of cancer risk has yet to be fully evaluated. The interpretation of previously reported human studies has been complicated by diverse dietary sources, including provitamin A (beta-carotene); limitations of quantifying dietary intake of vitamin A; and tissue distribution of vitamin A. Precancerous lesions that have shown response to retinoids include actinic keratosis, dysplastic nevi, leukoplakia, bronchial metaplasia, laryngeal papillomatosis, and cervical dysplasia. Ongoing chemoprevention trials will provide added information on the full role of retinoids in cancer prevention.

Introduction

The projected increase in the number of cancer cases during the next 50 years will result in unnecessary mortality and morbidity, reduced quality of life, and substantial cost (1). The evaluation of cancer prevention and control interventions provides new opportunities to contain and reduce the burden of cancer (2). Retinoids (vitamin A and its synthetic derivatives) and carotenoids are widely viewed as providing an opportunity for immediate application as chemopreventive compounds in human carcinogenesis (3). The continuing interest in these groups of compounds results from three types of studies: a number of epidemiologic studies that report the inverse association between dietary intake or blood levels of vitamin A or carotenoids and risk of cancer at several epithelial sites; a large number of clinical studies that demonstrate remission or reduction of epithelial proliferative lesions (precancers) or cancers with intake of these compounds; and an even larger number of laboratory studies that demonstrate the antiproliferative and differentiation-inducing effects of these compounds (4–7).

History of Vitamin A in Disease Prevention

Not well documented at the time was the apparently wide use of vitamin A as the treatment for night blindness. Egyptian papyrus records dating back to approximately 1000 BC illustrate that the "essence of fish liver," a source of highly concentrated vitamin A, was the standard treatment for night blindness (8). Contemporary scientific reports in 1909 and in 1920 led to the identification of vitamin A as the fat-soluble compound necessary for normal growth (9, 10). The 1925 publication of Wolbach and Howe was the first to report a relationship between vitamin A and metaplasia in rats (11).

The chemical structure of retinol, first reported in 1931 and consisting of a cyclic end group, a polyene side chain, and a polar end group, provides insight into its relationship to carotenoids (12). The chemical structure of beta-carotene was originally reported in 1930 and later observed to be two molecules of retinol joined at the polar end groups (12). The carotenoids, especially beta-carotene, can be converted to retinal during absorption through the mucosa and then converted to retinol (12). Thus, beta-carotene and to some extent other carotenoids can have the biological properties of vitamin A. However, there continues to be controversy whether the major anticancer properties of carotenoids are due to their antioxidant role or their conversion to retinoids (13). Thus, dietary carotenoids have been included in the following summary tables. The association of vitamin A deficiency with human cancer was first reported in 1941 and further supported the role of vitamin A in human cancer (14).

The observation that vitamin A deficiency was related to cutaneous epithelial lesions resulted in numerous therapeutic studies to treat cutaneous lesions (15). However, clinical observations reidentified that excessive intake of retinol, greater than 100 000 IU by adults, results in hypervitaminosis A, in which the intake of retinol exceeds the liver's ability to remove and store the retinoid (16, 17). The associated hepatic, mucocutaneous, gastrointestinal, and musculoskeletal side effects of excessive vitamin A intake led to the development of synthetic retinoids. By changing the chemical structure of vitamin A, the new synthetic retinoids were anticipated to have lower toxicity plus improved therapeutic or disease-prevention properties (18). One of the most widely studied and clinically effective synthetic retinoids, isotretinoin, is being evaluated in several human chemoprevention trials (3).

Biologic Properties

Retinoids and carotenoids have different pathways of absorption, transport, and storage (17). Naturally occurring retinol and its esters are converted to retinol and then to retinyl esters during absorption and passage through intestinal mucosa. Coupled with chylomicrons, retinyl esters are transported via the lymphatic system to the peripheral blood to the liver for storage (17). Beta-carotene is separated into retinal and converted to retinol in intestinal mucosa and, like dietary retinol, transported and stored in the liver (17). In contrast, retinoic acid is absorbed directly through the venous portal route, metabolized, and not stored in the liver (17). Thus, plasma levels of retinyl esters can be expected to reflect dietary intake of naturally occurring vitamin A (retinol and retinyl esters) and beta-carotene (and some other carotenoids).

Naturally occurring vitamin A has critical biological activity in three areas: vision, reproduction, and growth (proliferation and differentiation) (15, 18, 19). In contrast, retinoic acid is only biologically active in reproduction and cellular growth, proliferation and differentiation (20). The synthetic retinoids are only active in proliferation and differentiation (20).

Laboratory animal studies have provided substantial evidence that retinoids have chemopreventive effects (21). Unfortunately, these studies also indicate that the effect of retinoids differs according to which retinoid and dose is evaluated, which carcinogen is used to produce a tumor, which animal model is used, and which tumor type or tumor site is generated (21). For example, isotretinoin has substantial effect in the mouse skin-cancer model but is considered inactive in the rat breast-cancer model (21). In addition, the potential spectrum and magnitude of side effects associated with retinoids in human chemoprevention trials cannot be evaluated using animal models.

Human Studies

Epidemiologic studies indicate that for a wide range of predominantly epithelial cancer sites an inverse correlation exists between dietary intake or blood levels of vitamin A (or carotenoids) and cancer risk (4). In interpreting the results of these studies, we must keep in mind that dietary sources of vitamin A may be correlated, either positively or negatively, with other nutritive and nonnutritive components in foods. Table 1 summarizes the association between lung cancer risk and vitamin A. Twelve case-control or cohort studies have consistently reported an inverse association between lung cancer and dietary sources of vitamin A. These include two studies that evaluated vegetable intake in general, six studies that evaluated total dietary intake of vitamin A, and four studies that evaluated dietary intake of beta-carotene. Consistent results between vitamin A and lung cancer risk were not observed when serum measures of vitamin A were evaluated. Table 1 also shows that five of eleven studies that evaluated serum retinol or serum beta-carotene indicated an inverse association with lung cancer risk.

The associations of breast, bladder, and colorectal cancers with

Table 1. Epidemiologic Studies of Vitamin A and Lung Cancer Risk

		Association		
Site	Design	Yes	No	Foods/Nutrients
		Diet		
Lung	Case-control	1	0	Vegetables
		4	0	Total Vitamin A
		3	0	Carotene
	Cohort	1	0	Vegetables
		2	0	Total Vitamin A
		1	0	Carotene
		Serum/Plasma		
Lung	Case-control	2	0	Retinol
	Cohort	1	4	Retinol
		2	2	Beta-carotene

Table 2. Epidemiologic Studies of Vitamin A and Breast, Bladder, and Colorectal Cancer Risk

Site	Design	Association: Yes	Association: No	Foods/Nutrients
		Diet		
Breast	Case-control	2	0	Total Vitamin A
Bladder	Case-control	1	0	Total Vitamin A
Colorectum	Case-control	2	1	Vegetable and/ or milk
	Cohort	1	0	Total Vitamin A
		Serum/Plasma		
Breast	Cohort	0	1	Retinol
		1	0	Beta-carotene
Bladder	Case-control	1	0	Retinol/Carotene

vitamin A are summarized in Table 2. Two dietary studies report an inverse association between breast cancer risk and total dietary intake of vitamin A. Using serum levels, one of two studies shows an inverse association between breast cancer risk and serum retinol or beta-carotene. For bladder cancer, Table 2 summarizes two studies that indicate an inverse association with total dietary intake of vitamin A or with serum retinol or serum beta-carotene. Four studies regarding colorectal cancer are summarized in Table 2. Three of the four studies show an inverse association between colorectal cancer and total dietary intake of vegetables and/or milk or total vitamin A intake.

The reports of epidemiologic studies concerning other cancer sites are summarized in Table 3. Four separate studies have shown an inverse association between total dietary intake of vitamin A and cancer of the larynx, esophageal cancer, stomach cancer, and cervical cancer. Of substantial interest is the report of three studies of a positive correlation between total dietary intake of vitamin A and prostate cancer risk. Table 3 also shows that three of a total of nine case-control studies indicate an inverse association between vegetable intake and esophageal cancer, four of five studies show an association between vegetable intake and stomach cancer, and one study shows an inverse association with pancreatic cancer. Also, three cohort studies indicate an inverse association between vegetable intake and stomach cancer,

Table 3. Epidemiologic Studies of Vitamin A and Other Cancer Risks

Site	Design	Association		
		Yes	No	Foods/Nutrients
		Diet		
Larynx	Case-control	4	0	Total Vitamin A
Esophagus				
Stomach				
Cervix				
Prostate		(3)	0	
		Serum/Plasma		
Esophagus	Case-control	8	1	Vegetables
Stomach				
Pancreas				
Stomach	Cohort	3	0	Vegetables
Prostate				
General				

Table 4. Epidemiologic Studies of Vitamin A and Cancer Risks

Site	Design	Association		
		Yes	No	Foods/Nutrients
		Diet		
Gastrointestinal tract	Case-control	0	1	Retinol/Carotene
Prostate		1	0	Liver, Carrots
Ovary		1	0	Carotenes
		Serum/Plasma		
Esophagus	Case-control	1	0	Retinol
Stomach	Cohort	2	0	Retinol
General		3	2	Retinol

prostate cancer, and several cancers in general. Table 4 summarizes case-control studies that illustrate that gastrointestinal-tract cancers combined were not associated with dietary retinol or dietary beta-carotene. However, in a case-control study, prostate cancer was shown to be inversely associated with dietary liver and dietary carrot intake.

Ovarian cancer, in a case-control study, was also shown to be inversely associated with dietary beta-carotene intake. In addition, a case-control study showed an inverse association between serum retinol and esophageal cancer. Also shown in the table, two cohort studies have reported an inverse association between serum retinol and stomach cancer, and three of five cohort studies have reported an inverse association between serum retinol and a composite group of cancers. Thus, epidemiologic studies provide substantial evidence of an inverse association between dietary or serum vitamin A levels and cancer risk (4).

Many synthetic retinoids accumulate preferentially in the skin (22). Thus, a number of studies evaluating retinoids in the treatment of cutaneous, precancerous skin lesions, skin cancer, and other epithelial lesions have been carried out (4, 5, 20). Table 5 summarizes the response of subjects with precancerous cutaneous lesions. Actinic keratosis was treated topically with tretinoin in a total of 153 subjects, of which 70 had a complete response and 74 had a partial response. Etretinate was used to treat 105 subjects with actinic keratosis, resulting in 59 complete responses and 36 partial responses. Also, 16 patients with actinic keratosis were treated with arotinoid, which elicited 10 partial responses. Retinoid treatment was used with subjects with a diagnosis of keratoacanthoma. Nine of these patients were treated with etretinate, which yielded 6 complete responses and 3 partial responses. Also, 2 patients were treated with isotretinoin yielding 1 complete response and 1 partial response.

The treatment of patients with several different skin cancers is

Table 5. Retinoid Trials in Humans with Precancerous Cutaneous Lesions

Site	Cancer	Retinoid	Response[a] CR	PR	Subjects (No.)
Skin	Actinic Keratosis	Tretinoin (topical)	70	74	153
		Etretinate	59	36	105
		Arotinoid	0	10	16
	Keratoacanthoma	Etretinate	6	3	9
		Isotretinoin	1	1	2

[a]CR = complete response; PR = partial response.

Table 6. Retinoid Trials in Humans with Several Skin Cancers

Site	Cancer	Retinoid	Response[a] CR	PR	Subjects (No.)
Skin	Basal cell	Isotretinoin	3	0	3
		Tretinoin (topical)	14	19	34
		Isotretinoin	39	162	11
			248 lesions		
		Etretinate	3	14	40
	Squamous cell	Isotretinoin	2	5	9
		Etretinate	1	1	4
	Melanoma	Isotretinoin (topical)	1	1	2
		Isotretinoin	0	3	20
	T-Cell lymphoma	Isotretinoin	9	24	60
		Etretinate	12	12	31

[a]CR = complete response; PR = partial response.

summarized in Table 6. Three subjects were treated with isotretinoin in one of its first therapeutic applications for the treatment of basal-cell cutaneous cancer. All three obtained a complete response. Several other studies also treated basal-cell cutaneous cancer with 3 different retinoids. Thirty-four patients were topically treated with tretinoin, yielding 14 complete responses and 19 partial responses. Isotretinoin was used to treat 11 subjects with a total of 248 basal-cell cancers, of which 39 lesions had a complete response and 162 lesions had a partial response. Also, 40 patients with basal-cell cancer were treated with etretinate, of which 3 had a complete response and 14 had a partial response. Squamous-cell cutaneous cancers were also treated using retinoids. Of these, 9 patients were treated with isotretinoin, of which 2 obtained complete responses and 5 partial responses. In addition, 4 patients were treated with etretinate, of which 1 had a complete and 1 had a partial response. Isotretinoin was also used in the treatment of cutaneous melanoma. Two patients received topical application of isotretinoin, which yielded 1 complete response and 1 partial response. In addition, 20 patients with melanoma received isotretinoin, of which 3 obtained a partial response. Retinoids were

Table 7. Retinoid Trials in Humans with Oral and Lung Precancerous Lesions

Site	Cancer	Retinoid	Response	Subjects (No.)
Oral	Leukoplakia	Tretinoin	16	27
		Isotretinoin (topical)	14	16
		Isotretinoin	37	48
		Etretinate	38	48
	Laryngeal papillomatosis	Isotretinoin	4	6
		Etretinate	39	42
Lung	Bronchial metaplasia	Etretinate	36	36

used to treat a total of 91 patients with T-cell, lymphoma, and mycosis fungoides. Sixty patients were treated with isotretinoin, which yielded 9 complete responses and 24 partial responses. In addition, 31 patients received etretinate, which yielded 12 complete and 12 partial responses.

The information gathered in evaluating the effect of retinoids on oral and lung precancerous lesions is summarized in Table 7. Three different retinoids were used to treat patients with oral leukoplakia. Twenty-seven patients received tretinoin, of which 16 obtained at least a partial response. Topical isotretinoin was used on 16 oral leukoplakia patients, of which 14 had an objective response. In addition, 48 patients received isotretinoin, systemically yielding 37 objective responses. Also, 38 of 48 patients that received etretinate obtained an objective response. Patients with a diagnosis of laryngeal papillomatosis were treated with retinoids. Six patients received isotretinoin, of which 4 had at least a partial response. Also, 42 patients received etretinate, of which 39 had at least a partial response. Of 36 patients with a diagnosis of bronchial metaplasia who were treated systemically with etretinate, all 36 had an objective response.

Table 8 summarizes the evaluation of retinoid use among patients with cervical dysplasia or bladder cancer. Of the 74 patients with a diagnosis of cervical dysplasia who were treated topically with tretinoin, 51 had an objective response. Also, 74 patients with bladder cancer were given etretinate, which yielded 38 objective responses.

Table 8. Retinoid Trials in Humans with Cervical Dysplasia or Bladder Cancer

Site	Cancer	Retinoid	Response	Subjects (No.)
Cervix	Cervical dysplasia	Tretinoin (topical)	51	74
Bladder	Bladder	Etretinate	38	74

Human Cancer Prevention Trials

Natural and synthetic vitamin A agents are being evaluated in several ongoing or recently completed chemopreventive trials. The results of these trials, indicating the ability of retinoids to reduce cancer risk and their spectrum of side effects, will have a substantial impact on the future role of retinoids in cancer prevention research and public health.

Retinol (50 000 IU) plus zinc (50 mg) and riboflavin (200 mg) was provided in capsules once per week to 610 residents of Huixian Province, China (22). The subjects were considered at high risk of esophageal cancer by virtue of the high prevalence of esophageal cancer in the province. The chemoprevention-intervention trial involved a comparison with the use of placebo capsules for a median duration of 13.5 months. The initial report of the results of this trial concluded that there was no improvement in esophageal lesions in subjects receiving the vitamin A plus other nutrients compared with subjects receiving the placebo (23). The interpretation of the results of this trial is difficult in part because of the limited 13.5-month median duration of the trial. The trial was substantially reanalyzed as an observational case-control study. Cases were defined as those subjects that had an increase in their plasma retinol between the initial and final points of the 13.5-month examination period, whereas controls were defined as subjects that had no change or a decrease in plasma retinol over that period. The apparent concern was that there were confounding factors, such as dietary intake or metabolic differences, that were not measured during the trial but may have reduced the power of the primary analysis of the trial. The second report, based upon the case-control analysis, concluded that cases with an increase in plasma retinol had a statistically lower prevalence of esophageal metaplasia as compared with controls. Such an insightful analysis provides new evidence for the effect of vitamin A, in combination with zinc and riboflavin, as a chemopreventive agent for esophageal and aerodigestive-tract cancers.

The recent report by Hong *et al.* also provides evidence for retinoids as chemopreventive agents against *aerodigestive*-tract, epithelial cancers (24). Isotretinoin, at 50–100 mg per meter squared of body surface area per day, compared with a placebo, was administered for 12 months to subjects with a recent definitive surgery for head and neck cancer. One hundred subjects were considered disease free at entry on trial, and 49 were given isotretinoin. Newly diagnosed head and neck lesions were the primary end point for the trial. The results of the trial indicate a statistically lower incidence of head and neck lesions for subjects given isotretinoin than subjects given placebos.

Beta-carotene has been reported to result in complete or partial (> 50%) reduction of oral leukoplakia (25). Twenty-five subjects with a clinical diagnosis of oral leukoplakia were administered 30 mg of beta-carotene per day for 3 months, with responders continued on 30 mg of beta-carotene per day for an additional 3 months. Follow-up continued for an added 6 months. A comparison, placebo, group was not part of the trial design. Of the 25 subjects enrolled, 17 were classified as responding after 3 months of beta-carotene: 2 complete responses plus 15 partial responses. Of the 11 responding patients, 8 relapsed within 3 months after completion of the intervention, indicating a high recurrence rate.

Another recent report indicates that very high doses of vitamin A (retinyl palmitate) were well tolerated and that side effects appeared not to reduce subject adherence significantly (26). Study subjects had a recent diagnosis of primary lung cancer with definitive surgery rendering them apparently disease free. Retinyl palmitate (300 000 IU per day) was randomly assigned to 138 eligible subjects, and 145 additional subjects received standard observation, a placebo. No one was removed from the 28-month median follow-up intervention because of side effects. The chemoprevention effect of such high doses of vitamin A has yet to be published. However, a preliminary report suggests that a lower incidence of newly diagnosed lung cancer was initially observed in subjects assigned retinyl palmitate compared with those assigned a placebo (U. Pastorino, personal communication, April, 1991).

Retinoids are being evaluated in a number of ongoing trials (3). The evaluation of topical transretinoic acid, tretinoin, versus a placebo by investigators at the University of Arizona provides important information on the role of topical, and thus higher-dose delivery, retinoids in squamous epithelial cervical dysplasia (3). Prior reports suggested that transretinoic acid has an effect in reversing cervical dysplasia (27).

The evaluation of retinoids and carotenoids in the prevention of skin cancer is also ongoing. Nonmelanoma skin cancers are the most common cancers, resulting in substantial morbidity and cost. Many synthetic retinoids and beta-carotene are stored in the skin or subcutaneous fat. However, the dose of retinoids chosen for evaluation in all of the ongoing or recently completed trials was lower than that given in the above-noted trials in chemoprevention of aerodigestive-tract cancer. The lower dosage was due to the cutaneous side effects observed for the therapeutic doses used for aerodigestive-tract cancers and cutaneous lesions observed by dermatologists. The trial of isotretinoin, 10 mg per day, compared with a placebo in the reduction of risk of newly diagnosed nonmelanoma skin cancer was recently reported (28). High-risk subjects with a history of at least two prior basal-cell skin cancers consumed the retinoid for up to three years but, compared with the placebo, demonstrated no difference in subsequent nonmelanoma skin cancer incidence. The design of the trial cannot be addressed if the dose was too low, the subjects had too high a risk for this natural agent, or dose duration was too short. Cutaneous side effects were commonly observed even at the low dose. A similar negative result has been reported for beta-carotene versus a placebo in a similar population at high risk of nonmelanoma skin cancer (29). The dose of beta-carotene, 50 mg per day, significantly increased plasma beta-carotene concentrations. Thus, there was little doubt that an adequate dose was provided. Unfortunately, there were minimal data specific for skin cancer prevention from prior reports of laboratory or human studies at the time this trial was begun. Subsequent research has not provided substantial added rationale for beta-carotene to lower risk of nonmelanoma skin cancer in such high-risk subjects. An evaluation of the primary prevention effect of nonmelanoma skin cancer in a somewhat lower risk group, such as subjects with a clinical history of actinic keratosis but no prior skin cancer, may provide better information on the role of the common food constituents beta-carotene and vitamin A in the chemoprevention of skin cancer.

This is precisely the approach currently being evaluated for retinol versus a placebo in the primary prevention of nonmelanoma skin cancer (7). Subjects with a clinical history of more than 10 actinic keratoses have been enrolled and continued on the intervention for up to 5 years. The retinol dose, 25 000 IU per day, was selected to provide a substantial increase in the recommended daily allotment but was lower than has been associated with hypervitaminosis A or other side effects. The rationale for retinoids as chemopreventive agents for epithelial and especially cutaneous cancers was substantiated when the trial began in 1983.

Conclusion

A substantial literature, both laboratory and human, indicates that natural and synthetic retinoids may have cancer-risk reduction effects in a variety of epithelial sites. Initial chemopreventive trials generally suggest a role for retinoids and possibly for beta-carotene in the prevention of aerodigestive-tract cancers. The value of retinoids as chemopreventive agents against other types of cancers and levels of cancer risk has yet to be fully evaluated.

ACKNOWLEDGMENTS

The research for this paper was supported in part by grants from the United States Public Health Service (CCR905033, CA34256, CA27502, CA09629), the National Dairy Board, and trials were administered in cooperation with the National Dairy Council and the Arizona Disease Control Research Commission (8277-0-1-0-930).

REFERENCES

1. Janerick DT. Forecasting cancer trends to optimize control strategies. *J Natl Cancer Inst.* 1984;72:1317–1321.
2. Greenwald P, Cullen JW, McKenna JW. Cancer prevention and control: from research through applications. *J Natl Cancer Inst.* 1987;79:389–400.
3. Boone CW, Kelloff GJ, Malone WE. Identification of candidate cancer chemopreventive agents and their evaluation in animal models and human clinical trials: a review *Clin Res.* 1990;50:2–9.
4. Bertram JS, Kolonel LN, Meyskens FL. Rationale and strategies

for chemoprevention of cancer in humans. *Cancer Res.* 1987;47: 3012–3031.

5. Lippman SM, Meyskens FL. Retinoids for the prevention of cancer. In: Moon T, Micozzi M, eds. *Investigating the Role of Micronutrients.* New York: Marcel Dekker, Inc. 1989:243–272.
6. Ip C, Ip MM. Chemoprevention of mammary tumorigenesis by a combined regimen of selenium and vitamin A. *Carcinogenesis.* 1981;2:915–918.
7. Moon TE. Retinoids as cancer prevention agents. *American Society of Preventive Oncology Proceedings.* 1989:6.
8. Ragab Papyrus Institute. *Treating Eye.* Giza, Egypt, 1984.
9. Stepp W. Versuche uber futterung mit lipoidfreir nahrung. *Biochem Z.* 1909;22:452–460.
10. Drummond JC. The nomenclature of the so-called accessory food factors (vitamins). *Biochem J.* 1920;14:660–666.
11. Wolbach SB, Howe PR. Tissue changes following improvation of fat soluble A vitamin. *J Exp Med.* 1925;42:753–777.
12. Williams SR. Nutrition and diet therapy. St. Louis: Times Mirror/ Mosby, College Publishing; 1985:117–124.
13. Burton GW, Ingold KU. Beta-carotene: an unusual type of lipid antioxidant. *Science.* 1984;224:569–573.
14. Abels JC, Gorhman AT, Pack GT, Rhoads CP. Metabolic studies in patients with cancer of the gastrointestinal tract, I: plasma vitamin A levels in patients with malignant neoplastic diseases, particularly of the gastrointestinal tract. *J Clin Invest.* 1941;20:749–753.
15. Peck GL. Retinoids in clinical dermatology. In: Fleischmajer R, ed. *Progress in Diseases of the Skin.* San Francisco: Grune and Stratton, Inc; 1981;1:227–269.
16. Winghorst DV, Nigra T. General clinical toxicology of oral retinoids. *J Am Acad Dermatol.* 1982;6:675–683.
17. Wolf G. Multiple functions of Vitamin A. *Physiol Rev.* 1984;64: 873–879.
18. Bollag W. Vitamin A and retinoids: from nutrients to pharmacotherapy in dermatology and oncology. *Lancet.* 1983;1:360–362.
19. Moore T. Effect of vitamin A deficiency in animals: pharmacology and toxicology of vitamin A. In: Sebrell WH, Harris RS, eds. *The Vitamin.* 2nd ed. New York: Academic Press; 1967:245–294.
20. Lippman SM, Kessler JF, Meyskens FL. Retinoids as preventive and therapeutic anticancer agents (II). *Cancer Treat Rep.* 1987;71: 493–515.

21. Moon RC, McCormick DL, Mehta RG. Inhibition of carcinogenesis by retinoids. *Cancer Res.* 1983;43:2469–2474.
22. Wahrendorf J, Munoz N, Jian-Bang L, Thurnham DI, Crespi M, Bosch FX. Blood retinol and zinc riboflavin status in relation to precancerous lesions of the esophagus: findings from a vitamin intervention trial in the People's Republic of China. *Cancer Res.* 1988;48:2280–2283.
23. Munoz N, Wahrendorf J, Lu JB, *et al.* No effect of riboflavin, retinol and zinc on prevalence of precancerous lesions of esophagus. *Lancet.* 1985;2:111–114.
24. Hong WK, Lippman SM, Itri LM, *et al.* Prevention of second primary tumors with Isotretinoin in squamous-cell carcinoma of the head and neck. *N Engl J Med.* 1990;323:795–801.
25. Garewal HS, Meyskens ML, Killen D, *et al.* Response of oral leukoplakia to beta carotene. *J Clin Oncol.* 1990;8:1715–1720.
26. Pastorino U, Chiesa G, Infante M, *et al.* Safety of high dose vitamin A: randomized trial on lung cancer chemoprevention. *Oncology.* 1991;48:131–137.
27. Graham V, Surwit ES, Weiner S, Meyskens FL. Phase II trials of beta-all-trans retinoic acid for cervical intraepithelial neoplasia delivered by a collagen sponge and cervical cap. *West J Med.* 1986;145:192–195.
28. Tangrea JA. The Isotretinoin—basal cell carcinoma prevention trial: results of the three year intervention phase. *American Society of Preventive Oncology Proceedings.* 1991:36.
29. Greenberg ER, Barron JA, Stukel TA, *et al.* A clinical trial of beta carotene to prevent basal-cell and squamous-cell cancers of the skin. *N Engl J Med.* 1990;323:789–795.

NORMAN I. KRINSKY

Actions of Carotenoids in Cells and Animals

ABSTRACT

Many studies have indicated that carotenoid pigments can prevent mutagenesis, genotoxic effects, and malignant transformation in bacteria and mammalian tissue, either in cell culture or in organ culture. In addition, multiple papers have reported that carotenoids act as anticarcinogenic agents in animals treated with ultraviolet light, ultraviolet light with chemicals, or chemical carcinogens alone. The early experiments used pharmacological doses of carotenoids, but more recent reports indicate that relatively small doses can be effective. Since these effects are seen with both provitamin A and nonprovitamin A carotenoids, it would appear that these effects are intrinsic to the carotenoid molecule and are not due to the metabolic conversion to retinoids. Partially based on these observations, the suggestion has been made that carotenoid pigments may function as chemopreventive agents for reducing the risk of cancer in humans. Numerous human intervention studies are under way to test this hypothesis.

Introduction

Olson has tried to persuade the scientific community to differentiate among the biological activities of carotenoids with respect to their functions, actions, and associations (1). In the case of animals on vitamin A–deficient diets, the metabolism of the provitamin A carotenoids such as beta-carotene to retinol and retinoic acid would be a biological *function*. However, the functional role of carotenoids in the primate fovea is not yet established. *Actions* of carotenoids would include their role as tissue and plasma antioxidants (2), their ability to inhibit either UV-induced or chemically induced tumors in rodents (3), and their inhibition of malignant transformation of cells in culture (4). Finally, an example of an *association* would be the mounting epidemiological evidence that an inverse relationship exists between dietary or plasma carotenoid levels and a variety of human cancers (5, 6). Some of these activities are depicted in Figure 1. This paper reviews the actions and associations of carotenoids as anticarcinogens that served as the original basis for the proposal that beta-carotene might function to reduce human cancer rates (7). Evidence continues to accumulate that in many systems carotenoids are effective in delaying the onset of or in preventing tumorigenesis in animals, and in inhibiting genotoxity or malignant transformation in cell and organ cultures. In addition, more evidence has appeared that carotenoids exhibit immunoenhancing action. Since these reports include observations that carotenoids without any provitamin A activity, such as canthaxanthin, lutein, crocetin, fucoxanthin, and lycopene (Fig. 2), have similar activities, it would appear that the results are attributable to properties of the intact carotenoid molecule and not necessarily to metabolities, such as the retinoids, retinol, retinal, and retinoic acid. Such observations suggest that the activities reported here involve the known chemical and biological functions of carotenoids, which include, among others, photoprotection, radical quenching, and antioxidant behavior. The connections between the known functions and the activities reported here, however, remain to be elucidated.

Antimutagenic Actions in Bacteria

Some of the earliest reports of a protective action of carotenoids against photosensitized damage came from bacterial studies (8). In addition, carotenoids can prevent mutagenesis in *Salmonella typhimurium*. This system has been used to demonstrate the protective effects of beta-carotene against the mutagenic potential of 8-methoxypsoralen (8-MOP) and UV-A (9), or of cyclophosphamide (10). Several other carotenoids were tested in this system, using aflatoxin B_1 (AFB_1) to induce mutagenesis. Cryptoxanthin was reported to be more effective than beta-carotene or canthaxanthin, but lycopene had no effect (11).

Actions on Cells and Cell Cultures

The interesting observation that both beta-carotene and canthaxanthin could inhibit malignant transformation caused by either methylcholanthrene (MCA) or x-radiation in C3H10T1/2 cells was reviewed

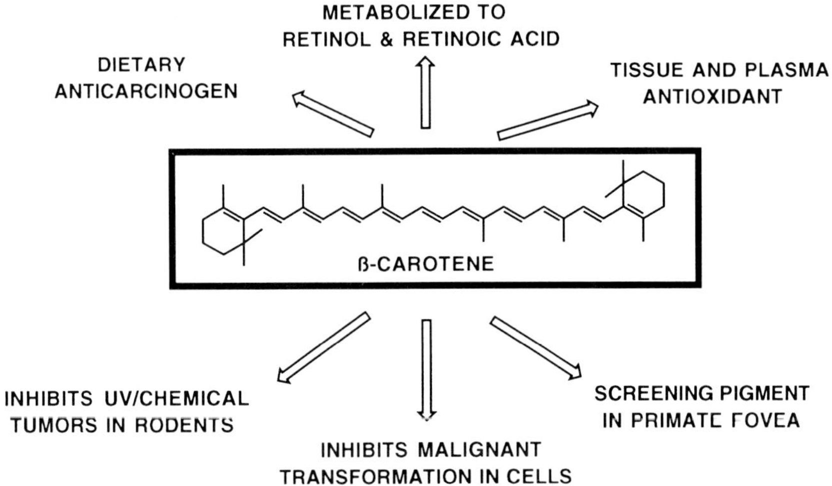

Figure 1. Several biological activities of carotenoids.

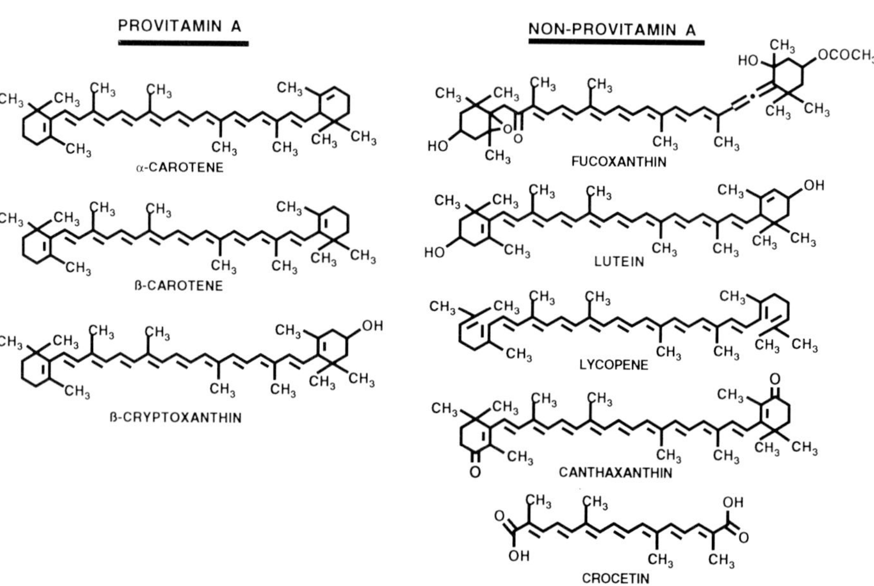

Figure 2. Structures of some of the carotenoids reported to prevent tumor formation or malignant transformation.

recently (4), and the work has been extended to other carotenoids. In addition to beta-carotene and canthaxanthin, alpha-carotene and lycopene (Fig. 2) were effective in inhibiting MCA-induced malignant transformation (12). Lutein was inhibitory at 10 μM, but this dihydroxy-xanthopyll increased the number of transformants at lower concentrations. Alpha-tocopherol also inhibited malignant transformation but was only about 10% as active as lycopene.

Following an earlier report of a modest effect of crocetin in animals (13), this carotenoid was tested in C3H10T1/2 cells exposed to AFB_1. At 100 μM, crocetin treatment results in an elevation in the concentration of cytosolic GSH and an increase in the activity of GSH S-transferase and GSH peroxidase (14). These effects might explain the action of crocetin in altering the activity of microsome-activated AFB_1, resulting in decreased cytotoxicity, and a decrease in AFB_1-DNA adducts.

Fucoxanthin (Fig. 2), derived from brown algae, has also been reported to inhibit tumor cell growth (15). Over a three-day period, fucoxanthin inhibited the growth of the human neuroblastoma cell line, GOTO. N-myc expression was inhibited within four hours of exposure to fucoxanthin.

There is some additional evidence that carotenoidss can specifically inhibit the growth of tumor cells in culture. For example, 70 μM of beta-carotene or canthaxanthin inhibited the proliferation of both SK-MES lung carcinoma and SCC-25 oral carcinoma, two cultured human squamous-cell lines (16). This concentration of carotenoid had no effect on the growth of normal human keratinocytes. Additionally, researchers reported that the beta-carotene effect in tumor cells was accompanied by a rapid appearance of a unique 70 kD protein, analogous to heat shock proteins (16).

Confusion still exists with respect to the mechanisms of action of the carotenoids in these systems. Since prostaglandins (PG) have been demonstrated to be strong tumor promoters (17), the effect of carotenoids and retinoids on PG formation has been studied. The conversion of ^{14}C-arachidonic acid to PG was monitored in squamous-carcinoma cells of the tongue (SCC-25), in the presence of retinoic acid, N-4-hydroxyphenyl retinamide, canthaxanthin, and beta-carotene (18). Both the retinoids and canthaxanthin inhibited the formation of PG, thus appearing to have anticarcinogenic activity. However, beta-carotene increased the conversion of arachidonic acid to PG, acting therefore to stimulate tumor promotion.

Actions in Animal Systems

I have recently reviewed some of the early studies on the effects of carotenoids in preventing tumor formation in rats and mice induced with either ultraviolet (UV) light alone or UV light in combination with chemicals (19, 20). Tumors are induced in mice or rats by UV light alone (21, 22), a combination of UV light and carcinogens such as dimethylbenzanthracene (DMBA) (23), benzo[a]pyrene (24, 25), or 8-MOP (26). UV-B light has continued to be used as a carcinogenic insult, and canthaxanthin, at 10 g/kg, can reduce the tumor burden without influencing the tumor incidence (27). This effect is even more striking when a combination of canthaxanthin and retinyl palmitate (120 IU/g) is added to the diet.

Other groups have used dietary or environmental carcinogens in experimental animals supplemented with carotenoids, and have observed protection against DMBA (28–30), dimethylhydrazine (DMH) (31, 32), or N′-N-methylnitro-nitrosoguanidine (33) with beta-carotene or canthaxanthin. Topical administration of beta-carotene not only inhibits (34) but also reverses (35) squamous-cell carcinoma produced in the hamster buccal pouch by treatment with topical DMBA. Similar results were reported with oral administration of beta-carotene, canthaxanthin, or an algal extract containing carotenoids (36). This work has been confirmed and extended by two independent laboratories. One report indicates that topically applied beta-carotene not only prevents DMBA-induced cheek tumors in hamsters but also prevents the accompanying stomach tumors (37). Also, the beta-carotene–treated animals retained a normal SDS-polyacrylamide electrophoretic pattern of cheek pouch keratin, whereas keratin from DMBA-treated hamsters had an abnormal pattern. In another report, a similar decrease was observed in tumor incidence in DMBA-treated hamsters, as well as a decrease in polyamine levels in erythrocytes and urine in the beta-carotene–treated animals (38).

There have been other examples of beta-carotene acting as an anticarcinogen. It is possible to induce tumors fairly rapidly by using the carcinogen DMBA as well as the tumor promoter phorbol myristyl acetate (PMA). Skh or Sencar mice treated with DMBA/PMA and supplemented with 3% beta-carotene in their diets, either in the form of beadlets (containing 10% beta-carotene) or by adding the crystalline pigment directly to the chow, develop skin tumors. Both carotenoid preparations protect Skh mice, but not the Sencar strain (39). These experiments point out the great importance of strain differences in animals, and these differences may be exaggerated when one compares experiments in different species. A similar protocol with DMBA/PMA-induction of skin tumors in Skh mice, using beta-carotene at 175 μg per day, reported a significant decrease in the number of skin papillomas but no effect on the ultimate development of malignant tumors (40). The researchers concluded that beta-carotene was working during the PMA-induced promotional phase of tumor formation.

In addition to the beta-carotene experiments reported above, canthaxanthin at 1.1 mg to 3.4 mg (2–6 mmol) per kilogram was fed to rats for three weeks before treatment with DMBA, and a 65% decrease in the incidence of mammary tumors was observed (41). These doses of canthaxanthin have been compared with 1 mmol/kg of retinyl acetate after methylnitrosourea (MNU) treatment, and since no difference was observed, the authors concluded that the carotenoid pigment does not inhibit promotion (41). Crocetin has also been tested, resulting in a report that intraperitoneal injection of this carotenoid inhibited the growth of C-6 glial cells in rats (42). Crocetin has also been tested against AFB_1, in which test a three-day oral treatment with 2 mg/kg to 6 mg/kg prevented the formation of AFB_1-DNA adducts and increased the liver levels of GSH, GSH-transferase, and GSH peroxidase (43).

Action on Drug Metabolism

It has been hypothesized that carotenoids might act by affecting the metabolism of carcinogens, either by increasing the normal metabolic pathways or by inducing new pathways that render the carcinogen inactive (44–46). A variation of that hypothesis has appeared recently (47), indicating that benzopyrene treatment in rats leads to a decrease in the retinol levels in the liver and small intestine, and that beta-carotene administration at 2 g/kg prevents this depletion. This observation suggests that it is the retinoid depletion that is associated with carcinogenesis, and that would certainly indicate the need for a followup experiment with the nonprovitamin A canthaxanthin.

Failure to Demonstrate Activity

As noted earlier, supplementation with 3% beta-carotene did not significantly protect Sencar mice from DMBA/PMA-induced tumors (39). Using DMH followed by MNU in F344 rats, beta-carotene (0.2%) had only weak, organ-specific effect in preventing tumor formation (48). In addition, two reports have appeared on the effects of carotenoids on BBN-induced bladder cancer. In one case, beta-carotene fed to rats at 1.6 g/kg for 42 weeks colored the organs but did not protect against tumor formation (49). In another report, beta-carotene or canthaxanthin was fed at 1 g/kg for 5 weeks before and 26 weeks after treatment with hydroxy-BBN, and only the mice receiving the beta-carotene supplement showed significant protection against the development of bladder cancer (50). The different results reported in these two papers may be a result of species differences in response to either the carotenoid or the carcinogen.

Immunological Activities

In a preliminary report, liposomes containing beta-carotene induced active inflammatory infiltrates in oral tumor–bearing hamsters that were not observed in hamsters lacking tumors (51). These infiltrates, which consisted of macrophages, lymphocytes, mast cells, and polymorphonuclear leukocytes, stained positively TNF-α, and that observation could partially explain the cytotoxicity associated with the carotenoids. An extensive review of carotenoids and immune function has appeared recently (52).

Conclusions

I have reviewed some of the available evidence indicating that carotenoid pigments can act as antimutagenic, chemopreventive, and immunoenhancing agents. The animal studies supporting carotenoid involvement as anticarcinogenic agents continue to appear, although there are occasional negative findings reported. In most of these studies, investigators are working with animals that do not absorb carotenoids readily from their diets, and high concentrations of the pigments are added to the diet to elevate plasma and tissue levels. Even in the bacterial and cell systems reported here, the delivery of the extremely lipophilic carotenoids is problematic, and it is difficult to determine the concentrations of the pigments in the medium bathing the cells.

Nevertheless, the actions observed in many of the reports are striking. What will be more striking will be the results from human intervention studies, which should finally enable us to determine whether the anticarcinogenic activities are a true biological action or merely an association awaiting confirmation.

ACKNOWLEDGMENT

Much of the work in the author's laboratory has been supported by the National Cancer Institute, grant number CA 51506.

REFERENCES

1. Olson JA. Biological actions of carotenoids. *J Nutr.* 1989;119: 94–95.
2. Krinsky NI. Antioxidant functions of carotenoids. *Free Radic Biol Med.* 1989;7:617–635.
3. Krinsky NI. Carotenoids as chemopreventive agents. *Prev Med.* 1989;18:592–602.
4. Bertram JS, Rundhaug JE, Pung A. Carotenoids inhibit chemically- and physically-induced neoplastic transformation during the post-initiation phase of carcinogenesis. In: Prasad KN, Meyskens FL Jr, eds. *Nutrients and Cancer Prevention.* Clifton, NJ: Humana Press; 1990:99–111.
5. Ziegler RG. Vegetables, fruits, and carotenoids and the risk of cancer. *Am J Clin Nutr.* 1991;53:251S–259S.
6. Byers T, Perry G. Dietary carotenes, vitamin C, and vitamin E as protective antioxidants in human cancers. *Annu Rev Nutr.* 1992;12: 139–159.
7. Peto R, Doll RJ, Buckley JD, Sporn MB. Can dietary β-carotene materially reduce human cancer rates? *Nature.* 1981;290:201–208.
8. Mathews-Roth MM. Photoprotection by carotenoids. *Fed Proc.* 1987;46:1890–1893.
9. Santamaria L, Bianchi L, Bianchi A, Pizzala R, Santagati G, Bermond P. Photomutagenicity by 8-methoxypsoralen with and without singlet oxygen involvement and its prevention by beta-

carotene: relevance to the mechanism of 8-MOP photocarcinogenicity and to PUVA application. *Med Biol Environ.* 1984;12:541–546.

10. Belisario MA, Pecce R, Battista C, Panza N, Pacilio G. Inhibition of cyclophosphamide mutagenicity by β-carotene. *Biomed Pharmacother.* 1985;39:445–448.
11. He Y, Campbell TC. Effects of carotenoids on aflatoxin B_1-induced mutagenesis in *S. typhimurium* TA 100 and TA 98. *Nutr Cancer.* 1990;13:243–253.
12. Bertram JS, Pung A, Churley M, Kappock TJ IV, Wilkins LR, Cooney RV. Diverse carotenoids protect against chemically induced neoplastic transformation. *Carcinogenesis.* 1991;12:671–678.
13. Mathews-Roth MM. Effect of crocetin on experimental skin tumors in hairless mice. *Oncology.* 1982;39:362–364.
14. Wang C-J, Shiah H-S, Lin J-K. Modulatory effect of crocetin on aflatoxin B_1 cytotoxicity and DNA adduct formation in C3H10T1/2 fibroblast cells. *Cancer Lett.* 1991;56:1–10.
15. Okuzumi J, Nishino H, Murakoshi M, *et al.* Inhibitory effects of fucoxanthin, a natural carotenoid, on N-*myc* expression and cell cycle progression in human malignant tumor cells. *Cancer Lett.* 1990;55:75–81.
16. Schwartz JL, Singh RP, Teicher B, Wright JE, Trites DH, Shklar G. Induction of a 70 kD protein associated with the selective cytotoxicity of beta-carotene in human epidermal carcinoma. *Biochem Biophys Res Commun.* 1990;169:941–946.
17. Cerutti PA. Oxidant tumor promoters. In: Coburn NH, Moses HL, Stanbridge EJ, eds. *Growth Factors, Tumor Promoters, and Cancer Genes.* New York: Alan R. Liss; 1988:239–247.
18. ElAttar TMA, Lin HS. Effect of retinoids and carotenoids on prostaglandin formation by oral squamous carcinoma cells. *Prostaglandins Leukot Essent Fatty Acids.* 1991;43:175–178.
19. Krinsky NI. Carotenoids in medicine. In: Krinsky NI, Mathews-Roth MM, Taylor RF, eds. Carotenoids: chemistry and biology. New York: Plenum Press; 1989:279–292.
20. Krinsky NI. Effects of carotenoids in cellular and animal systems. *Am J Clin Nutr.* 1991;53:238S–246S.
21. Mathews-Roth MM. Carotenoid pigment administration and delay in development of UV-B-induced tumors. *Photochem Photobiol.* 1983;37:509–511.
22. Mathews-Roth MM, Krinsky NI. Carotenoids affect development

of UV-B induced skin cancer. *Photochem Photobiol.* 1987;47:507–509.

23. Mathews-Roth MM. Antitumor activity of β-carotene, canthaxanthin and phytoene. *Oncology.* 1982;39:33–37.
24. Santamaria L, Bianchi A, Arnaboldi A, Andreoni L. Prevention of the benzo[a]pyrene photocarcinogenic effect by β-carotene and canthaxanthin. *Med Biol Environ.* 1981;9:113–120.
25. Santamaria L, Bianchi A, Arnaboldi A, Andreoni L, Bermond P. Benzo[a]pyrene carcinogenicity and its prevention by carotenoids: relevance in social medicine. In: Meyskens FL, Prasad KN, eds. *Modulation and Mediation of Cancer by Vitamins.* Basel: Karger; 1983:81–88.
26. Santamaria L, Bianchi A, Andreoni L, Santagati G, Arnaboldi A, Bermond P. 8-Methoxypsoralen photocarcinogenesis and its prevention by dietary carotenoids: preliminary results. *Med Biol Environ.* 1984;12:533–537.
27. Gensler HL, Aickin M, Peng YM. Cumulative reduction of primary skin tumor growth in UV-irradiated mice by the combination of retinyl palmitate and canthaxanthin. *Cancer Lett.* 1990;53: 27–31.
28. Alam BS, Alam SQ, Weir JC Jr, Gibson WA. Chemopreventive effects of β-carotene and 13-*cis*-retinoic acid on salivary gland tumors. *Nutr Cancer.* 1984;6:4–12.
29. Alam BS, Alam SQ. The effect of different levels of dietary β-carotene on DMBA-induced salivary gland tumors. *Nutr Cancer.* 1987;9:93–101.
30. Alam BS, Alam SQ, Weir JC Jr. Effects of excess vitamin A and canthaxanthin on salivary gland tumors. *Nutr Cancer.* 1988;11: 233–241.
31. Temple NJ, Basu TK. Protective effect of β-carotene against colon tumors in mice. *JNCI.* 1987;78:1211–1214.
32. Basu TK, Temple NJ, Hodgson AM. Vitamin A, beta-carotene and cancer. In: Tryfiades GP, Prasad KN, eds. *Nutrition, Growth, and Cancer.* New York: Alan R. Liss; 1988:217–228.
33. Santamaria L, Bianchi A, Ravetto C, Arnaboldi A, Santagati G, Andreoni L. Supplemental cartenoids prevent MNNG induced cancer in rats. *Med Biol Environ.* 1985;13:745–750.
34. Suda D, Schwartz J, Shklar G. Inhibition of experimental oral carcinogenesis by topical beta-carotene. *Carcinogenesis.* 1986;7: 711–715.

35. Schwartz J, Suda D, Light G. Beta carotene is associated with the regression of hamster buccal pouch carcinoma and the induction of tumor necrosis factor in macrophages. *Biochem Biophys Res Commun.* 1986;136:1130–1135.
36. Schwartz J, Shklar G, Reid S, Trickler D. Prevention of experimental oral cancer by extracts of Spirulina-Dunaliella algae. *Nutr Cancer.* 1988;11:127–134.
37. Gijare PS, Rao KVK, Bhide SV. Modulatory effects of snuff, retinoic acid, and β-carotene on DMBA-induced hamster cheek pouch carcinogenesis in relation to keratin expression. *Nutr Cancer.* 1990;14:253–259.
38. Hibino T, Shimpo K, Kawai K, *et al.* Polyamine levels of urine and erythrocytes on inhibition of DMBA-induced oral carcinogenesis by topical beta-carotene. *Biogenic Amines.* 1990;7:209–216.
39. Lambert LA, Koch WH, Wamer WG, Kornhauser A. Antitumor activity in skin of Skh and Sencar mice by two dietary β-carotene formulations. *Nutr Cancer.* 1990;13:213–221.
40. Steinel HH, Baker RSU. Effects of β-carotene on chemically-induced skin tumors in HRA/Skh hairless mice. *Cancer Lett.* 1990; 51:163–168.
41. Grubbs CJ, Eto I, Juliana MM, Whitaker LM. Effect of canthaxanthin on chemically induced mammary carcinogenesis. *Oncology.* 1991;48:239–245.
42. Wang C-J, Chou M-Y, Lin J-K. Inhibition of growth and development of transplantable C-6 glioma cells inoculated in rats by retinoids and carotenoids. *Cancer Lett.* 1989;48:135–142.
43. Wang C-J, Shiow S-J, Lin J-K. Effects of crocetin on the hepatotoxicity and hepatic DNA binding of aflatoxin B_1 in rats. *Carcinogenesis.* 1991;12:459–462.
44. Menon R, Bartley J, Som S, Banerjee MR. Metabolism of 7,12-dimethylbenz[a]anthracene by mouse mammary cells in serum-free organ culture medium. *Eur J Cancer Clin Oncol.* 1987;23:395–400.
45. Basu TK, Temple NJ, Ng J. Effect of dietary β-carotene on hepatic drug-metabolizing enzymes in mice. *J Clin Biochem Nutr.* 1987;3: 95–102.
46. Edes TE, Thornton W Jr, Shah J. β-carotene and aryl hydrocarbon hydroxylase in the rat: an effect of β-carotene independent of vitamin A activity. *J Nutr.* 1989;119:796–799.
47. Edes TE, Gysbers DG, Buckley CS, Thornton WH Jr. Exposure to

the carcinogen benzopyrene depletes tissue vitamin A: β-carotene prevents depletion. *Nutr Cancer.* 1991;15:159–166.

48. Imaida K, Hirose M, Yamaguchi S, Takahashi S, Ito N. Effects of naturally occurring antioxidants on combined 1,2-dimethylhydrazine- and 1-methyl-1-nitrosourea-initiated carcinogenesis in F344 male rats. *Cancer Lett.* 1990;55:53–59.
49. Pedrick MS, Turton JA, Hicks RM. The incidence of bladder cancer in carcinogen-treated rats is not substantially reduced by dietary B-carotene (BC). *Int J Vitam Nutr Res.* 1990;60:189–190.
50. Mathews-Roth MM, Lausen N, Drouin G, Richter A, Krinsky NI. Effects of carotenoid administration on bladder cancer prevention. *Oncology.* 1991;48:177–179.
51. Schwartz JL, Flynn E, Shklar G. The effect of carotenoids on the antitumor immune response *in vivo* and *in vitro* with hamster and mouse immune effectors. *Ann N Y Acad Sci.* 1990;587:92–109.
52. Bendich A. Antioxidant micronutrients and immune responses. *Ann N Y Acad Sci.* 1990;587:168–180.

REGINA G. ZIEGLER, GISKE URSIN, NEAL E. CRAFT, AMY F. SUBAR, BARRY I. GRAUBARD, and BLOSSOM H. PATTERSON

Does Beta-Carotene Explain Why Reduced Cancer Risk Is Associated with Vegetable and Fruit Intake? New Research Directions

ABSTRACT

Increased intake of vegetables, fruits, and carotenoids and elevated blood levels of beta-carotene are consistently associated with reduced risk of lung cancer in epidemiologic studies. Epidemiologic research also suggests that carotenoids may reduce the risk of other cancers, although the evidence is less extensive and consistent. The simplest explanation is that beta-carotene is protective. However, the possible roles of other carotenoids, other constituents of vegetables and fruits, and associated dietary patterns have not been adequately explored.

To evaluate these other hypotheses, we are undertaking three lines of research. First, with dietary data from the 1982–84 Epidemiologic Followup Study of the first National Health and Nutrition Examination Survey and the 1987 National Health Interview Survey, we have determined which food groups and nutrients are highly correlated with vegetable and fruit intake. Second, we have developed and characterized a liquid chromatography method for optimal recovery and resolution of the common carotenoids in blood, specifically lutein, zeaxanthin, beta-cryptoxanthin, lycopene, alpha-carotene, and beta-carotene. Third, in a population-based case-control study of lung cancer among white men in New Jersey, we are assessing whether estimates of the intake of the individual carotenoids might produce stronger inverse associations than estimates of provitamin A carotenoids based on current food composition tables.

Introduction

The hypothesis that beta-carotene can reduce the risk of cancer is relatively recent. Previously, attention focused on vitamin A because of its recognized role in normal cell differentiation and because high doses of retinoids (vitamin A analogues) limited carcinogenesis in animal experiments. In the 1980s interest in beta-carotene escalated for several reasons. First, beta-carotene is the most abundant and the most efficiently converted of the provitamin A carotenoids (vitamin A precursors) in vegetables and fruits. Second, a protective role for beta-carotene explained the early epidemiologic evidence that increased vegetable and fruit intake reduced cancer risk. Third, serum levels of beta-carotene are responsive to dietary intake, unlike serum levels of vitamin A, which are maintained within a narrow range in well-nourished populations by vitamin A stored in the liver. Finally, a plausible mechanism, as an antioxidant, was postulated for beta-carotene that did not require its conversion to vitamin A.

Prospective Studies of Carotenoid Intake and Cancer

Before questioning whether the beta-carotene hypothesis really explains the epidemiologic findings, we must review the evidence. Prospective studies and then a limited number of retrospective studies will be considered. In a prospective study, dietary information and/or blood samples are collected from a group of nondiseased people, and this cohort is followed over time. When a sufficient number of cancer diagnoses or deaths have occurred, the data collected earlier are compared for the cases and the noncases in the cohort, or for the cases and matched controls selected from the cohort. Thus exposure, whether measured by dietary intake or blood nutrient levels, is ascertained before clinical disease.

Seven prospective studies of carotenoid intake and cancer have been published (1–8), with the earliest appearing in 1979 (1), in locations including Japan (1, 2), Norway (4), the Netherlands (8), and the United States (3, 5–7). The exposure most frequently evaluated was vegetable and fruit intake. Only three studies (3, 7, 8) actually assessed carotenoid intake by including in the interview most of the major sources of carotenoids in the diet and developing a quantitative index by weighting the frequencies of consumption of these foods by their measured carotenoid content, based on food composition tables.

Not all these studies looked at the same cancers; only two (3, 7) systematically investigated the most prevalent cancers in their cohort. Three (1, 2, 5, 7) of the five studies (1, 2, 3, 5, 7, 8; note: some references deal with the same studies) that analyzed all cancers combined found a reduced risk with increased intake of vegetables and fruits and/or carotenoids. Five (1–4, 6, 8) of six studies (1–4, 6–8) found a reduced risk of lung cancer with increased intake. A reduced risk of breast (7), cervical (1, 2), stomach (1, 2), and oral-pharyngeal (3) cancer was noted in the one study that investigated the cancer. However, risk of bladder cancer was decreased in only one (7) of two (3, 7) studies; and no protective effect was seen for intake of vegetables and fruits or of carotenoids for prostate cancer in three studies (1–3, 7), for colon cancer in two studies (3, 7), or for nonmelanoma skin cancer in one study (3).

Thus in these prospective studies of diet and cancer, high levels of vegetable and fruit intake are consistently associated with a reduced risk of lung cancer, and possibly other cancers. However, the protective factor is difficult to identify. Only one study systematically investigated the relationship of all the common nutrients to risk of lung cancer; carotenoid intake alone was significantly associated with reduced risk (3). The roles of nonnutrient constituents of vegetables and fruits and of individual carotenoids were not evaluated in any of these studies. In addition, the one study that compared the impact of vegetable, fruit, and carotenoid intake found that fruit was the most predictive of reduced lung cancer risk (8). Dietary retinol (preformed vitamin A) was not protective in three (3, 7, 8) of four lung cancer analyses (3, 4, 7, 8), which suggests that beta-carotene does not first have to be metabolized into retinol to be effective.

Prospective Studies of Blood Carotenoid Levels and Cancer

Prospective studies have looked not only at vegetable and fruit and carotenoid intake but also at carotenoid concentrations in serum or plasma before the onset of cancer. Seven such studies have been published (9–20), with locations including the continental United States (9, 13–17, 19), Hawaii (12), England (18), Switzerland (10, 11), and Finland (20). In the seven years since the first of these studies was published, evaluation of exposure has become more sophisticated. The earliest study measured total carotenoids by colorimetry (9); later studies have used liquid chromatography (LC) to separate and measure beta-carotene (10–14, 18–20). Recently blood levels of other individual carotenoids, such as lycopene, have also been quantitated (15–17).

All of these studies systematically tested for associations with each of the common cancers in their cohorts. A reduction in risk of all cancer with high blood beta-carotene levels was noted in two (18, 20) of the three studies (18–20) that analyzed all sites combined. A reduction in lung cancer risk was associated with elevated blood beta-carotene levels in five (10–13, 18, 19) of six studies (10–13, 18–20); the inverse associations were statistically significant in four of these studies (10–13, 18); trends were seen in all five. Also, a reduced risk of stomach cancer was consistently associated with high beta-carotene levels in three (10–12, 18) of four studies (10–12, 18, 20). However, for bladder cancer there was no apparent effect of high beta-carotene in two (12, 16) of four studies (12, 16, 18, 20), or for colon cancer in three (10, 11, 14, 19) of five studies (10–12, 14, 18, 19). The three analyses of prostate cancer indicated no protection associated with high beta-carotene (17, 20) or total carotenoid (9) concentrations.

Although the simplest explanation of these prospective studies is that beta-carotene can reduce the risk of lung and stomach cancer, other carotenoids and other constituents of vegetables and fruits were not evaluated in a systematic fashion; and elevated blood beta-carotene levels may simply indicate increased consumption of vegetables and fruits. It is provocative that in one cohort subjects with high serum lycopene levels had significantly reduced risks of pancreatic and bladder cancer and a nonsignificantly reduced risk of prostate cancer, but no comparable beta-carotene effects were seen (15, 16, 17). Serum beta-carotene levels were inversely associated with risk of lung cancer in this cohort, but lycopene was not measured in these blood samples (13). Like beta-carotene, lycopene is an antioxidant and may be more effective in certain tissues (21); however, it may also be simply an indicator of vegetable and fruit intake. In the one study that assayed for micronutrients shortly after blood collection, plasma vitamin C was more strongly associated with reduced risk of stomach cancer than was beta-carotene (10, 11), which is consistent with other evidence that vitamin C plays a role in the etiology of stomach cancer (22). However, only plasma beta-carotene, not vitamin C, was inversely associated with lung cancer risk in this study. In general, vitamin C, which like beta-carotene is concentrated in vegetables and fruits, has not been evaluated adequately in studies of nutrition and cancer because of the liability of vitamin C in blood. However, methods are now available to stabilize this micronutrient for long-term storage (23). In six (9, 10–13, 19, 24) of the seven analyses of lung cancer outcomes in these cohorts (9, 10–13, 19, 20, 24), strong and/or consistent associations for retinol (vitamin A) similar to those for beta-carotene were not seen, suggesting that beta-carotene need not first be converted to retinol to be active.

Retrospective Studies of Carotenoid Intake and Lung Cancer

In addition to the prospective studies just reviewed, a number of retrospective studies of carotenoids and specific cancers have been conducted. In a retrospective case-control study, patients with a particular cancer are identified and comparable control subjects selected. Then information about usual diet prior to signs of disease, blood samples, or both are collected and compared for the cases and controls. Although there is a possibility for bias when cancer cases recall usual dietary patterns, no clear evidence for bias exists in a number of well-conducted studies. The lung has been the site studied most intensively in retrospective studies because of the prevalence of lung cancer and the increasing evidence from epidemiologic studies that diet may be involved in its etiology. Fifteen retrospective studies of carotenoid intake and lung cancer have appeared since 1977 (25–40). The investigations have been conducted in the continental United States (27–30, 32, 33, 35, 37), Hawaii (26, 36), Canada (39), Italy (31, 34), France (40), Australia (38), and Singapore (25). Retrospective studies of blood carotenoid levels and lung cancer will not be considered here. The severity of this particular cancer and its treatment suggests that appetite and metabolism would be altered and would complicate the interpretation of nutrient levels in blood drawn after diagnosis.

Twelve (26–30, 32–37, 39, 40) of these fifteen retrospective studies of lung cancer formed a quantitative index of carotenoid intake; the others evaluated vegetable and fruit intake. Fourteen (25–37, 39, 40) of the fifteen studies demonstrated a decreased risk of lung cancer with increased intake of carotenoids or green or yellow-orange vegetables. In all fourteen analyses inverse associations or trends were statistically significant. This consistency among epidemiologic studies is remarkable.

Risk of lung cancer was inversely associated with dietary vitamin

C in four of these studies (26, 32, 35, 36) and with dietary fiber in two (32, 36). However, the associations were generally weaker than those with carotenoid intake. Intake of retinol seemed unrelated to risk in nine (26–30, 32, 33, 36, 38, 39) of twelve (26–30, 32–36, 38–40) studies that considered it, once again suggesting that beta-carotene need not first be converted to retinol to be protective. Only four of the studies compared the influence of vegetables and fruits with estimated carotenoid intake. Three found that vegetable intake was more predictive of reduced lung cancer risk than the carotenoid estimate (27, 28, 36, 39), whereas the fourth found that fruit intake was more predictive (35). As will be discussed later, these results suggest that beta-carotene may not explain why vegetables and fruits are protective; but their interpretation is complicated by the lack of reliable food composition data for individual carotenoids, such as beta-carotene.

Seven of these retrospective studies of dietary carotenoids and lung cancer used general population (26–29, 36, 39) or neighborhood (30, 32) controls, not hospital controls. Thus the dietary patterns among their controls are representative of those of healthy, typical populations. When the controls in these studies were stratified into quartiles or tertiles on the basis of vegetable and fruit and carotenoid intake, smoking-adjusted relative risks of lung cancer ranged from 1.4 to 2.2 in low consumers relative to high consumers. From a public health perspective, this implies that adoption of the levels of vegetable and fruit and carotenoid intake characteristic of the upper 30% of a typical community might be sufficient for a noticeable (29%–55%) reduction in lung cancer risk among the lower 30% of vegetable and fruit consumers. Were all members of the community to adopt the levels of vegetable and fruit consumption characteristic of the upper 30%, the risk of lung cancer in the community might be reduced 15% to 31%.

Based on these and other findings, the National Cancer Institute (NCI) recommends eating five or more servings of vegetables and fruits a day (41). Optimal intake of vegetables and fruits has not yet been determined scientifically. Nonetheless, approximately 9% of Americans presently consume five or more servings of vegetables and fruits a day (42). Thus this level of consumption typifies the upper range of vegetable and fruit intake in the United States and is feasible as well as prudent.

Retrospective Studies of Carotenoid Intake and Other Cancers

Retrospective studies indicate that vegetable and fruit intake may also reduce the risk of other cancers. But because of fewer studies and/or less consistency among studies, the epidemiologic evidence for a role for carotenoids is at present less persuasive than the evidence for lung cancer. Other cancers for which there is suggestive evidence from retrospective studies of the protective effect of vegetables, fruits, and possibly carotenoids are cancer of the mouth, pharynx, larynx, esophagus, stomach, colon, rectum, bladder, cervix, and breast.

Alternatives to the Beta-Carotene Hypothesis

To summarize, a reduced risk of lung cancer is consistently observed with increased dietary intake of vegetables and fruits and carotenoids in prospective and retrospective studies. In addition, a reduced risk of lung cancer is consistently associated with high blood levels of beta-carotene in prospective studies. The simplest explanation is that beta-carotene is protective. However, alternative hypotheses have not been adequately explored. Other plausible explanations for reduced risk include other carotenoids, other constituents of vegetables and fruits, and dietary patterns tightly correlated with frequent vegetable and fruit consumption.

Dietary Patterns Associated with Vegetable and Fruit Consumption

To help evaluate these alternative hypotheses, we are undertaking three lines of research. First, we are attempting to identify the dietary patterns associated with high vegetable and fruit consumption. From the perspective of cancer etiology, this effort may suggest alternatives to the beta-carotene hypothesis that need to be evaluated in epidemiologic and experimental studies. In addition, from a public health perspective, it will point to correlated dietary patterns whose nutritional and health consequences must be considered when NCI advocates a diet rich in vegetables and fruits (41).

We are currently utilizing two nationally representative dietary surveys to identify the nutrients, food groups, and food preparation practices associated with high vegetable and fruit intake. We are using the 115-item food frequency interview administered to 10,000 adults, aged 32 to 75, in the 1982–84 Epidemiologic Followup Study (EFS) of the first National Health and Nutrition Examination Survey (NHANES I) (43, 44) and the 60-item food frequency interview administered to 20,000 adults, aged 19 to 90, in the 1987 National Health Interview Survey (NHIS) (45). Both surveys focused on diet during the preceding year. Preliminary results from the two data sets were similar, and only the NHANES I EFS findings are presented here.

When nutrient intake was evaluated (Table 1), vitamin C, dietary fiber, potassium, folate, and vitamin A (presumably the provitamin A carotenoids) were highly associated with servings per week of vegetables and fruits, with the correlation coefficients (r's) ranging from 0.8 to 0.6. Percent of calories from fat was inversely correlated with vegetable and fruit intake ($r = -0.28$), although absolute intake of saturated fat, monounsaturated fat, and cholesterol seemed unrelated. When food group consumption was considered (Table 2), certain vegetable and fruit subgroups, such as dark green vegetables, yellow-orange vegetables, and citrus fruits, were only moderately correlated with total vegetable and fruit intake ($r = 0.4–0.6$). Red meat (beef and pork) intake was not associated; however, poultry and fish, which in a recent study was related to a reduced risk of colon cancer (46), and whole grains were weakly positively associated.

Effects of exposures that were highly correlated, such as vegetable and fruit intake and vitamin C intake ($r = 0.81$), would be difficult to

Table 1. Correlation Between Vegetable and Fruit Intake and Nutrient Intake in the 1982–84 NHANES I Epidemiologic Followup Study

Macronutrients	r[a]	Micronutrients	r[a]
Calories	.29	Vitamin A	.56
% calories from fat	−.28	Vitamin C	.81
% calories from carbohydrates	.41	Thiamin	.40
% calories from protein	−.12	Riboflavin	.29
Saturated fat	.08	Folate	.57
Oleic acid	.07	Calcium	.29
Linoleic acid	.22	Iron	.39
Cholesterol	.06	Sodium	.28
Dietary fiber	.76	Potassium	.61

[a] Pearson's correlation coefficient.

Table 2. Correlation Between Vegetable and Fruit Intake and Food Group Intake in the 1982–84 NHANES I Epidemiologic Followup Study

Food Group	r[a]	Food Group	r[a]
Vegetables	.82	Dairy products	.18
Dark green vegetables	.41	Starches	.16
Yellow-orange vegetables	.54	Cereals	.14
Fruits	.83	Breads	.08
Citrus fruits	.60	Whole grains	.20
Beef/pork	−.003	Desserts	−.0007
Poultry/fish	.23	Sodas	−.06
Processed meats	−.007	Alcohol	.07

[a] Pearson's correlation coefficient.

Table 3. Categorization of 1982–84 NHANES I EFS Participants by Intake of Vegetables and Fruits and of Vitamin C

Vitamin C	Vegetables and Fruits			
	Lowest Quartile	Quartile 2	Quartile 3	Highest Quartile
Lowest quartile	18%	5.3%	1.6%	0.3%
Quartile 2	6.0%	11%	6.2%	1.5%
Quartile 3	1.0%	6.8%	11%	6.2%
Highest quartile	0.2%	1.4%	6.3%	17%

evaluate separately in an epidemiologic study of typical Americans. As shown in Table 3, 57% of the population ranked in the same quartile for both these exposures (Q1/Q1 + Q2/Q2 + Q3/Q3 + Q4/Q4), and only 6% differed by more than one quartile (Q1/Q3 + Q1/Q4 + Q2/Q4 + Q3/Q1 + Q4/Q1 + Q4/Q2). Vegetable and fruit intake and percent of calories from fat were only moderately correlated ($r = -0.28$), and their effects should be separable in a large-enough epidemiologic study. As demonstrated in Table 4, only 33% of the population ranked in the equivalent quartiles for both exposures (25% would be expected if the exposures were statistically independent), and almost as much of the population, 27%, differed by more than one quartile.

Table 4. Categorization of 1982–84 NHANES I EFS Participants by Vegetable and Fruit Intake and Percent of Calories from Fat

Percent Calories from Fat	Vegetables and Fruits			
	Lowest Quartile	Quartile 2	Quartile 3	Highest Quartile
Highest quartile	9.8%	7.3%	5.1%	2.9%
Quartile 3	6.2%	7.0%	6.4%	5.4%
Quartile 2	4.8%	6.0%	6.8%	7.4%
Lowest quartile	4.3%	4.7%	6.7%	9.3%

Table 5. Median Intake of Nutrients and Food Groups by Quartile of Vegetable and Fruit Intake in the 1982–84 NHANES I Epidemiologic Followup Study

Nutrient or Food Group	Vegetable and Fruit Intake			
	Lowest Quartile	Quartile 2	Quartile 3	Highest Quartile
Vitamin C, mg	71	128	166	230
Dietary fiber, g	8.4	11.5	14.2	19.2
Folate, μg	181	229	265	333
Dark green vegetables, servings/week	.50	.75	1.00	1.75
Yellow-orange vegetables, servings/week	.83	1.26	2.00	3.24

Table 5 demonstrates the striking gradient in absolute intake of selected nutrients and food groups across quartiles of vegetable and fruit consumption and suggests the potential public health impact of programs targeting vegetables and fruits. For vitamin C, dietary fiber, folate, dark green vegetables, and yellow-orange vegetables, the median absolute intake in the highest quartile of vegetable and fruit consumption was two to four times the median intake in the lowest quartile. Thus it is prudent to investigate whether the dietary patterns associated with high vegetable and fruit intake suggest any nutritional or medical concerns, especially in vulnerable subgroups.

Development of an LC Method with Improved Separation and Recovery of Individual Carotenoids

Our second line of research concerns the consistently observed increase in subsequent incidence of lung and stomach cancers among those with low serum or plasma beta-carotene levels. Although these observations point to a protective role for beta-carotene, low blood beta-carotene levels may simply be an indicator of decreased intake of all carotenoids, and vegetables and fruits in general. Additional individual carotenoids and other constituents of vegetables and fruits need to be measured in these studies.

More than 600 carotenoids, all yellow to red in color (47), exist in biological materials; five to ten separable, structurally distinct carotenoids are typically identified in serum or plasma collected from United States populations (48). Beta-carotene is the most abundant, and the most efficiently converted, of the provitamin A carotenoids in vegetables and fruits. However, lycopene is often the carotenoid at highest concentrations in serum in the United States (48). Many of the carotenoids, not just beta-carotene, are effective antioxidants. In fact, carotenoids probably evolved to protect plants from reactive oxygen species generated in photosynthesis.

As we began to evaluate LC methods for separating the major individual carotenoids in human serum and plasma, it became apparent that there was little information published on recovery of the individual carotenoids. One reason was the lack of availability of pure reference materials for carotenoids other than beta-carotene. Another was that cancer research was focused on beta-carotene. Poor recovery during measurement of a carotenoid could lead to an imprecise estimate of exposure, and thus obscure an association. In addition, spurious associations could be generated by differential recovery between cases and controls.

The Environmental Epidemiology Branch of the NCI, in collaboration with the National Institute of Standards and Technology (NIST), decided to develop an LC method for measurement of individual carotenoids in human serum and plasma that would give both excellent resolution and recovery. In addition, the method had to be reproducible and practical so that it could be used by a variety of laboratories on the large numbers of samples collected in epidemiologic studies. Research indicated that a polymeric octadecylsilane stationary phase

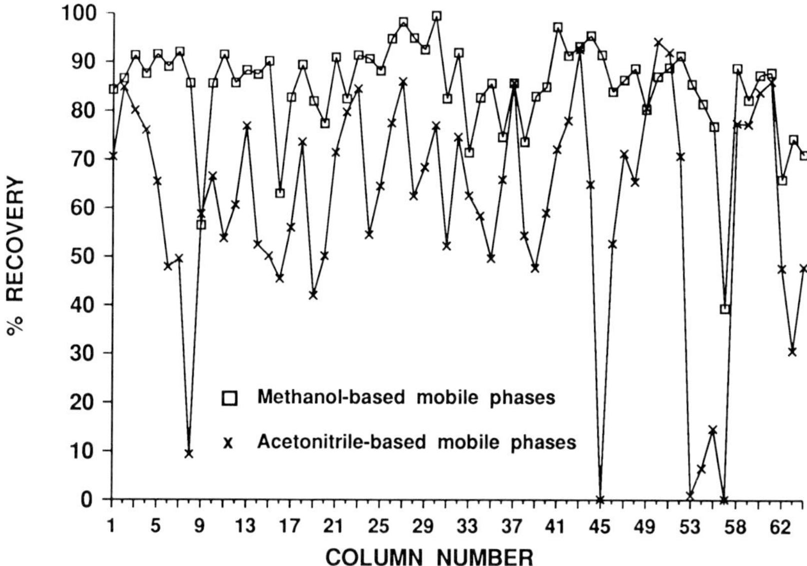

Figure 1. Total recovery of a mixture of seven carotenoids (lutein, zeaxanthin, beta-cryptoxanthin, echinenone, lycopene, alpha-carotene, and beta-carotene) from 64 commercially available reversed-phase LC columns using methanol- and acetonitrile-based mobile phases.

gave better resolution than a monomeric octadecylsilane phase, narrow pore packings were more reproducible than wide pore, and methanol or buffered acetonitrile mobile phases and biocompatible frits produced the highest recoveries (49). Among the multiple parameters evaluated, switching from an unbuffered acetonitrile-based mobile phase to a methanol-based one gave the most striking increase in recovery. Figure 1 demonstrates the improved recovery of carotenoids obtained on 58 out of 64 LC columns by using a methanolic mobile phase.

Percent recovery of the common serum carotenoids—lutein, zeaxanthin, beta-cryptoxanthin, lycopene, alpha-carotene, and beta-carotene—with the new NIST/NCI LC method and with three accepted LC methods that have been used in epidemiologic studies are presented in Table 6. The columns and mobile phases used in replicating these three LC methods were those published in the literature. Recovery was measured by flow injection analysis (50). The NIST/NCI method gives 93% to 99% recovery of each of the six carotenoids. Recovery drops to 70% or less for lycopene and to 80% or less for at

Table 6. Percent Recovery of Individual Carotenoids with the New NIST/NCI LC Method and Three Other LC Methods

Method	Lutein[a]	Zeaxanthin[a]	Beta-Cryptoxanthin	Lycopene	Alpha-Carotene	Beta-Carotene
NIST/NCI	95	94	93	97	99	99
A	80	75	82	68	89	91
B	99	98	85	70	77	84
C	99	91	96	101	94	91

[a]Lutein and zeaxanthin coelute in all methods except NIST/NCI.

least one additional carotenoid with methods A and B. Method C gives quite good recovery of all six carotenoids, but its resolution of individual carotenoids is limited. Of the four methods, only the NIST/NCI method can resolve the structural isomers lutein and zeaxanthin.

The ability of the NIST/NCI method to separate individual serum carotenoids is demonstrated in Figure 2. Not only are structural isomers that frequently coelute (alpha-cryptoxanthin/beta-cryptoxanthin and lutein/zeaxanthin) resolved, but geometric isomers are as well. The two small peaks trailing the all-trans beta-carotene peak are the 9-*cis* and 13-*cis* isomers, which together make up approximately 10% of total serum beta-carotene. The two peaks after all-trans lycopene and the peak before it contain its geometric isomers. Analysis time for this separation is 20 minutes; total run time including reequilibration is 30 minutes.

Although optimizing the recovery and resolution of the measurement techniques for individual carotenoids in human serum reduces the possibility of obscured or biased associations in prospective studies of blood carotenoids and cancer, carotenoid degradation during storage of blood samples can lead to similar problems. Even with storage under optimal conditions, at −70° C, evidence suggesting loss of beta-carotene has been reported (12, 13). Other carotenoids, such as lycopene, may be more labile than beta-carotene. At present epidemiologists compensate for degradation by matching noncases to cases on length of storage of serum samples or by standardizing for length of storage in analysis. Nonetheless, more thought should be given to practical ways to protect individual carotenoids from oxidative degradation during long-term storage of biological samples.

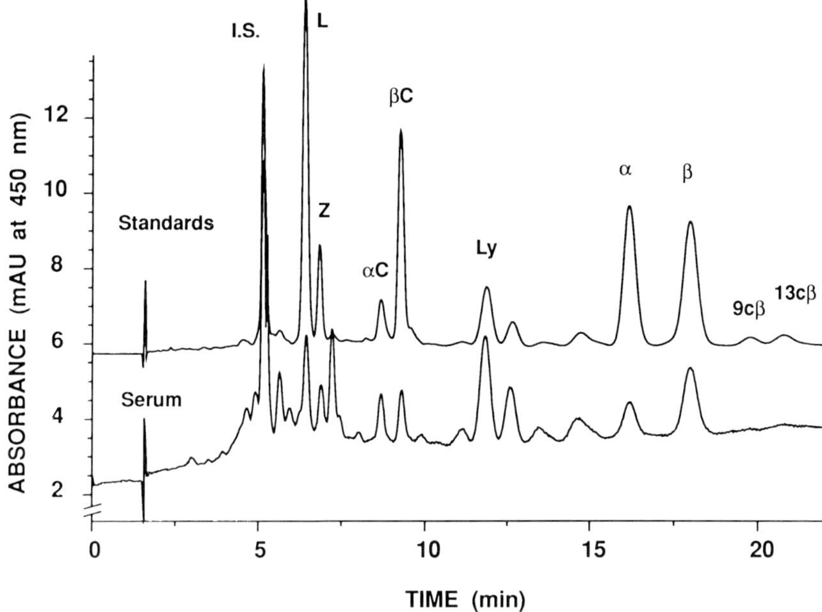

Figure 2. Resolution of serum cartoenoids with the NIST/NCI LC method. The upper tracing is of a mixture of the six most common serum carotenoids [lutein (L), zeaxanthin (Z), beta-cryptoxanthin (βC), lycopene (Ly), alpha-carotene (α), and beta-carotene (β)]; also seen are alpha-cryptoxanthin (αC), several unlabeled geometric isomers of lycopene, 9-*cis*-beta-carotene (9cβ), and 13-*cis*-beta-carotene (13cβ). The lower tracing is of an extract of human serum. The internal standard (I.S.) is beta-apo-8′-carotenal. LC conditions: Bakerbond C_{18} column, gradient elution at 2.0 mL/min, 27°C, detection at 450 nm. Solvent A = 90% acetonitrile/10% ethyl acetate; solvent B = 90% methanol/10% ethyl acetate containing 100 mM ammonium acetate; gradient = 100% A for 2 min, linear to 50% A/50% B over 4 min, linear to 100%B over 14 min.

Comparison of Food Groups, Indices of Total Carotenoid Intake, and Individual Carotenoid Measures in Cancer Studies

Our third research direction involves the incorporation of the individual carotenoid composition of various foods into analyses of the relationships between diet and cancer in retrospective and prospective studies. Up to now, epidemiologic studies have had to rely on the estimates of provitamin A carotenoids in United States Department of Agriculture (USDA) food composition tables (51). These values are not measures of beta-carotene or of total carotenoids. They reflect the content of alpha-carotene, beta-carotene, lycopene, cryptoxanthin, and several other chemically similar hydrocarbon carotenoids, since the Association of Official Analytical Chemists' approved method for identifying provitamin A carotenoids in foods does not usually resolve these compounds. The USDA and NCI will soon publish a list of the major individual carotenoids in the common foods that is based on a scientific evaluation of literature values and new research. Once these data become available, they can be used in the analysis of published and ongoing epidemiologic studies to refine hypotheses about the role of vegetables, fruits, and carotenoids.

It is provocative that of the four retrospective studies of diet and lung cancer that compared the influence of carotenoids and food groups, all four found stronger inverse associations with vegetable and fruit intake than with quantitative estimates of carotenoids (27, 28, 35, 36, 39). One study was a population-based case-control study of incident lung cancer conducted among white men in New Jersey (28); results are shown in Table 7. More pronounced trends in lung cancer risk are seen with vegetables in general, dark green vegetables, and yellow-orange vegetables than with carotenoids. Similarly, in a population-based case-control study of incident lung cancer conducted among multiethnic men and women in Hawaii (36), total

Table 7. Smoking-Adjusted Relative Risks of Lung Cancer Among Current and Recent Cigarette Smokers: New Jersey White Males[a]

	Level of Consumption			
Nutrient or Food Group	Upper 25%	Middle 50%	Lower 25%	*P*
Retinol	1.0	1.1	1.0	.48
Carotenoids	1.0	1.5	1.7	.02
Vitamin A	1.0	1.2	1.2	.26
Dairy products	1.0	0.8	0.9	.26
Vegetables and fruit	1.0	1.7	1.8	.005
Fruit	1.0	1.4	1.2	.28
Vegetables	1.0	1.3	1.7	.004
Dark green vegetables	1.0	1.4	1.8	.002
Yellow-orange vegetables	1.0	1.6	2.2	<.001

Adapted from Ziegler *et al.* (28).

[a]Included are 524 cases and 354 controls.

Table 8. Adjusted Relative Risks of Lung Cancer Among Multiethnic Hawaiians[a]

Nutrient or Food Group	Level of Consumption				P
	Upper 25%	Quartile 3	Quartile 2	Lower 25%	
Men					
Beta-Carotene	1.0	1.5	2.4	1.9	.001
Vegetables	1.0	1.9	2.3	2.7	<.001
Women					
Beta-Carotene	1.0	1.9	2.4	2.7	.01
Vegetables	1.0	3.2	3.0	7.0	<.001

Adapted from Marchand *et al.* (36).

[a]Included are 230 male cases, 597 male controls, 102 female cases, and 268 female controls.

vegetable intake was more predictive of reduced risk in both men and women than a beta-carotene estimate (Table 8). Two explanations of these findings are possible. One, beta-carotene is indeed protective; but food groups rich in beta-carotene are better measures of its intake than an approximate index of the hydrocarbon carotenoids. Alternatively, the protective agent may be another carotenoid or another constituent of vegetables. With more valid measures of the individual carotenoids, including beta-carotene, in foods, we hope to distinguish these hypotheses.

Conclusion

Epidemiologic studies have consistently associated increased intake of vegetables and fruits and carotenoids and elevated blood levels of beta-carotene with reduced risk of lung cancer. Epidemiologic research also suggests that vegetables and fruits and carotenoids may be involved in the etiology of certain other cancers, although fewer studies have been conducted and the results are less consistent. The simplest explanation is that beta-carotene is protective, and a number of clinical trials of beta-carotene supplements have been initiated to evaluate this specific hypothesis. However, other carotenoids, other constituents of vegetables and fruits, and dietary patterns closely associated with vegetable and fruit intake need to be explored further as alternatives to the beta-carotene hypothesis.

REFERENCES

1. Hirayama T. Diet and cancer. *Nutr Cancer.* 1979;1:67–81.
2. Hirayama T. A large-scale cohort study on cancer risks by diet—with special reference to the risk reducing effects of green-yellow vegetable consumption. In: Hayashi Y, Nagao M, Sugimura T, eds. *Diet, Nutrition and Cancer.* Tokyo: Japan Sci. Soc. Press; 1986:41–53.
3. Shekelle RB, Lepper M, Liu S, Maliza C, Raynor WJ, Jr, Rossof AH. Dietary vitamin A and risk of cancer in the Western Electric Study. *Lancet.* 1981;2:1185–1190.
4. Kvale G, Bjelke E, Gart JJ. Dietary habits and lung cancer risk. *Int J Cancer.* 1983;31:397–405.
5. Colditz GA, Branch LG, Lipnick RJ, *et al.* Increased green and yellow vegetable intake and lowered cancer deaths in an elderly population. *Am J Clin Nutr.* 1985;41:32–36.
6. Wang L, Hammond EC. Lung cancer, fruit, green salad, and vitamin pills. *Chin Med J.* 1985;98:206–210.
7. Paganini-Hill A, Chao A, Ross RK, Henderson BE. Vitamin A, β-carotene, and the risk of cancer: a prospective study. *J Natl Cancer Inst.* 1987;79:443–448.
8. Kromhout D. Essential micronutrients in relation to carcinogenesis. *Am J Clin Nutr.* 1987;45:1361–1367.
9. Willett WC, Polk BF, Underwood BA, *et al.* Relation of serum vitamins A and E and carotenoids to the risk of cancer. *N Engl J Med.* 1984;310:430–434.
10. Stahelin HB, Rosel F, Buess E, Brubacher G. Cancer, vitamins, and plasma lipids: Prospective Basel Study. *J Natl Cancer Inst.* 1984; 73:1463–1468.
11. Stahelin HB, Gey KF, Eichholzer M, Ludin E. β-carotene and cancer prevention: the Basel Study. *Am J Clin Nutr.* 1991;53: 265S–269S.
12. Nomura AMY, Stemmermann GN, Heilbrun LK, Salkeld RM, Vuilleumier JP. Serum vitamin levels and the risk of cancer of specific sites in men of Japanese ancestry in Hawaii. *Cancer Res.* 1985;45:2369–2372.
13. Menkes MS, Comstock GW, Vuilleumier JP, Helsing KJ, Rider AA, Brookmeyer R. Serum beta-carotene, vitamins A and E, se-

lenium, and the risk of lung cancer. *N Engl J Med.* 1986;315: 1250–1254.

14. Schober SE, Comstock GW, Helsing KJ, *et al.* Serologic precursors of cancer, I: prediagnostic serum nutrients and colon cancer risk. *Am J Epidemiol.* 1987;126:1033–1041.
15. Burney PGJ, Comstock GW, Morris JS. Serologic precursors of cancer: serum micronutrients and the subsequent risk of pancreatic cancer. *Am J Clin Nutr.* 1989;49:895–900.
16. Helzlsouer KJ, Comstock GW, Morris JS. Selenium, lycopene, α-tocopherol, β-carotene, retinol, and subsequent bladder cancer. *Cancer Res.* 1989;49:6144–6148.
17. Hsing AW, Comstock GW, Abbey H, Polk, BF. Serologic precursors of cancer: retinol, carotenoids, and tocopherol and risk of prostate cancer. *J Natl Cancer Inst.* 1990;82:941–946.
18. Wald NJ, Thompson SG, Densem JW, Boreham J, Bailey A. Serum beta-carotene and subsequent risk of cancer: results from the BUPA study. *Br J Cancer.* 1988;57:428–433.
19. Connett JE, Kuller LH, Kjelsberg MO, *et al.* Relationship between carotenoids and cancer: the Multiple Risk Factor Intervention Trial (MRFIT) Study. *Cancer.* 1989;64:126–134.
20. Knekt P, Aromaa A, Maatela J, *et al.* Serum vitamin A and subsequent risk of cancer: cancer incidence follow-up of the Finnish mobile clinic health examination survey. *Am J Epidemiol.* 1990; 132:857–870.
21. Di Mascio P, Kaiser S, Sies H. Lycopene as the most efficient biological carotenoid singlet oxygen quencher. *Arch Biochem Biophys.* 1989;274:532–538.
22. Forman D. The etiology of gastric cancer. In: O'Neill IK, Chen J, Bartsch H, eds. *Relevance to Human Cancer of N-Nitroso Compounds, Tobacco Smoke, and Mycotoxins.* Lyon, France: IARC; 1991:22–32.
23. Margolis SA, Paule RC, Ziegler RG. The measurement of ascorbic and dehydroascorbic acid in sera preserved in dithiothreitol or metaphosphoric acid. *Clin Chem.* 1990;36:1750–1755.
24. Wald N, Boreham J, Bailey A. Serum retinol and subsequent risk of cancer. *Br J Cancer.* 1986;54:957–961.
25. MacLennan R, Da Costa J, Day NE, Law CH, Ng YK, Shanmugaratnam K. Risk factors for lung cancer in Singapore Chinese, a population with high female incidence rates. *Int J Cancer.* 1977; 20:854–860.

26. Hinds MW, Kolonel LN, Hankin JH, Lee J. Dietary vitamin A, carotene, vitamin C and risk of lung cancer in Hawaii. *Am J Epidemiol.* 1984;119:227–237.
27. Ziegler RG, Mason TJ, Stemhagen A, *et al.* Dietary carotene and vitamin A and risk of lung cancer among white men in New Jersey. *J Natl Cancer Inst.* 1984;73:1429–1435.
28. Ziegler RG, Mason TJ, Stemhagen A, *et al.* Carotenoid intake, vegetables, and the risk of lung cancer among white men in New Jersey. *Am J Epidemiol.* 1986;123:1080–1093.
29. Samet JM, Skipper BJ, Humble CG, Pathak DR. Lung cancer risk and vitamin A consumption in New Mexico. *Am Rev Respir Dis.* 1985;131:198–202.
30. Wu AH, Henderson BE, Pike MC, Yu MC. Smoking and other risk factors for lung cancer in women. *J Natl Cancer Inst.* 1985; 74:747–751.
31. Pisani P, Berrino F, Macaluso M, Pastorino U, Crosignani, Baldasseroni A. Carrots, green vegetables, and lung cancer: a case-control study. *Int J Epidemiol.* 1986;15:463–468.
32. Byers TE, Graham S, Haughey BP, Marshall JR, Swanson MK. Diet and lung cancer risk: findings from the Western New York Diet Study. *Am J Epidemiol.* 1987;125:351–363.
33. Bond GG, Thompson FE, Cook RR. Dietary vitamin A and lung cancer: results of a case-control study among chemical workers. *Nutr Cancer.* 1987;9:109–121.
34. Pastorino U, Pisani P, Berrino F, *et al.* Vitamin A and female lung cancer: a case-control study on plasma and diet. *Nutr Cancer.* 1987;10:171–179.
35. Fontham ETH, Pickle LW, Haenszel W, Correa P, Lin Y, Falk RT. Dietary vitamins A and C and lung cancer risk in Louisiana. *Cancer.* 1988;62:2267–2273.
36. Marchand LL, Yoshizawa CN, Kolonel LN, Hankin JH, Goodman MT. Vegetable consumption and lung cancer risk: a population-based case-control study in Hawaii. *J Natl Cancer Inst.* 1989;81: 1158–1164.
37. Mettlin C. Milk drinking, other beverage habits, and lung cancer risk. *Int J Cancer.* 1989;43:608–612.
38. Pierce RJ, Kune GA, Kune S, *et al.* Dietary and alcohol intake, smoking pattern, occupational risk, and family history in lung cancer patients: results of a case-control study in males. *Nutr Cancer.* 1989;12:237–248.

39. Jain M, Burch JD, Howe GR, Risch HA, Miller AB. Dietary factors and risk of lung cancer: results from a case-control study, Toronto, 1981–1985. *Int J Cancer.* 1990;45:287–293.
40. Dartigues J-F, Dabis F, Gros N, *et al.* Dietary vitamin A, beta-carotene and risk of epidermoid lung cancer in South-western France. *Eur J Epidemiol.* 1990;6:261–265.
41. National Cancer Institute. *Diet, Nutrition, and Cancer Prevention: The Good News.* Rev ed. Bethesda, Md: NCI; 1992.
42. Patterson BH, Block G, Rosenberger WF, Pee D, Kahle LL. Fruit and vegetables in the American diet: data from the NHANES I survey. *Am J Public Health.* 1990;80:1443–1449.
43. Cornoni-Huntley J, Barbano HE, Brody JA, *et al.* National Health and Nutrition Examination I—Epidemiologic Followup Survey. *Public Health Rep.* 1983;98:245–251.
44. Madans JH, Kleinman JC, Cox CS, *et al.* 10 years after NHANES I: report of initial followup, 1982–84. *Public Health Rep.* 1986;101: 465–473.
45. National Center for Health Statistics. *The National Health Interview Survey Design, 1973–1984, and Procedures, 1975–1983.* Hyattsville, Md: DHHS; 1985. DHHS publication PHS 85-1320. Ser. 1, no. 18.
46. Willett WC, Stampfer MJ, Colditz GA, Rosner BA, Speizer FE. Relation of meat, fat, and fiber intake to the risk of colon cancer in a prospective study among women. *N Engl J Med.* 1990;323: 1664–1672.
47. Britton G, Goodwin TW. *Carotenoid Chemistry and Biochemistry.* Elmsford, NY: Pergamon Press; 1982.
48. Stacewicz-Sapuntzakis M, Bowen PE, Kikendall JW, Burgess M. Simultaneous determination of serum retinol and various carotenoids: their distribution in middle-aged men and women. *J Micronutr Anal.* 1987;3:27–45.
49. Epler KS, Sander LC, Ziegler RG, *et al.* Evaluation of reversed-phase liquid chromatography columns for recovery and selectivity of selected carotenoids. *J Chromatogr.* 1992;595:89–101.
50. Craft NE, Wise SA, Soares JH. Optimization of an isocratic liquid chromatographic separation of carotenoids. *J Chromatogr.* 1992; 589:171–176.
51. United States Department of Agriculture. *Composition of Foods: Raw, Processed, Prepared.* Washington, DC: USDA; 1978–89: revised sections 8-1–8-2. USDA Agriculture Handbook no. 8.

Contributors to Volume 3

DONITA L. ABANGAN
Dermatology Branch
National Cancer Institute
National Institutes of Health
Building 10, Room 12N238
Bethesda, MD 20892

ADRIANNE BENDICH
Human Nutrition Research
Hoffmann-La Roche, Inc.
340 Kingsland Street
Nutley, NJ 07110-1199

JOHN S. BERTRAM
Molecular Oncology Program
Cancer Research Center of Hawaii
University of Hawaii at Manoa
1236 Lauhala St.
Honolulu, HI 96813

GLADYS BLOCK
Public Health Nutrition Program
Department of Social and Administrative Health Sciences
419 Warren Hall
University of California at Berkeley
Berkeley, CA 94720

JULIE E. BURING
Departments of Medicine and Preventive Medicine
Brigham and Women's Hospital
Harvard Medical School
900 Commonwealth Avenue East
Boston, MA 02215

C. E. BUTTERWORTH, Jr.
Department of Nutrition Sciences
University of Alabama at Birmingham
School of Medicine and School of Health-Related Professions
Birmingham, AL 35294-3360

T. COLIN CAMPBELL
Division of Nutritional Sciences
Cornell University
Martha Van Rensselaer Hall
Ithaca, NY 14853-4401

JUNSHI CHEN
Institute of Nutrition and Food Hygiene
Chinese Academy of Preventive Medicine
Beijing
People's Republic of China

CAROLYN CLIFFORD
Diet and Cancer Branch
National Cancer Institute
6130 Executive Boulevard
Executive Plaza North, Suite 212
Rockville, MD 20852

PELAYO CORREA
Section of Epidemiology
Department of Pathology
Louisiana State University Medical Center
1901 Perdido Street
New Orleans, LA 70112

NEAL E. CRAFT
Organic Analytical Research Division
Chemical Science and Technology Laboratory
National Institute of Standards and Technology
Gaithersburg, MD 20899

JOHN J. DiGIOVANNA
Dermatology Branch
National Cancer Institute
National Institutes of Health
Building 10, Room 12N238
Bethesda, MD 20892

ELIZABETH T. H. FONTHAM
Section of Epidemiology
Department of Pathology
Louisiana State University Medical Center
1901 Peridido Street
New Orleans, LA 70112

HARINDER S. GAREWAL
Section of Hematology-Oncology (111D)
Tucson VA Medical Center
3601 South 6th Avenue
Tuscon, AZ 85723

DAVID F. C. GIBSON
Molecular Oncology Program
Cancer Research Center of Hawaii
University of Hawaii
1236 Lauhala Street
Honolulu, HI 96813

MARC T. GOODMAN
Epidemiology Program
Cancer Research Center of Hawaii
1236 Lauhala Street
Honolulu, HI 96813

BARRY I. GRAUBARD
Biometry Branch
Division of Cancer Prevention and Control
National Cancer Institute
Bethesda, MD 20892

PETER GREENWALD
Director, Division of Cancer Prevention and Control
National Institutes of Health
Bethesda, MD 20892

JEAN H. HANKIN
Epidemiology Program
Cancer Research Center of Hawaii
1236 Lauhala Street
Honolulu, HI 96813

DOUGLAS C. HEIMBURGER
Department of Nutrition Sciences
UAB Station
Birmingham, AL 35294-3360

CHARLES H. HENNEKENS
Departments of Medicine and Preventive Medicine
Brigham and Women's Hospital
Harvard Medical School
900 Commonwealth Avenue East
Boston, MA 02215

MOHAMMAD Z. HOSSAIN
Molecular Oncology Program
Cancer Research Center of Hawaii
University of Hawaii
1236 Lauhala Street
Honolulu, HI 96813

DAVID J. HUNTER
Department of Epidemiology
Harvard School of Public Health
900 Commonwealth Avenue East
Boston, MA 02215

CLEMENT IP
Department of Surgical Oncology
Roswell Park Memorial Institute
666 Elm Street
Buffalo, NY 14263

MICHAEL A. JONAS
Channing Laboratory
Departments of Medicine and Preventive Medicine
Harvard Medical School
Brigham and Women's Hospital
900 Commonwealth Avenue East
Boston, MA 02215

PAUL KNEKT
Research Institute for Social Security
Social Insurance Institution
P.O. Box 78
SF-00381 Helsinki, Finland

LAURENCE N. KOLONEL
Epidemiology Program
Cancer Research Center of Hawaii
1236 Lauhala Street
Honolulu, HI 96813

KENNETH H. KRAEMER
Dermatology Branch
National Cancer Institute
National Institutes of Health
Building 10, Room 12N238
Bethesda, MD 20892

NORMAN I. KRINSKY
Department of Biochemistry
Tufts University School of Medicine
136 Harrison Avenue
Boston, MA 02111-1837

BRET A. LASHNER
University of Chicago Medical Center
Box 400n, 5841 S. Maryland Avenue
Chicago, IL 60637

LOÏC LE MARCHAND
Epidemiology Program
Cancer Research Center of Hawaii
1236 Lauhala Street
Honolulu, HI 96813

MING LI
Division of Nutritional Sciences
Cornell University
Ithaca, NY 14853

GERALD LITWACK
Department of Pharmacology
Jefferson Medical College
908 Bluemle Life Sciences Building
233 South 10th Street
Philadelphia, PA 19107

LAWRENCE J. MACHLIN
Department of Human Nutrition Research
Hoffmann-LaRoche, Inc.
340 Kingsland Street
Nutley, NJ 07110-1199

JoANN E. MANSON
Channing Laboratory
Department of Medicine
Brigham and Women's Hospital
Harvard Medical School
900 Commonwealth Avenue East
Boston, MA 02215

RICHARD C. MOON
Life Sciences Department
IIT Research Institute
10 West 35th Street
Chicago, IL 60616-3799

THOMAS E. MOON
Arizona Disease Prevention Center and Arizona Cancer Center
University of Arizona Health Sciences Center
1515 N. Campbell, Rm. 2942
Tucson, AZ 85724

ABRAHAM M. Y. NOMURA
Epidemiology Program
Cancer Research Center of Hawaii
1236 Lauhala Street
Honolulu, HI 96813

BANOO PARPIA
Division of Nutritional Sciences
Cornell University
Ithaca, NY 14853

BLOSSOM H. PATTERSON
Biometry Branch
Division of Cancer Prevention and Control
National Cancer Institute
Bethesda, MD 20892

GARY L. PECK
Dermatology Branch
National Cancer Institute
National Institutes of Health
Building 10, Room 12N238
Bethesda, MD 20892

WILLIAM A. PRYOR
Biodynamics Institute
Louisiana State University
Baton Rouge, LA 70803-1800

DONNA H. RYAN
Pennington Biomedical Research Center
6400 Perkins Road
Baton Rouge, LA 70808

GEORGE M. SOBALA
Gastroenterology Unit
The General Infirmary
Leeds, West Yorkshire
LS1 4EX
United Kingdom

BARRY STARR
Harvard College
Kirkland House, No. 382
95 Dunster Street
Cambridge, MA 02138-5912

AMY F. SUBAR
Applied Research Branch
Surveillance Program
Division of Cancer Prevention and Control
National Cancer Institue
Bethesda, MD 20892

GISKE URSIN
Department of Epidemiology
School of Public Health
University of California
Los Angeles, CA 90024

LYNNE R. WILKENS
Epidemiology Program
Cancer Research Center of Hawaii
1236 Lauhala Street
Honolulu, HI 96813

LI-XIN ZHANG
Molecular Oncology Program
Cancer Research Center of Hawaii
University of Hawaii
1236 Lauhala Street
Honolulu, HI 96813

LUE PING ZHAO
Epidemiology Program
Cancer Research Center of Hawaii
1236 Lauhala Street
Honolulu, HI 96813

REGINA G. ZIEGLER
Environmental Epidemiology Branch
Epidemiology and Biostatistics Program
Division of Cancer Etiology
National Cancer Institute
Executive Plaza North, No. 443
Bethesda, MD 20892

Index